Neighborhood Health Centers

Neighborhood Health Centers

Edited by

Robert M. Hollister
Bernard M. Kramer
Seymour S. Bellin

Lexington Books
D.C. Heath and Company
Lexington, Massachusetts
Toronto   London

Library of Congress Cataloging in Publication Data

Hollister, Robert M.   comp.
Neighborhood health centers.

Bibliography: p.
1. Community health services—Addresses, essays, lectures. I. Kramer,
Bernard M., joint comp. II. Bellin, Seymour S., joint comp. III. Title.
[DNLM: 1. Community health services. WA525 H744n 1974]
RA425.H579   362.1'2   73-19791
ISBN 0-669-92510-1

Published simultaneously in Canada.

Printed in the United States of America.

International Standard Book Number: 0-669-92510-1

Library of Congress Catalog Card Number: 73-19791

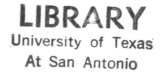

Contents

List of Tables   ix

Preface   xiii

Part I   Introduction   xv

Chapter 1 — Neighborhood Health Centers as Demonstrations
Robert M. Hollister   1

Chapter 2 — Neighborhood Health Centers as a Social Movement
Robert M. Hollister, Bernard M. Kramer, and
Seymour S. Bellin   13

**Part II   Precursors of the Present Generation of Neighborhood
Health Centers**   25

Chapter 3 — The Neighborhood Health Center — Reform Ideas
of Yesterday and Today
John D. Stoeckle and *Lucy M. Candib*   29

Part III   Evolution of the Neighborhood Health Centers of the 1960s   41

Chapter 4 — Background, Context and Significant Issues in
Neighborhood Health Center Programs
Lisbeth Bamberger Schorr and *Joseph T. English*   45

Chapter 5 — Healing the Poor in Their Back Yard
Sar A. Levitan   51

Part IV   Perspectives of Evaluation   65

Chapter 6 — Some Accomplishments and Findings of
Neighborhood Health Centers
Daniel I. Zwick   69

Chapter 7 — A Political Scientist's View of the Neighborhood
Health Center as a New Social Institution
Eugene Feingold   91

Chapter 8 — Neighborhood Health Centers
   Health/PAC Bulletin   101

Part V   Consumer Participation and Community Control   105

Chapter 9 — The Politics of Community Medicine Projects:
   A Conflict Analysis
   Jeoffry B. Gordon   107

Chapter 10 — A Sociomedical View of Neighborhood
   Health Centers
   Jack Elinson and *Conrad E. A. Herr*   123

Chapter 11 — Community Control — or Community Conflict?
   H. Jack Geiger   133

Chapter 12 — NENA: Community Control in a Bind
   Des Callan and *Oliver Fein*   143

Part VI   Administration   157

Chapter 13 — Administrative Problems of Neighborhood
   Health Centers
   Paul R. Torrens   161

Part VII Costs and Financing   175

Chapter 14 — Cost of Services at Neighborhood Health Centers:
   A Comparative Analysis
   Gerald Sparer and *Arne Anderson*   179

Chapter 15 — An Economist's View of the Neighborhood
   Health Center as a New Social Institution
   Rashi Fein   189

Part VIII Patients' Use and Response   195

Chapter 16 — Actual Public Acceptance of the Neighborhood
   Health Center by the Urban Poor
   Seymour S. Bellin and *H. Jack Geiger*   199

Chapter 17 — The Impact of a Neighborhood Health Center on
      Patients' Behavior and Attitudes Relating to Health Care:
      A Study of a Low-Income Housing Project
      Seymour S. Bellin and *H. Jack Geiger*   213

Chapter 18 — Basic Utilization Experience of OEO Comprehensive
      Health Services Projects
      Mark A. Strauss and *Gerald Sparer*   231

Chapter 19 — A Neighborhood Health Center: What the Patients
      Know and Think of Its Operation
      Bruce Hillman and *Evan Charney*   243

Part IX Quality of Care   253

Chapter 20 — Comparisons Between OEO Neighborhood Health
      Centers and Other Health Care Providers of Ratings of the
      Quality of Health Care
      Mildred A. Morehead, Rose S. Donaldson, and
      Mary R. Seravalli   257

Part X   Allied Health Workers and Health Teams   275

Chapter 21 — The Family Health Worker
      Harold B. Wise, E. Fuller Torrey, Adrienne McDade,
      Gloria Perry, and *Harriet Bograd*   281

Chapter 22 — Factors Influencing the Effectiveness of Health Teams
      Irwin M. Rubin and *Richard Beckhard*   291

Part XI Neighborhood Health Centers as Instruments of Change —
      Relationships with, and Impacts on, Other Health Institutions   305

Chapter 23 — Impact of Ambulatory-Health-Care Services on the
      Demand for Hospital Beds: A Study of the Tufts Neighborhood
      Health Center at Columbia Point in Boston
      Seymour S. Bellin, H. Jack Geiger, and *Count D. Gibson*   309

Chapter 24 — Effect of the Neighborhood Health Center on the
      Use of Pediatric Emergency Departments in Rochester,
      New York
      Louis I. Hochheiser, Kenneth Woodward, and
      Evan Charney   317

Chapter 25 — Relating a Neighborhood Health Center to a
General Hospital: A Case History
Anthony R. Kovner, Gerald Katz, Stanley B. Kahane,
and *Cecil G. Sheps*   325

Bibliography   333

Index   345

About the Editors   351

List of Tables

5-1 Estimated OEO Allocations for Health, Fiscal 1965–68 (Millions)   52
5-2 Grantees and Administering Agencies of Neighborhood Health
    Centers, July 1968   61
6-1 Amounts of OEO and HEW Grants for Neighborhood Health
    Centers and Other Local Projects   72
6-2 HEW Grants for Local Projects to Develop Comprehensive Health
    Care of Preschool and School Age Children   72
6-3 Projects Receiving OEO Grant Support   73
6-4 Administering Agencies of Operational Projects Receiving OEO
    and HEW Financial Assistance, 1965–1971   74
6-5 Administering Agencies of Projects Aided by OEO at Time of
    Initial Grant Award   78
14-1 General Characteristics of Centers Included in the Study   181
14-2 Percentage Distribution of Costs at Selected Neighborhood Health
    Centers by Level of Care, 1970   183
14-3 Unit Cost of Services Including General–Services Costs, 1970   184
14-4 Cost in Dollars per Unit of Medical Service According to Type of
    Encounters in Neighborhood Health Centers, 1970   185
14-5 Annual Cost per Registered Person at Selected Neighborhood
    Health Centers According to Level of Care, 1970   187
16-1 Encounters With All Health Center Professionals in 1968 by
    Continuity of Residence   202
16-2 Average Annual Encounters With Health Center Physicians in
    1968   203
16-3 Regular Source of Care   204
16-4 Evaluations of Different Sources of Health Care in Four Criteria
    by Regular Source of Care Prior to Advent of Center   205
16-5 Evaluation of Different Sources of Health Care in Four Criteria
    by Current Regular Source of Care   207
17-1 Selected Social Characteristics of the Columbia Point Survey
    Samples: Wave I Health Survey (November 1965) and Wave II
    Health Survey (November 1967)   215
17-2 Conditions for Which a Doctor Should Be Seen   218
17-3 Selected Aspects of the Columbia Point Community Which Are
    Rated "Very Good" or "Good" in the Baseline and Follow-up
    Surveys   219
17-4 Reasons Given for Liking and Disliking Health Center by
    Columbia Point Residents, 1967 Survey   221
17-5 Evaluation of Physicians   223
17-6 Sources of Regular Health Care Which Would Be Chosen if All
    Sources Were Cost-free   224

18-1 Comprehensive Health Services Projects Selected for Study 233
18-2 Encounters at Clinic per Year per "Registrant," Observed Active Registrant and User of Clinical Services 234
18-3 Encounters at Clinic per Year per "Registrant" and per User of Clinical Services 240
19-1 Description of Job Role of Team Nurse by Patient and Nurse 247
19-2 Description of Job Role of Family Health Assistant by Patient and FHA 247
19-3 Comparative Perceived Quality of Care vs. Knowledge of Their Physician's Name 250
19-4 Comparison of Where Patient Would Go "If All Care Were Free" With Knowledge of Physician's Name 250
19-5 Satisfied and Dissatisfied Families: Visits to Health Center 251
19-6 Satisfied and Dissatisfied Families: Outreach Staff Contacts and Social Evaluation 251
20-1 Number of Patient Records Reviewed by Type of Provider and Specialty in Baseline Medical Audit 261
20-2 Baseline Medical Audit Scores of Selected Health Providers as Per Cents of the Over-all Average for Medical School Affiliated Hospital Outpatient Departments 262
20-3 Components of Average Baseline Adult Medicine Scores of Selected Health Providers as Per Cents of the Average for Medical School Affiliated Hospital Outpatient Departments 262
20-4 Components of Adult Medicine Baseline Audit 263
20-5 Components of Average Baseline Obstetrical Scores of Selected Health Providers as Per Cents of the Average for Medical School Affiliated Hospital Outpatients Departments 264
20-6 Components of Obstetrical Baseline Audit 265
20-7 Components of Average Baseline Pediatric Scores of Selected Health Providers as Per Cent of the Average for Medical School Affiliated Hospital Outpatients Departments 266
20-8 Components of Pediatric Baseline Audit 267
23-1 Annual Number of Hospital Admissions and Total Hospital Days per Hundred Persons for Columbia Point (Boston) and the United States 310
23-2 Annual Admissions to and Total Days Spent in Boston City Hospital According to Type of Medical Condition for Columbia Point Families Continuously in Residence for Persons under 65 Years of Age 311
23-3 Annual Admissions to and Total Days Spent at All Hospitals, for 61 Households Continuously on Welfare, for 296 Persons Under Age of 65 313

24-1 Sample Sizes and Total Numbers of Pediatric Emergency-
Department Visits During the Periods Studied   318
24-2 Yearly Percentages of Sampled Pediatric Emergency-Department
Visits from Center Area, According to Complaint   319
24-3 Percentage Changes in Pediatric Emergency-Department Visits
from Different Areas   320
24-4 Percentage Changes in Pediatric Emergency-Department Visits
from Center Area to Individual Hospitals and Percentage Changes
in Total Pediatric Emergency-Department Visits   321
24-5 Number of Pediatric Emergency-Department Visits from Health
Center Census Tracts During Periods Studied   322

Preface

This collection of articles about neighborhood health centers assembles some of
the more important discussions and evaluations of the centers at a time when
these attempts to improve primary health care in poor areas are under increasingly vigorous attack. Conservative critics of the centers cry they are too expensive, that they deliver poor quality care. Critics from the left view them as "too
little too late," and charge they impede prospects for more thoroughgoing
change by providing symbolic responses to real needs and by draining off
pressures for larger changes.

How effective have the centers been? The evidence remains fragmentary,
but there now exist enough fragments of sufficient quality to begin to piece
together answers to the hard evaluative questions which will determine the form
in which the centers will survive and the content of the lessons which they provide. The collection of articles which follows is an attempt to sift the existing
evidence and to contribute to the process of digestion and diffusion of the
experience of the neighborhood health centers.

This volume seeks to inject more factual information into discussions of the
merits of centers now in existence and of the neighborhood health centers as
delivery system models. It aims to help restructure the conceptual framework of
these debates and insists that persons critical of the centers deal more squarely
with the hard evidence of solid accomplishments.

Clear-headed analysis helps to describe the roots and direction of social
change. The neighborhood health center movement has its roots in simple good
sense. It makes good sense to offer services to people where they live and in tune
with how they live. A heartless national administration has been doing all in its
power to abandon the poor—Black, White, Spanish-speaking and Indian. Yet
no amount of technocratic slight of hand nor sanctimonious sermons about
efficiency will change the fundamental requirement that a wealthy nation provide health care for all its people. And it remains desirable that this be done in
the context of people's neighborhoods. The analysis that follows attempts to
place the health center movement in perspective and to provide a framework for
assessing its current status.

We are not uncritical of the performance of neighborhood health centers,
but we see them as being partially successful with regard to many of their initial
goals. The growth and development of this set of new institutions is threatened;
it is therefore critically important that those aspects of the centers which are
working well, or which can work, be identified, sustained and spread. The
accomplishments of the health centers have not been communicated as widely
as they deserve to be. We view the most effective defense of the centers as one
that candidly admits shortcomings, but assembles the relevant evidence and
interprets it in an organized framework. To date the neighborhood health centers
have been defended in specific conflicts with governmental agencies and others,

but a broader defense based on the growing volume of reports and studies of the centers has not existed. We seek to fill this gap.

The book begins with two introductory chapters by the editors. The first describes how the health centers have played out themes inherent in the demonstration project model for attempting social change. The second analyzes the current generation of neighborhood health centers as a social movement stimulated by the intersection of several supportive trends and then promptly undermined by the dispersion of these individual forces.

The reprinted articles which follow enable the reader to explore more deeply some of the themes discussed in the introductory chapters. The collection of articles is designed to be a reference or a source book of materials on neighborhood health centers. It is very selective. The bibliography at the end of the book is a guide to other material. The selection of the articles included here attempts to cover a broad range of issues about neighborhood health centers and to remain of a manageable size. Some of the articles were chosen because they present important empirical evidence, others because they articulate a particular point of view or argument. Some quite useful papers have had to be omitted because they were too long or because they duplicate material found in other pieces. The papers are organized into sections which cover the major dimensions of the experience of the health centers. Short essays by the editors introduce the issues covered by, and the articles in, each section.

The reader is not a how-to-do-it manual, but by reporting the experiences of the neighborhood health centers it supplies information which should be directly useful to persons working with neighborhood health centers and related attempts to improve primary health care services.

Bernard Kramer had the initial idea and did the preparatory work for this book. He sought the collaboration of Robert Hollister and Seymour Bellin. Robert Hollister prepared first drafts of all the freshly written material and brought the volume to its final form. We gratefully acknowledge the assistance of The Medical Foundation, Inc., which supported part of Robert Hollister's work on this project. We express our deep appreciation to Susan Sudman, Phyllis Bagwell Cater and Pamela Morgan who helped with bibliographical and other research.

Part I
Introduction

1 Neighborhood Health Centers as Demonstrations

Robert M. Hollister

The current generation of neighborhood health centers started as demonstration projects. OEO's foray into health began in 1965 under the "research and development" authority of the Community Action Program. In 1966, OEO was granted specific authority to establish comprehensive health services projects by an amendment to the Economic Opportunity Act sponsored by Senator Edward Kennedy. HEW's support for neighborhood health centers was based on Section 314 (e) of the Partnership for Health Act of 1967, entitled "Project Grants for Health Services Development." This section of the law included authority to fund demonstration projects. HEW sponsorship of health centers was enabled further by a December 1967 statement by the Surgeon General giving priority under Section 314 (e) to projects which would serve poor areas.

Proponents' views of the centers as demonstrations varied in terms of their assumptions about what would be demonstrated and how the process of demonstration would occur. Some felt that the centers would demonstrate the efficacy of a model which they favored and were confident would work well when implemented. They believed that the success of neighborhood health centers would stimulate the creation of other centers across the country, hopefully enough to serve all poor persons. Another major conception of the demonstration function maintained that the experience of the centers would help answer questions and to resolve policy dilemmas.[1] A third was more rationalistic: what was demonstrated by the centers would be determined and communicated by the results of formal evaluations of efficiency and effectiveness.

It was rarely the case that persons active in the health center movement made explicit their conceptions of the demonstration process. Their notions about this process were not very carefully formulated. They stressed one or another conception, balancing them in different combinations. The centers were sold as demonstrations when that tack was expedient. In terms of agency posture, the dominant vision was a combination of the first two conceptions, but OEO staff members paid lip service to the more rationalistic model in their dealings with the Office of Management and Budget.

The experience to date of the federally-sponsored health centers has been influenced greatly by the fact that they have been established and financed as demonstrations rather than as regular, continuing programs. They have accrued the benefits of the demonstration project approach to reform—being "fashion-

1

able, politically attractive, rationally appealing, inexpensive and not binding."[2]
Inevitably, the centers have also suffered from the problems inherent in this
approach.

Arguments for and against the centers amount to a series of disagreements
about what they demonstrate. It is particularly important to ask evaluative questions in the context of a demonstration process because this cast to the inquiry
implies a commitment to taking a broader look. It suggests the importance of
looking at a wide range of accomplishments, documenting both their intended
and their unintended consequences. It insists on surveying the results on all
objectives expressed for the centers, not just in relation to those goals subjected
to the most systematic or most recent formal evaluation efforts.

This collection of readings attempts to correct a general failure to recognize
and communicate significant accomplishments of the centers. It is essential to
revive the demonstration purposes of the centers in order to draw the lessons
they hold and to recognize and to sustain their accomplishments and strengths,
as well as to correct their deficiencies.

The centers discussed in this book are those sponsored by OEO and by HEW
under Section 314 (e) of the Partnership for Health Act. Many other neighborhood health units resemble these centers to varying degrees in terms of location,
scope of services and other aspects. To the extent that they are similar, some of
the findings with regard to the OEO and HEW 314 (e) centers may apply to
them also.

Through 1971, OEO had sponsored approximately 100 comprehensive
health services projects, many of them neighborhood health centers. Another
50 or so had been funded by HEW. The total federal outlay for these projects
was approximately $400 million.[3] Three-fourths of the centers are located in
urban areas, one-fourth in rural. They serve upwards of one million patients.

The centers provide comprehensive primary health care services in one-stop
facilities. A full range of preventive, curative, and rehabilitative services are
delivered to service populations of between 6,000 and 50,000. Eligibility for
services has been handled variously at different times. At present, the centers
offer free services for persons who are poor according to OEO or state Medicaid
guidelines. Many offer services to the "near poor" at fees determined on a
sliding scale. About one-half of the employees of the centers are residents of the
service areas. The centers attempt to offer family-oriented care and to maintain
continuous personalized relationships between patients and health professionals.
Consumer participation in the planning and management of the centers is provided by arrangements which vary widely. They include the selection of
consumer representatives to serve on advisory committees and boards of directors
as well as the employment of area residents.

The health centers originally sponsored by the Office of Economic Opportunity have been transferred for continuing support to HEW. It is uncertain how
long HEW will continue to fund the centers on a project grant basis. HEW cut

the budgets of centers for fiscal year 1973 and more substantial reductions are promised in the future. The department is pressing the centers to become more financially self-sufficient. No money is being spent to establish new centers.[a]

What Do Demonstration Projects Demonstrate?

The articles reprinted in this reader offer a set of partial answers to the broad question, what do the health centers demonstrate? Taken together, these reports document the considerable merits of the centers. The health services which they provide represent very real improvements to the patients who use them. Their experiences yield important lessons with respect to approaches that have been successful and should be sustained as well as those that should be avoided in future attempts to improve ambulatory care systems.

Although the accomplishments of the health centers have not met the highest expectations expressed by some, the improvements for which they are responsible represent substantial achievement. These improvements were not easy to come by and cannot be casually dismissed simply because they are not as complete as would be desired. They are not complete because improving health care in poor areas is difficult and takes time. So does progress toward other important goals of the centers: employing poor residents, training persons for new health career roles, securing consumer involvement in planning and running health services, and demonstrating and refining new modes of organization, finance, and management.

Some critics claim that the centers are too costly, use resources inefficiently, maintain a dual system of health care, provide poor quality health care, stimulate unproductive community conflict, drain off pressures for more substantial, more permanent changes in the health care system. How true are these claims? Proponents argue that the neighborhood health centers are succeeding in providing comprehensive, high quality care, at a reasonable cost, training significant numbers of new professionals and paraprofessionals in health, devolving political power to community groups, making substantial and lasting changes in the health care system. How true are these contentions? The material in this reader presents and weighs the evidence—favorable as well as unfavorable. On balance, the evidence testifies to the fundamental soundness of the neighborhood health center concept.

---

[a]The most recent set of units resembling neighborhood health centers to be established were the Family Health Centers of HEW, created to try out the package of benefits included in President Nixon's Family Health Insurance Plan, no longer an active proposal. The Family Health Centers are smaller and offer a much more restricted set of services than do the original neighborhood health centers sponsored by OEO and HEW.

The articles in this book address the question of what the health centers demonstrate with regard to development, structure and operation, i.e., precursors of the present generation of neighborhood health centers; evolution of the neighborhood health centers of the 1960s; perspectives of evaluation; consumer participation and community control; administration; costs and financing; patients' use and response; quality of care; allied health workers and health teams; neighborhood health centers as instruments of change—relationships with, and impacts on, other health institutions.

In spite of their record of substantial accomplishment, the neighborhood health centers appear to demonstrate very different things to different people in different places with different personal or institutional agendas. The centers have evoked varied interpretations of finite experiences, which one would think from the variety of perceptions were designed more as a Rorscharch test than a controlled experiment. There is a rampant Rashomon effect in perceptions of what the centers have accomplished.

We can no more force uniform consumption and assimilation of the working experience of the centers than we can produce universal values and shared knowledge by making students read the same textbook. To some extent the differing conclusions with regard to the performance of the health centers are based in divergent philosophies of change. There is a strong tendency toward ignoring evidence of real change unless it appears in favored forms which are associated with (and held to be the only effective ways of approaching) the goals of the centers. Donald Schon has observed:

> We conceive of our institutions—nations, religions, business organizations, industries—as enduring. Change of values is seen as deviance, undependability, flightiness. Values are presumed to be firm and constant. To the extent that we admit historical change, we see it according to the model of *progress*—steady change occurring within a stable framework of value. . . .
>
> Yet institutions, laws, actions, occupations, professions and even our concept of character can be seen, after the fact, to have changed; it is only that we are somehow protected from awareness of these changes while they are occurring. And we are all historical revisionists. Magically, we forget the earlier institutions and values, and the assumptions of stability that surrounded them.[4]

Since the health centers differ significantly in terms of organizational structure, scope of services, size, structures of governance, and styles of medical practice, what can centers as a group demonstrate? The larger truth is that the centers share a great many characteristics, and therefore it is accurate and useful to consider them collectively. It is the case that they have significant variations, but the varied experiences of individual centers have validity in their own right. Many of the articles included in this volume refer to the experience of single centers. It is important to be cautious about generalizing on the basis of these individual experiences. On the other hand, the particular experiences are often quite similar to those of other centers and so have general applicability.

It is useful to view the centers not solely as institutions delivering health services, but also as collections of characteristics which are separable from the health center organizational framework. The experience of the centers indicates the potentialities and limitations of these separate characteristics as well as those of the centers per se. In addition, the neighborhood health centers were seen by their initial sponsors and supporters as being institutions which would accomplish a number of ends logically separate from the *neighborhood* character of the places. Today, a few short years later, the significance of this distinction is more apparent. As the loose alliance of national constituencies which supported neighborhood health centers has eroded, and other approaches to improving primary health care have grown in popularity, there is increasing scrutiny of the performance of the centers. What aspects of their operation are necessarily linked to each other? What aspects are mutually reinforcing and therefore essential components of the model? Are there goals of the neighborhood health centers that could be accomplished or approached more efficiently and more effectively by other service delivery models? Or—another way of stating the same questions—are there elements of the neighborhood health center concept that can be successfully extracted from the model and implemented in other settings, in other combinations of components? More specifically, can prepaid group practices or reorganized hospital outpatient departments successfully improve the continuity of care and its acceptability? Is there anything in the makeup of neighborhood health centers that gives them superiority as a vehicle for achieving these reform ends?

These questions underlie current attacks on the health centers. It was hard to see in 1966, but patently obvious today, that the neighborhood health center is a vulnerable concept. The diffuse alliance of reformers who supported their development held a set of objectives for the new institutions which masked a number of important conflicts. A prominent medical historian noted with regard to an earlier generation of neighborhood health centers:

> As is not infrequently the case when a professional development or trend is in "fashion," the name by which it is designated acquires an aura of approval, and is used to describe activities and enterprises that differ widely, so that they may share some of the aura. This was also the fate of the health center concept, and is in part responsible for its decline.[5]

In addition, the initial designs of the neighborhood health centers were not always a logically tight model. There is no reason why they should have been (even though individuals' conceptions may have been internally consistent). The point is that the neighborhood health centers became a *focus* of a number of reform ideas in health care which were related, but not inextricably so. The neighborhood center concept attracted a number of ideas for change which lived happily under the same umbrella for a while and in some cases perhaps even matured a bit. But the longer range future of some of these reformist notions is not inextricably linked to other components of the model. Therefore, some common aspects of the original design of neighborhood health centers have faded out—emphasis on team practice of medicine, environmental causes of poor health, and social services related to health care—and others are being successfully appropriated by other ambulatory care models which are increasingly competitive with the neighborhood centers.

Again, there is nothing "wrong" with this phenomenon. It is a natural kind of evolution. But it is, from some perspectives, a distressing set of developments. To some observers, it appears that the most important aspects of the centers are being lost in the shuffle. They are being discarded as third party payers refuse to reimburse the centers for including them in the services which they offer. And to those individuals who have labored hard for years to make the existing neighborhood health centers work, it seems that some important parts of their operations are being jettisoned without ever being given a fair trial.

How Does the Process of Demonstration Occur?

In weighing the experience of the centers, it is essential to understand how the demonstration process which they stimulate actually occurs. It is impossible to further the demonstration process or to influence it effectively without a clearer collective understanding of how it takes place.[6]

In the most important ways, collective digestion of the working experience of the centers has occurred quite informally. Influential assessments of the efficacy, the potentialities and limitations of the centers are often molded with very little support from the available facts. Are the facts not available enough? Or in the wrong form? Or are persons unwilling to perceive them or to accept them as factual? To a very real extent, we see what we want to see, we learn what we want to learn. There are a host of common sense reasons, for example, to support the contention that neighborhood health centers are inefficient and cost too much. The existence of systematic information which refutes the claim proves to be only a minor obstacle to sustaining the belief.

In part, the proponents and employees, supporters of the centers, have done an inadequate job of building and communicating their case. After the initial flush of innovative creation, the more recent period of criticism has elicited a rather defensive response from persons associated with the centers. They are too busy and too battle weary to fight back effectively. They know all too well some of their own shortcomings and they accept the validity of criticisms on these scores, even though these attacks are often grossly inappropriate and evidence a highly discriminatory double standard of evaluation. To some extent, they are hamstrung by shifts in political forces that have rearranged the constellation of objectives attached to the centers. The political muscle has atrophied behind some of those objectives on which the centers can show real accomplishment.

The process of demonstration of the results and experiences of the neighborhood health centers occurs simultaneously by several different routes. Other health agencies and institutions observe the progress of the centers and are also touched more directly by the centers in some instances when the centers want something from, and therefore negotiate and otherwise interact with them. By virtue of their continued existence, the centers indicate that comprehensive, personalized, family-oriented health care is desirable and possible. The existence of the centers permits comparison of their effectiveness and efficiency with alternative sources of ambulatory health services. The comparison may not be made carefully or accurately, but the basis for solid measurements is provided. Thousands of persons with various levels of training and various professional roles and attachments gain direct experience through working for the centers. It is impossible to generalize about what they take away, but surely their personal beliefs are modified somewhat by the experience. Those who move on to other jobs carry with them altered conceptions of what is desirable and possible and how improvements in primary health care services can be designed and implemented. The media of demonstration are not only published reports, but volumes of individual conversations, speeches, films, and every other type of communication.

The actual process of demonstration differs radically from the rationalistic demonstration project model. The persons setting up the neighborhood health centers were doers more than believers in the rationalistic conceptions of the demonstration process. Nonetheless, they and others following the progress of the centers did adhere to some elements of it. The rationalistic model bears repeating because it is not entirely a straw man. It perhaps overstates what any one individual believes, but it does represent some of our collective myths about how reform proceeds.

The rationalistic view of the demonstration project approach prescribes: Implement a defined model in a few instances that will provide good tests of its key features. Carefully evaluate how well the model achieves its objectives. Use these results to decide whether or not the model merits being extended in other areas and to determine which aspects of it work and which should be changed.

Reality distorts and denies each feature of this conception of the demonstration process. The demonstration model proves to be an effective cover for starting new programs, but the elements of the formal model do not hold true. The mental model of the demonstration project approach bears very little

resemblance to the actual experience of the centers. The history of the neighborhood health centers sponsored by OEO and HEW gives the lie to this approach,
just as other federal programs of the sixties have done. The model is not
implemented in just a few places, but in many. The model itself varies considerably and in ways which defy any possibility of controlling many important
variables. Formal evaluation efforts are sponsored and implemented conscien-
tiously, but they contribute only very indirectly to the more dominant, highly
political and less factually based process of evaluation which occurs outside of
the sponsoring agencies. (The collection of papers in this reader includes the
results of some of the formal evaluations of the centers with the intention of
injecting them more forcefully into the informal, politically charged process of
assessing the centers.) The informal evaluative looks at the centers have applied
unreasonably high standards which are not applied to other health care facilities.
In addition, the formal evaluation efforts tend to focus on only a few of the
important original objectives of the centers, overlooking some of those objectives
on which the centers have demonstrated real accomplishment, but for which
they now find little political support.

Paying lip service to the demonstration project model proved to be a useful
tactic at a number of points in the development of the centers. Where there are
anticipated opponents to a new program, one way of circumventing them is to
portray the proposed program as a set of demonstration projects. Potential
criticism is defused because the demonstration approach entails setting up only
a few projects which will not be so great a threat as would be a program with
total coverage of all eligible persons. In addition, the demonstration approach
presents the projects as only possible solutions. They are established tentatively,
with a commitment to evaluating how well they do.

The centers were run by a wide variety of organizations—local departments
of public health, medical societies, antipoverty agencies, and medical schools.
OEO explained that this variation in sponsorship would enable testing of which
type worked best, but the political advantages of the spread are obvious. The
fact of some variation in the managing agencies was more important than any
aims of carrying out an experiment. In 1968, when the Office of Management
and Budget was trying to limit the number of new health centers being created
by OEO, the latter agency argued that the demonstration function of the centers
required the establishment of a dozen more centers in parts of the country where
none were in existence. An OEO memorandum stated that those geographic
areas with the greatest concentrations of poor people and greatest deficiencies in
health services existed in twenty-nine states, only seventeen of which had
neighborhood health centers. It concluded, "Although OEO has brought
national attention to Neighborhood Health Center concepts, states without at
least one such demonstration programs (sic) will move very slowly, if at all,
toward improving ambulatory service to the poor."[7]

The problem is that one cannot have the benefits of the demonstration project approach without falling prey to its vicissitudes as well. The short-run benefits include side-stepping potential opponents of the new programmatic thrust and attracting the involvement of energetic, talented persons interested in being a part of a demonstration—something new and promising. The problems inherent in the approach stem from the fact that the short history of the present generation of centers traces the unfortunate, by now classic scenario of governmentally-sponsored demonstration projects. Many points of the scenario distort the process of demonstration both during the development of the centers and later on when they have had some years of operating experience. The scenario—not unique to neighborhood health centers—goes as follows: Initial expectations are unrealistically high, objectives (which conflict with one another) are oversold in order to gather political support, projects are heralded as successful immediately after they are underway (or even earlier). The projects are given woefully inadequate technical assistance, which contributes to administrative and other problems. Evaluation efforts are soft-pedalled early on and are slow to be started. The model is implemented in additional communities. Administrative and managerial difficulties appear and fuel criticisms of the projects' performance. Proud promises are replaced by calls for hard-nosed evaluations, which when undertaken, ignore many of the initial objectives—the conflicts among which are now painfully apparent. The evaluation results which are produced turn out to be largely irrelevant to later decisions about levels of governmental support. Projects which were trumpeted as successful innovations at the start are a few short years later forced to discontinue some of their services and face the very real possibility of having to close down.

At about the same time as the optimistic glow of initial periods of implementation was rapidly fading in many of the centers, the national constituencies that supported the health centers were growing considerably less interested in them. And the national supporting agencies—OEO and HEW—began to pressure the centers for hard documentation of the results of their investment in order to impress the Administration and Congress with the necessity of maintaining and increasing the appropriations for these programs. The demonstration notion—of trying out a model, systematically evaluating it, then building new programs based upon the results of the evaluation—was perverted every step of the way. The broad outlines of the initial model were clear enough. But the evaluation efforts were inevitably skewed by the changing pressures felt by the national sponsoring institutions. The evaluations have tended not to assess the performance of the centers as vehicles for providing employment and job training to residents of poor communities, for devolving political power to health consumers in poor communities in health and related fields, or for stimulating broader changes in health care systems.

Another curious affliction of the demonstration project dynamic has been the tendency for observers and evaluators of the projects to apply ridiculously high standards to them. It has been expected by some, for example, that the health centers would demonstrate a measurable decline in the infant mortality rate of their service areas. Of course, this is a totally unreasonable expectation in the short run. But it follows naturally from the demonstration project principle of overpromise by initial sponsors, undersupport by funding sources and pressures for premature evaluation.[b] Another example–neighborhood health centers like other antipoverty programs have been criticized for their loose adherence to democratic ideals in the conduct of elections for consumer representatives on the advisory and governing boards of the centers. The elections have not been as tightly monitored as one might like, but they have not been scandalous either. The rate of voter participation by those eligible has usually been "low"–ranging from below 1 percent to above 30 percent in a few cases where massive efforts were made to turn out service populations who lived in a single housing project. The critics rarely stop to compare the rate of participation to that in the primaries of an off-year election in a large central city dominated by one party. Consumer elections at neighborhood health centers compare more favorably to this more reasonable standard.

The creation of the complicated new institutions which are the neighborhood health centers involved a series of pressing conflicts and crises in each locality. The persons responsible for establishing the health centers were totally preoccupied with dealing with these immediate problems. They were extremely impatient with suggestions that it was important to set up data systems that would generate information for eventual evaluation. This understandable, perhaps inevitable, resistance to implementing the bases for solid evaluation was to hurt the centers later on. One perscient observer of the early development of the centers wrote:

> In the beginning, it was assumed that the neighborhood health centers *should* be established, that they would be expensive to establish and operate, and that their newness prevented any meaningful examination of costs with other medical care mechanisms; as a result, relatively little concrete data are available on the neighborhood health center's effectiveness in relation to costs. Administrators of neighborhood health centers have not yet had to be coldly analytical about the benefits and costs of their new programs, but someday soon, they will have to begin. Indeed, the future of their centers may depend upon it.[8]

When the centers badly needed data which would support continued public funding of their operations, it was, with few exceptions, not available.

---

[b]Program evaluation staff at the OEO Office of Health Affairs resisted pressure to measure the effect of the health centers on health status of the groups being served, but the expectation that the centers would accomplish such a result has persisted along with desire to see the effects documented.

The resounding cry of failure has been ringing down the curtain on many of the dramas of the Great Society. These dramas may have played to favorable critical reviews at the start, but awkwardnesses of timing, staging and uneven performances added to "producer's panic" have caused many of them to close after short runs in spite of stellar individual performances and aspects of the productions which were more than redeeming. Above all, however, conservatism triumphed over compassion.

The charges that the centers have failed, that they do not measure up, come in large part from quarters which have never supported the centers or whose support for them has been inadequate. Critics of this ilk include local medical societies and private practitioners, medical school faculty, and bureaucrats interested in preserving other approaches to delivering care. These criticisms are basically dishonest in that they rue shortcomings for which they are partly responsible and decry failure to reach objectives to which they have never before demonstrated any great allegiance.

Another group of critics are persons who have supported many of the goals of the centers and have often worked for the centers themselves. These are staunch advocates of the centers, persons who have supported them for years, but who now voice criticisms because they feel that the centers have fallen short in their accomplishments. In some cases, people are disenchanted, having seen the obvious problems of the centers by being so close to them. Sometimes the individuals most deeply committed to the centers see failure in the fact that they have been blocked from establishing more neighborhood health centers and from sustaining initial ones in their original form. These purists—people who "cling to the dream," as one former administrator in the OEO office of Health Affairs put it—do not believe that the centers have achieved lasting improvements in the health system.

Both vectors of criticism fail to distinguish clearly enough between evaluating a program as a failure on the one hand, and, on the other, admitting to problems candidly, diagnosing them and calling for modifications and sustained or increased support.

The lessons for future demonstration projects are clear: Invest heavily early on—from Day One—in evaluation systems that will generate information in time to wage a more effective fight for survival a few years later. Sit hard on the coat-tails of colleagues eager to preach the myriad virtues of the new approach and to promise quick rewards from the requested public investments. Build in incentives for efficiency. Watch out for faint-hearted friends. Know the opposition.

References

1. See Lisbeth B. Schorr and Joseph T. English, "Background and Context of Significant Issues in Neighborhood Health Center Programs," *Milbank*

Memorial Fund Quarterly 66, 3, Part I (July 1968): 289–296, reprinted on pp. 45–50 of this reader.

2. Martin Rein, "The Demonstration as a Strategy of Change," in Martin Rein, *Social Policy* (New York: Random House, 1970), p. 140. This chapter by Rein, pp. 138–152 of his book, presents a comprehensive analysis of the assets and liabilities of the demonstration project approach. His findings with regard to demonstration projects in juvenile delinquency, employment training, vocational rehabilitation, education and other fields square well with experience of neighborhood health centers.

3. Daniel I. Zwick, "Some Accomplishments and Findings of Neighborhood Health Centers," *Milbank Memorial Fund Quarterly 50,* 4, Part I (October 1972): 390.

4. Donald A. Schon, *Technology and Change: The New Heraclitus* (New York: Delacourte Press, 1967), pp. xii–xiii.

5. George Rosen, "The First Neighborhood Health Center Movement—Its Rise and Fall," *American Journal of Public Health 61,* 8 (August 1971): 1630.

6. See Martin Rein, "Demonstration as a Strategy."

7. Memorandum by William Plissner, "Proposed New Efforts in Comprehensive Health Services," Nov. 5, 1969, p. 5.

8. Paul R. Torrens, "Administrative Problems of Neighborhood Health Centers," *Medical Care 9,* 6 (Nov.–Dec. 1971): 495.

2

Neighborhood Health Centers as a Social Movement

Robert M. Hollister, Bernard M. Kramer, and Seymour S. Bellin

Persons active in setting up and running neighborhood health centers talk about themselves and their programs as being part of a movement. The centers are not merely projects that implement a series of improvements in primary health care. They also express and carry a social movement defined by several impulses toward change that converged in the 1960s. It is impossible to understand the current generation of centers without viewing them as a social movement; its development was stimulated by the intersection of several supporting trends and then undermined by the divergence and weakening of these individual trends.

The health centers constitute a movement because they are in large part the product of several streams of reform that have not stood still while the centers were implemented. The debates pro and con the centers have proceeded in terms of competing political and reformist ideologies. It is important to analyze the health centers at least in part in terms of the extent to which they represent a playing out of larger political themes. Their fortunes are determined to a great extent by shifting balances in these ongoing conflicts waged by institutions and interest groups forming fluid alliances.

Why did neighborhood health centers come on the scene when they did, in the middle 1960s? The answer can be found by tracing strands of reformist thinking and social change. The neighborhood health centers were spawned by a particular confluence of events and forces: the decreasing quality of health care in poor areas; evolving popular definitions of the "health crisis"; changes in the institutional structure of the health care system; development of the civil rights movement; emergence of the "cycle of poverty" concept; evolution of the federal antipoverty program; revival of interest in concepts of neighborhood and community, and enthusiasm for administrative and political decentralization.

But the intersecting trends have evolved in such a way as to diffuse the very sources that gave rise to the centers. We may ask then whether the original sources of the movement have been dissipated beyond the point of productive convergence. This chapter traces these developments and relates each to the shifting fortunes of the neighborhood health center movement.

13

*1. The Decreasing Quality of Health Care in
Poor Areas*

The new neighborhood health centers responded to trends in health care that
adversely affected the poor. A major trend was the decreasing number of physicians practicing in poor neighborhoods across the country.[1] Poor, often black,
neighborhoods of some tens of thousands of residents in 1965 had perhaps half
a dozen remaining medical practitioners, most of whom were semi-retired. The
neighborhood health center filled a gap left by the departure of the general
practitioner from urban core areas.

A second factor supporting the development of the centers was the declining
quality of the municipal hospital systems.[2] Their physical facilities were old and
visibly decaying. The city hospitals were in an increasingly disadvantageous competitive position vis-a-vis other hospitals in a given locality. University medical
centers, for example, had grown substantially since World War II. These hospitals
were better financed and more attractive to prospective interns, residents and
other staff. As the number of physicians practicing in neighborhoods declined
(and the proportion of physicians who were in general practice decreased), increasing numbers of poor urban residents were using hospital emergency rooms
or outpatient departments as their primary source of ambulatory care.[3] Crowd-
ing of hospital facilities meant that patients were likely to encounter long waits
and curt treatment.

Shifts in metropolitan demography contributed to these trends as well.
In-migration from rural areas, high birth rates, and decreased death rates yielded
changes in the economic and racial composition of inner-city populations.
Physicians, like other middle-class citizens, were moving to the suburbs to follow
their preferred patients and their pocketbooks. Residential segregation was increasing. Altogether, these trends fueled the development of the neighborhood
health centers.

By the early 1970s, none of these conditions had altered dramatically. Some
things have changed, however. The existing neighborhood health centers,
although they hardly cover all of the geographic areas needing better health care,
have succeeded in maintaining effective substitutes for solo practitioners in some
of those areas of greatest need. They have reduced this source of complaint in
areas that had been clamoring for improvement a few years earlier. The original
complaint, now dealt with, is not an impetus for expansion of the number of
neighborhood health centers, although it probably helps to protect those that
currently exist.

Vigorous efforts have been undertaken in a number of cities to improve the
municipal hospital systems.[4] This process of upgrading is a slow one, but there
is visible movement by government, tangible response to complaints about the
public hospitals. This apparent response has worked to improve, or at least to
promise to improve, the quality of health care in poor areas.

2. Evolving Popular Definitions of the "Health Crisis"

In the middle 1960s, medical professionals, middle-class citizens, and others were beginning to worry about the rising cost of medical care, but the "health crisis" was largely defined in terms of the special problems suffered by groups that had been neglected and had suffered discrimination.[5]

By the early 1970s, the "health crisis" was felt acutely by a much broader spectrum of the U.S. population. The dominant emphasis was on cost. What was the crisis? The universal answer: high costs—of hospitalization, visits to the doctor, drugs, and everything else. Complaints about not being able to find a doctor when needed comprise an important part of the popular sense of crisis; but it is clearly subordinate to the issue of cost. The special difficulties of minority groups have tended to be forgotten as well.[6] The popular definition of the crisis is an important commodity politically because it determines in great measure the kinds of governmental interventions that will be propounded. Consequently, there is at present a spate of proposals for national health insurance which include something for all socioeconomic classes, not just the worst off. This development follows closely the general rule of planned change in the United States—that it occurs in large packages which yield benefits to each of the constituencies whose support is needed to secure the necessary votes in Congress and support in other forums of government. Some analysts believe that the national health insurance schemes currently being proposed would do very little to help the poor, because they increase effective demand for services without increasing or otherwise adjusting supply, except in the long run.[7] This argument maintains that the resulting system will tend to serve the richer, more pleasant patients better and will have little remaining capacity with which to treat the poor.

The earlier definition of the "health crisis" in terms of the special problems of the poor and minority groups in central cities and rural areas supported the development of neighborhood health centers which were designed specifically to serve these groups. The more recent popular definition of the "health crisis" emphasizes the cost of medical care to all persons and, to a lesser extent, a variety of complaints about the health care system as it affects a broad range of classes, not just the poor. This more recent definition of the crisis stimulates congressional and administration support for measures other than, broader than, neighborhood health centers.

Another school of thought maintains that the "health crisis" is a constant state of affairs, and that public conceptions of health care have labeled it as crisis-ridden in essentially the same regards over a period of decades. For example, Robert Alford and other observers have noted the similarities between the 1932 report of the Committee on the Costs of Medical Care and contemporary criticisms of the health care system.[8] Alford argues that shifts in the health care system are most accurately characterized as "dynamics without change":

The overwhelming fact about the various reforms of the health system that have been implemented or proposed—more money, more subsidy of insurance, more manpower, more demonstration projects, more clinics—is that they are absorbed into a system which is enormously resistant to change. The reforms which are suggested are sponsored by different elements in the health system and advantage one or another element, but they do not seriously damage any interests. This pluralistic balancing of costs and benefits successfully shields the funding, powers, and resources of the producing institutions from any basic structural change.[9]

An extension of this analysis would suggest that public conceptions of the health crisis foster the development of neighborhood health centers, but only a limited number of them and only in forms which maintain the present balances of institutional power.

3. Changes in the Institutional Structure of the Health Care System

By the middle 1960s, the U.S. health care system had moved significantly away from an earlier political pattern in which physicians were the dominant force. Contemporary institutional structure is characterized by diffusion of influence and a complicated network of relationships among groups and agencies.[10] The dominant forces are now the major institutional actors—third party payers, hospitals, medical centers, and governmental agencies—rather than professional associations.[11] These institutions pursue self-interests which are immensely more complicated than those which motivate any single profession. By the middle sixties it was in the institutional self-interests of a number of major groups to support the development of the neighborhood health centers, or at least not to torpedo their development. These self-interests were perceived by the parties involved, and they were powerful enough to accomplish them by virtue of the more dispersed pattern of political influence. "The AMA had cried wolf too frequently and too shrilly to raise again the specter of 'socialized medicine' when OEO proposed the establishment of neighborhood health centers."[12]

The centers represented an opportunity for hospitals and medical schools to respond to growing pressures to serve their immediately surrounding communities,[13] and to respond without having to upset their own organizational arrangements closer to home.[14] The decreasing federal support for basic medical research was an additional inducement to look with favor on the growing pots of money being made available for community medicine.

Proponents of a number of changes in the organization of the delivery of health care saw the health centers as instruments for trying out and for implementing these innovations (in particular, the team practice of medicine and the creation of new paraprofessional and professional roles). Hospitals sought to reduce overcrowding of their outpatient clinics and emergency rooms. The Office of Economic Opportunity wanted to improve the health status of poor Americans; to attack the cycle of poverty by improving health services. In addition, OEO was looking for ways to pursue its broad goals without arousing opposition from local governments and other groups. The neighborhood health centers proved to be such a less politically vulnerable program.

The interests of the medical schools with regard to neighborhood health centers have now shifted somewhat, leaving the health center movement without an earlier ally and with a new competitor. The schools quickly discovered the hidden pitfalls of involvement in the management of neighborhood centers. The experience of becoming enmeshed in bitter controversies with community groups over governance of the centers had lead a number of school to phase out of these operations. In addition, hostile reaction within medical schools to the expanding role of community medicine units has weakened the position of these departments in medical school power relations.

Many hospitals are now in a position of worrying about their rising vacancy rates. They are less concerned about crowded outpatient facilities than they are about trying to balance their budgets by keeping higher proportions of their beds filled. Therefore, the hospitals' interests in the health centers have changed somewhat. The neighborhood centers are no longer valued for their potential to decrease hospitalization, but are seen as new sources of patients to fill empty hospital beds. Hospitals are now interested in serving as back-ups to the neighborhood units partly because the centers provide an additional pool of patients with third party payers attached.

4. The Development of the Civil Rights Movement

The civil rights movement, cresting in the middle 1960s, pressed for better health care along with other demands. In this period of intense agitation, mobilization of energies, and confrontations with agents of discrimination, millions of Black Americans were unwilling to stand for second class services, health care included. Support of the health centers movement was a natural outcome. Although most of the neighborhood health centers were initiated by health providers, in many cases their development was spurred or supported by Black protests and grievances against hospitals and other provider organizations. It is no accident that federally-funded health centers are concentrated in areas where the civil rights movement was strong. Many of the health professionals active in setting up neighborhood health centers had been in the civil rights movement where they gained in political education and activist motivation.

Today, in the early 1970s, progressives and conservatives alike declare the civil rights movement dead. Former proponents of integration carefully avoid some of their earlier stands. Blacks continue to struggle for a better deal, but the struggle is harder against stronger opposition. It is a period of retrenchment and of consolidation of whatever gains have been made. As a result, the neighborhood health center does not have call today on the impressive energies and inspiration of the civil rights movement.

5. Emergence of the "Cycle of Poverty" Concept

The "cycle of poverty" explanations of the plight of poor persons reached a peak of popular acceptance in the middle sixties.[15] Health was seen as a crucial link in the chain, and one about which something could be done. By the early seventies there was decreasing interest in this theory. It was not discarded exactly, but was accepted as a vague general truth, no longer offering a satisfying explanation to guide and inspire new interventions. Health as a lever in the "war against poverty" stands motionless along with the retrenched antipoverty warriors.

6. Evolution of the Federal Antipoverty Program

The neighborhood health centers sponsored by OEO were initiated by the agency's Community Action Program and to some extent grew out of the early experiences of local CAPs. Local attempts to improve education and employment opportunities indicated that poor health was a strong barrier to improvement in these areas.[16]

OEO received scores of applications from local communities to sponsor fragmentary health programs, extensions of existing categorical projects.[17] In most cases, OEO rejected these proposals. The agency resolved to underwrite more comprehensive projects, which it felt would have more of a chance of making a lasting dent in the health problems of poor communities.[18] The first set of health centers that OEO funded built upon the existing ideas, plans, and dreams of persons in different parts of the country. OEO proved to be a congenial vehicle for the nurturance of these plans.[19]

Case study accounts document that neighborhood activists involved in setting up local centers were involved in other fields of community action before getting into health issues. There is good evidence that this prior experience with antipoverty work served these persons well in their participation as health consumer representatives. The earlier involvements sharpened leadership skills, provided useful knowledge about the working of local institutions and ways of maneuvering within and around them, and taught basics of community organization—from the practicalities of running effective meetings to the requisites of successful negotiations with major institutions.[20]

The Public Health Service of HEW behaved in many ways similarly to OEO in its sponsorship of neighborhood health centers. HEW entered the field later, sponsoring fewer centers. There have been significant differences in their administration of the centers, but the similarities with the OEO-funded centers are probably more important. The centers financed by the two agencies look very much the same in most respects—size, scope of services, organizational structure, and so forth.

As OEO evolved since the middle sixties, it became less viable as a base of support for the health centers. As a result, the health centers shifted from anti-poverty programs—with attendant emphasis on economic and political development—to programs limited strictly to health services.

The first set of neighborhood health centers established by OEO totaled eight projects. These were followed by a second wave of centers after the Kennedy amendment authorized $50 million for comprehensive health services projects. Thirty additional facilities were funded in 1967 and 1968. OEO tried to set up as many demonstration health centers as was possible. The Bureau of the Budget, later the Office of Management and Budget, continued to ask the agency, how many demonstration projects were enough to demonstrate what the health centers could do? When President Johnson mentioned a figure of fifty health centers, that became the cutoff point for health center demonstrations.

But partisans of the health centers movement advocated establishing enough centers to serve all eligible patients in the entire country. A 1967 report by HEW stated that a total of 620 centers would be needed in order to cover the 15.5 million low-income persons who "can be realistically served by comprehensive neighborhood health centers."[21] OEO's justification of its 1966 budget requests to the Bureau of the Budget projected a total of 530 centers by 1970.[22]

Those persons responsible for launching the neighborhood health center programs at the federal level sincerely viewed the centers as demonstrations which could contribute to answering questions about the organization of service delivery systems and a host of other dilemmas. But they also realized that the periods of time conducive to major innovative thrusts are often short. There was an understandable, politically realistic, urge to seize the opportunity, to ride the crest of support for reform as long as it lasted and to accomplish as much as possible before the wave crashed to shore and washed back down the beach. Those persons most responsible for extending the health center model were hardly inclined to wait for the results to come in from a few experiments and then to contemplate extension of the model. They knew that by then it might be too late to do so. They were confident enough that what they were pushing constituted an improvement over the existing situation in local communities, so they plunged ahead.

When OEO and HEW had set up as many neighborhood health centers as they could, why was the model not emulated more widely by other agencies

and institutions? Why have there not been resources to support new neighborhood health centers per se or in other organizational guises? To some extent,
the pieces of the model have been implemented by others, but the resources
have not been released to enable other units of government and other institutions to create health centers of the same scale and offering the same scope of
services as the initial centers underwritten by OEO and HEW. Some persons
familiar with the centers refer to weaknesses such as the project grant method
of financing. Many proponents of the centers advocate the creation of prepaid
group practices to serve as neighborhood health centers with greater financial
stability. Health maintenance organizations replaced neighborhood health
centers at center stage, but they have not come into being in substantial numbers yet, and the future of this ideas is uncertain. In other words, the expansion
of neighborhood health centers has been arrested as has the extension of key
characteristics of the centers in other organizational forms.

7. Revival of Interest in Concepts of Neighborhood and Community, and Enthusiasm for Decentralization

The middle 1960s saw a peaking of what appears to be a cyclical popular interest in concepts of neighborhood and community. Following an earlier period of
disenchantment with these ideas, and skepticism with regard to their fit with
reality,[23] a number of theorists argued forcefully that urban neighborhoods did
in fact exist,[24] served useful functions,[25] and provided a suitable base for
decentralization of governmental functions.[26] Experiments in the field of
education were the first of recent attempts at instituting community control.
Neighborhood health centers, by virtue of their geographic location and commitment to consumer participation (and in some cases, community control),
were another affirmation of neighborhoods and communities. They were
another set of experiments in decentralization.

By the early 1970s, popular support for decentralization of governmental
and other functions to neighborhood scale units had subsided considerably. The
ideas seemed simpler, more practical before they were tried out, than after the
fact.

Viewing the neighborhood health centers as a social movement that is now
under attack suggests that the opponents are unlikely to make judgments
strictly on the merits of the centers. A broader understanding of the centers'
shifting support should help to balance the ongoing process of assessing their
accomplishments. Changes in the complexion of the centers' political base imply
distinct shifts in the criteria and standards applied to their performance.

While the initial sources of support for the centers have eroded, the movement has taken on a dynamic of its own. The individual centers seek to carry on

their services. They are understandably reluctant to see themselves as vehicles of transition toward longer-lasting reform which rests more stably in other organizational contexts or structures. They have formed associations to serve their collective interests. These associations—both regional and national—have recently begun to realize their potential for carrying ahead the health center movement. They should be an increasingly influential force as the nation moves toward a national health insurance program.

References

1. Joyce C. Lashof, "Medical Care in the Urban Center," *Annals of Internal Medicine 68*, 1 (Jan. 1968): 242; Julius B. Richmond, *Currents in American Medicine: A Developmental View of Medical Care and Education* (Cambridge, Mass.: Harvard University Press, 1969), p. 64; Howard H. Hiatt, "Medical Care for Northbridge: A Model for Teaching Hospital-Community Interaction," *New England Journal of Medicine 284*, 11 (March 18, 1971): 594; Joseph L. Dorsey, "Manpower Problems in the Delivery of Medical Care," *New England Journal of Medicine 282*, 15 (April 19, 1970): 871.

2. Julius B. Richmond, *Currents in American Medicine,* pp. 63–64.

3. David George Satin and Frederick J. Duhl, "Help?: The Hospital Emergency Unit as Community Physician," *Medical Care 10*, 3 (May–June 1972): 249; L. Kinnian, "Role of the Emergency Unit in a Community Hospital," *New England Journal of Medicine 283*, 25 (Dec. 17, 1970): 1367.

4. *Hospitals 44*, 13 (July 1, 1970): 40–92. Special issue: The plight of the public hospital. Reports on programs to improve public hospitals underway in several major cities.

5. Anselm Strauss, "Medical Ghettos," *Trans-action 4*, 6 (May 1967): 7–15.

6. Good examples of the range of contemporary definitions of the health crisis include: Health/PAC, "Your Health Care in Crisis," brochure, no date; Health/PAC; *The American Health Empire: Power, Profits, and Politics* (New York: Random House, 1970), chs. 1 and 2, pp. 3–39; Harry Schwartz, "Health Care in America: A Heretical Diagnosis," *Saturday Review* (Aug. 14, 1971), pp. 14–17+; David D. Rutstein, *The Coming Revolution in Medicine* (Cambridge, Mass.: MIT Press, 1967), pp. 9–48; Selig Greenberg, *The Quality of Mercy: A Report on the Critical Condition of Hospital and Medical Care in America* (New York: Atheneum, 1971), chs. 1 and 2, pp. 3–53; Edward Kennedy, *In Critical Condition: The Crisis in America's Health Care* (New York: Simon and Schuster, 1972).

7. John Ehrenreich and Oliver Fein, "National Health Insurance: The Great Leap Sideways," *Social Policy 1*, 5 (Jan./Feb. 1971): 5–9; Bruce C. Stuart, "National Health Insurance and the Poor," *American Journal of Public Health 62*, 9 (Sept. 1972): 1252–1259.
For more comprehensive comparisons of alternative proposals for national health insurance see: Robert D. Eilers, "National Health Insurance: What

Kind and How Much?," *New England Journal of Medicine* (April 22 and 29, 1971), pp. 881–886 and 945–954; U.S. Congress, The Committee on Ways and Means, *Analysis of Health Insurance Proposals Introduced in the 92d Congress* (Washington, D.C.: Government Printing Office, 1971).

8. Committee on the Costs of Medical Care, *Medical Care for the American People* (Chicago: University of Chicago Press, 1932); Sumner N. Rosen, "Change and Resistance to Change," *Social Policy 1*, 5 (Jan./Feb. 1971): 4.

9. Robert Alford, "The Political Economy of Health Care: Dynamics Without Change," *Politics and Society 2*, 2 (Winter 1972): 128.

10. Ray Elling, "The Shifting Power Structure in Health," *Milbank Memorial Fund Quarterly 66*, 1 Part 2 (Jan. 1968): 119–143.

11. See: Barbara and John Ehrenreich, *The American Health Empire: Power, Profits and Politics* (New York: Random House, 1970), ch. 7, "The Medical Industrial Complex"; Harold B. Meyers, "The Medical-Industrial Complex," in Editors of Fortune, *Our Ailing Medical System* (New York: Harper & Row), ch. 3, pp. 65–74.

12. Sar A. Levitan, "Healing the Poor in Their Back Yard," ch. 7 in Sar A. Levitan, *The Great Society's Poor Law: A New Approach to Poverty* (Baltimore: Johns Hopkins Press, 1969), pp. 200–202.

13. H. Jack Geiger, "The Neighborhood Health Center: Education of the Faculty in Preventive Medicine," *Archives of Environmental Health 14*, 6 (June 1967): 912–916; Count D. Gibson, Jr. "Education in the Neighborhood Health Center," Occasional Paper No. 6 of The Education Research Center, MIT, Cambridge, Mass., 1969, pp. 1–7.

14. See: Robert J. Glaser, "The University Medical Center and Its Responsibility to the Community," *Journal of Medical Education 43*, 7 (July 1968): 790–797. The author takes a different position on the responsibility of the university medical center to the community, but presents a thorough analysis of alternative ways of contruing and acting upon that responsibility.

15. Daniel Patrick Moynihan (ed.), *On Understanding Poverty: Perspectives From the Social Sciences* (New York: Basic Books, 1969). This collection of papers presents and analyzes different conceptions of poverty and offers evidence in support and in opposition to them. They focus on pros and cons of the culture of poverty approach; Kenneth Bancroft Clark. *Dark Ghetto: Dilemmas of Social Power* (New York: Harper & Row, 1965), pp. 106–110; Peter Marris and Martin Rein, *Dilemmas of Social Reform, Poverty and Community Action in the United States* (New York: Atherton Press, 1967), pp. 37–40.

16. Lisbeth B. Schorr and Joseph T. English, "Background and Context of Significant Issues in Neighborhood Health Center Programs," *Milbank Memorial Fund Quarterly 66*, 3 Part I (July 1968): 290.

17. Sar. A. Levitan, "Healing the Poor," p. 192.

18. Lisbeth B. Schorr and Joseph T. English, "Background and Context," pp. 290–192. Sar A. Levitin, "Healing the Poor," pp. 193–195.

19. Daniel I. Zwick, "Some Accomplishments and Findings of Neighborhood Health Centers," *Milbank Memorial Fund Quarterly 50*, 4 Part I (October 1972), p. 388.

20. Robert M. Hollister, "From Consumer Participation to Community Control of Neighborhood Health Centers," Ph.D. dissertation, MIT, 1971, chs. 6 and 7, pp. 144–282.

21. Department of Health, Education and Welfare, *Delivery of Health Services for the Poor* (Washington, D.C.: Government Printing Office, Dec. 1967), pp. 52–53.

22. Office of Economic Opportunity, *National Anti-Poverty Plan and 1967 Budget Request,* Oct. 1965, Attachment B, p. 1.

23. Reginald R. Isaacs, "The Neighborhood Theory," *Journal of the American Institute of Planners 14*, 2 (Spring 1948): 15–23.

24. Herbert Gans, *The Urban Villagers: Group and Class in the Life of Italian-Americans* (New York: Free Press of Glencoe, 1962).

25. Jane Jacobs, *The Death and Life of Great American Cities* (New York: Random House, 1961); Suzanne Keller, *The Urban Neighborhood* (New York: Random House, 1968).

26. Milton Kotler, *Neighborhood Government: The Local Foundations of Political Life* (New York: Bobbs-Merrill, 1969).

Part II

Precursors of the Present Generation of
Neighborhood Health Centers

Introduction

It has become popular to point out that neighborhood health centers are not entirely new, that there have been earlier experiments in reorganizing ambulatory health services which were similar in a number of ways to those of the present generation of centers. The experience of these earlier health centers is instructive because of what it suggests about the prospects for continuation of today's centers and how the process of rejecting some parts of this collection of reforms and institutionalizing others may be occurring. The article by John D. Stoeckle and Lucy M. Candib which follows describes the factors which gave rise to the earlier centers and those which lead to their demise.[1] If the present generation of health centers is similar in some ways—location, interest in consumer participation, coordination of previously fragmented services—does this imply that they may be a short-lived set of innovations just as the earlier generation was? The reasons the authors offer for the decline of the movement are very much worth trying on for size by the present group of centers. Which apply and which do not? The reader of this article may find himself wondering whether some decades hence he will run across comparable articles that dust off for examination the experience of the health centers of the 1960s and 1970s.

The parallels with the earlier health centers are hardly complete; some argue that Stoeckle and Candib stretch the comparison too far. It is important to note the differences: The earlier centers were limited to preventive services; a key aspect of today's centers is their joining of a comprehensive range of both preventive and curative services. Today's centers are larger in size of staff, numbers of patients, and physical facilities. Many of today's centers operate under different auspices than the earlier ones, which were run by municipal health departments and private social agencies.

In any case, the experience of these historical predecessors, if it is accurate to call them that, stimulates a potentially productive line of inquiry and planning about the present centers. In addition, it places them in useful historical perspective. There is a strong tendency among social reformers to claim as totally new the measures they espouse. Heralding an approach as innovative is perhaps an inevitable trapping of attempts at reform. It can help to engender public enthusiasm for the idea. Who wants to spend public dollars on reforms which have been tried before and found wanting, or have faded out over time? There are real dangers to reform which ignores historical precedent. Historical analysis in this area can be an effective route to identifying potential supports and obstacles to reform which may exist in the present as well. For example, Stoeckle and Candib argue convincingly that some of the organizational goals of the earlier centers were contradictory, a theme that sounds all too familiar to persons monitoring the performance of the OEO- and HEW-sponsored centers. Historical knowledge can be a valuable means for avoiding pitfalls and building stronger approaches to reform, or it can breed cynicism and fuel attitudes that everything has been tried already, that no real change is possible without revolution.

The historical perspective with regard to the centers is important also in providing clearer benchmarks against which to guage the amount of change accomplished by the current generation of centers. This information about the earlier centers permits some to argue that it has all been tried before, but a careful digestion of the data allows us to point to ways in which the present set of centers are in fact unique and innovative.

Stoeckle and Candib do not really explain what happened to this earlier generation of neighborhood health centers. Did they cease to operate? Were they absorbed by other programs and modified in the process? The end of the story trails off, indicating an important topic for further research.

Reference

1. For a complementary treatment of the same issues, see: George Rosen, "The First Neighborhood Health Center Movement—Its Rise and Fall," *American Journal of Public Health* 61, 8 (August 1971): 1620–1637. While Stoeckle and Candib describe the earlier health center movement as originating in the period 1910–15 and note its decline in the late 1930's, Rosen distinguishes two periods of growth of the earlier centers—an initial group of experimental programs which were quite short-lived, and then a larger and more enduring group of centers which built on the experiences of the earlier set.

3

The Neighborhood Health Center—
Reform Ideas of Yesterday and Today

John D. Stoeckle and Lucy M. Candib

The neighborhood health center is now a popular solution to the care, or lack of it, of poor people. As it reappears again on the national scene, a brief account of its origins and history will recall earlier ideas about this innovation that are important not only for a perspective on the health center today but for any reappraisal of the goals of medical care and the organizations for it.

Since its early beginnings in the 1900's four ideas have dominated the health-center movement: district location; community participation; bureaucratic organization; and preventive care.[1-4] What were the health problems of the poor that the first centers proposed to solve? Undernutrition and infectious disease were prevalent in the slums. Rational preventive measures of infant feeding and immunization were on hand. However, preventive care on a mass basis was generally unavailable and inaccessible. The fault was medical organization. The existing community agencies for poor relief and medical care were separated, unco-ordinated and inefficient. A new institution, the health center, would solve these health problems by a program of prevention and an organization in which district location, community participation and bureaucratic arrangements would be emphasized. Some expected that the center might also become an institution for the reform of medical practice outside the hospital, for the renewal of community life and even for the rehabilitation of the poor out of poverty itself.

In the following account the meanings and interpretations that the early founders of health centers gave to the ideas of district location, community participation, bureaucratic organization and preventive care are reported. Experience with early health centers is briefly noted, and comparisons made between the rationale of the ideas and the actual work of centers. Against this historical background, the new interpretations and meanings of health-center plans are noted along with comments on the opportunities and contradictions of the new centers in dealing with modern health and social problems of the poor.

Reprinted from *New England Journal of Medicine* 280, 25 (June 19, 1969): 1385-1391.

District Location—Site of Care, Its Method and Meanings

The early health centers of 1910-1915, financed by local taxes or philanthropy, or both, and organized by voluntary agencies or municipal health departments, were located within city neighborhoods or districts, and their work was often confined to its population. Yet even then this district location was not entirely new or without historical antecedents in the settlement house, the "milk depots," relief agencies and clinics, and private practice itself.

Twenty years before, in the 1890's, settlement houses were located in immigrant slums, so too were the many charitable relief agencies that grew up around immigrant groups—the Hebrew, the Catholic and the special ethnic societies of Swedes, Germans, Italians and Irish. Somewhat later, health agencies, both public and private, also undertook neighborhood locations, following the settlement house and an even older, almost ancient tradition among medical practitioners in locating their separate offices in separate neighborhoods. One early voluntary effort, for example, the "milk depots" or "stations" for under-nourished children were first located in poor neighborhoods. Later, similar public clinics for infant feeding and those for tuberculosis and venereal disease did the same. By the time the health-center movement began in 1910-1915 the districts were by no means without some social or medical services.

The district location of centers was undertaken with several hopeful expectations. The first was that as a decentralization of the site of care, district location would bring health services closer to the residential life of the urban poor. Made more accessible by a more convenient local site and distance, health services would have greater use, a goal of public health then concerned with the great indifference of many slum dwellers to municipal health services in central locations at the city hall and municipal-hospital outpatient departments. Secondly, district location not only promised to make services more accessible, but also it would rationally limit the work of the health center's staff. If district boundaries could be prescribed, as they often were, the staff could personally reach all the people in the district, including the "recalcitrant" ones, by home and health-center visits. Indeed, some district health centers reported that 100 per cent of all new babies were visited. Writing about the child health stations of the New York Milk Committee, its secretary, Wilbur C. Phillips, stated the organizational strategy of district-based services in general:

> First, in order to reach and instruct every mother, the area covered by
> the work of the child welfare station would have to be definitely
> restrictive in size; it must become a "unit" for 100% effort, with every
> baby known to the doctors and nurses and both these agents kept free
> to center on keeping babies from falling ill.[5]

Prevention was to be applied to everyone, at least in the slums, where illness was more prevalent. Municipal authorities either implicitly or explicitly adopted the strategy of district-based services. However, as Phillips later learned, district location and limitation alone did not ensure "100% participation."

Thirdly, if the district location and limitation were good for the doctor and nurse in their visits with patients, it might also help the local residents to influence the staff. In everyday encounters with the middle-class professionals, slum residents might actually change the operation of the center and the attitudes of its staff. However, any benefit that the residents realized was never specifically recorded in opinion surveys or in commentaries of their own since the center was invariably described by its managers. Although Robert Woods, a settlement-house organizer and spokesman, did not report what slum dwellers actually thought and what they may have gained for themselves, he did not think informal contacts with them could be ignored:

> The local health center gathers under one head a group of services which in greater or less degree have been undertaken in the past by the settlement. In all their technical phases the settlement clearly and unquestionably must be ready to pass them over to the health center. It is, however, equally clear—and this the promoters of the health center do not always appreciate, that all the values of acquaintance and influence which the settlement has in its various organizations, up and down the streets, in the homes and conversational groups, must continue to be of indispensable importance to any local campaign.[6]

Fourthly, whereas some thought district location was only important for improving access and use, others viewed the district as a rational administrative arrangement for public financing and public control of services. Health services and districts should, in effect, be organized like public education and school districts. Such was the view of William O. White, an early founder of a health center in Pittsburgh:

> In the educational field there has gradually developed a knowledge of the equipment necessary for a given population, and this equipment has been apportioned so as to be easily accessible by those whom it is to serve. The management of these units is centered in a legally constituted governing body, which also controls the expenditure of funds collected by taxation. The same form of control is applicable throughout to tuberculosis and other health problems.[7]

The opinion that health care ought to be just like public schooling, similarly financed, organized and controlled, went into the planning, if not the actual organization of health services by municipal departments. Cities were divided into health districts and health centers set up, but the similarities ended there. If public schools provided the district all its educational services, the health center provided but a fraction of health care. Private practice would not permit competition by centers in care outside the hospital or to have treatment dominated by public authorities. The center's own limited preventive practice implied such restrictions; its opponents frankly stated them.[8,9] Neither did the administration of municipal health departments nor the governance of centers follow the school-board model of citizen representation. They remained largely in the hands of appointed municipal officials and the public-health professionals.

Finally, although it was not explicit in any of the commentaries on health centers, the district-based center contained still another meaning, an egalitarian ideal that there should always be one public institution in the community that would not deny a patient treatment. On such a principle, hospital care was always available at district hospitals in England and at municipal hospitals in the United States. Similarly, out-of-hospital care was available from and the responsibility of private practitioners, each doctor, in effect, having an outpatient department in his own office for the poor. The hospital outpatient department, in turn, was only a supplemental institution to private practice[10]; the district-based health center was another. Like the district hospital, the health center would always be available, at least for some "office care," if the district resident could not pay for it somewhere else.

All these features of the district concept were applicable to the organization of care for everyone. Yet, in real life, both public and private actions were confined only to districts full of poor people. The site of care of the health center meant only poverty "districts" and the "poor." That the district acquired this meaning was not hard to understand. The health center was only part of a general social reform of the Progressive Era aimed at the uplift of the poor. And health-center supporters shared the same political, ethical and even religious rationale[11] for dealing with the poor alone rather than with all of society.

Community Participation—For Use, Research, Advice and Governance

In Phillips's view district location was a means of ensuring "100% participation," meaning, in modern terms, 100 per cent utilization by all residents. By defining the district boundaries and the number of people in them, he hoped to give the doctor and nurse time to reach everyone. But dependence on district boundaries and on the population's natural inclination to use practitioners did not work. Mothers still stayed away, so that Phillips then turned to neighborhood residents for help. From his experience with milk stations for children in New York City and child-health centers in Milwaukee in 1912, he devised a program that enlisted neighborhood residents as "aides" to recruit patients, to take household surveys and to participate in the governance of the center.[5] From each neighborhood block a resident was selected to be a personal contact for all the mothers, bringing them to the center. By this means 100 per cent participation was achieved! Some neighborhood aides also helped in taking a home census, a research practice put into "nonprofessional" hands to counteract antagonism to the investigations by professionals of welfare agencies. The favorable response to "neighborhood aides" suggests that health work even then may have become "over-professionalized."

Later (in 1915), in Cincinnati, Phillips elaborated the social unit, a complex plan of community participation in the actual governance of the health center and of other community services. Neighborhood residents, chosen on the basis of the block in which they lived, and advisors from the district, chosen on the basis of their occupation, were to be on the board of management of the unit and its health center.[12] In the social unit Phillips anticipated contemporary community organizers such as Alinsky[13] as well as those responsible for directives on OEO-supported health centers. Participation in civic life was first a democratic ideal with religious origins[14] and second a motivating force for health action. Since civic participation of any kind was often absent, or, at best, minimal in lower-class communities, the health agency could be a focus for its development. The outcome would be twofold: greater sense of community and maximum use of health services. Participation itself was then almost a sign of community health.

But not every health center was designed for democratic participation. Most of them were bureaucratically run by municipal health departments and voluntary agencies. Innovative as Phillips's endeavors in Cincinnati were, they were also short-lived, not from lack of neighborhood participation but because they lacked political support within the municipal government and aroused public suspicions that the social unit might, in fact, really be socialistic, if indeed not communistic.[15] Even though participation in a health agency might also have civic benefits, such as greater community cohesion so important for the development of the sense of community itself, Michael M. Davis, a historian of the movement, judged the attempts in other centers on a purely practical basis as unsuccessful and not worth the effort expended.[1] He saw the failures as the result more of attitudes of indifference in American neighborhoods than of hostile political interference. Neighbors were presumably individualistic about health while collectively more interested in education.

Bureaucratic Organization—Efficiency and Co-ordination

If the health center was a decentralization designed to make care more accessible and available, others simultaneously viewed it quite differently: as a needed centralization of clinics and welfare agencies or even of solo medical practices. Since these were in scattered locations in the community and under diverse managements as a result of a multitude of spontaneous voluntary efforts, they should be brought together into one building and one organization for efficiency and co-ordination. Multiple community-health and welfare agencies with overlap in function and serving special clienteles were viewed as inefficient. Reformers thought both social and medical services could be treated like industry—made more efficient through common facilities, equipment, administration, organization and use of less skilled help. Arguments for private group practice and hospital outpatient departments often had the same basis.[16] Some early health centers were even referred to as "department stores," a timely analogy since the department store was just then emerging as a model of retail efficiency. Clearly, the argument was not that patients were handicapped by the fragmentation or specialization of care but simply that services could be more efficiently and less expensively managed under a better administrative scheme of a health center.

In founding the famous Blossom Street Health Center in 1912, Wilinsky, a community practitioner in Boston's West End, based it on the idea of co-ordinating the work of health and welfare agencies by common housing.[17] The Center's rationale was ". . . the correlation of all health and social agencies under one roof with the beneficent result derived from contact with workers." The Center included the "Consumptive Hospital Department, Instructive District Nursing Association, Milk and Baby Hygiene Association, Visiting Physician of Boston Dispensary, and Hebrew Federated Charities." Since it depended only on common housing with organization for co-ordination, it was uncertain whether the agencies or the treatment was co-ordinated. They certainly were not the same thing. However, others besides Wilinsky were more definite. For example, commenting on plans for rural health centers, Biggs, like Wilinsky, expected co-ordination but also efficiency.[18] He depended on organization rather than housing alone, and it was clearly agencies, not therapies, that were to be co-ordinated for efficiency. Centers "not only insure co-operation and co-ordination between various branches of public health work through increasing efficiency, reducing overhead expenses of each, and making more money available for the actual conduct of work."

Still another aspect of the efficiency goal was the health center as a common facility for several users each sharing the cost of fixed facilities and technology (for example, x-ray equipment). Thus, Mountin argued for rural health centers to provide costly modern "workshops" for doctors not naturally inclined to take up practice away from the city or to enter into group practice by themselves.[19] Also part of the efficiency goal was the use of feldshers, nurses, auxiliaries and "ancillary personnel," a common historical feature of the health-center movement in both rural and urban areas throughout the world. Nonphysician help would increase the clinical span and output of the doctor and, indeed, might even substitute for him. Just as complex industrial work could be broken down into a set of simpler jobs, so could the doctor's job—and then others, of course, could do part of it. Everywhere the reform was bureaucratic, and its goal efficiency if nothing else.[2] Efficiency itself was good, and the internal working of the center more important than its program.[3,4]

Although most centers were preoccupied with the efficiency and co-ordination of agencies and of traditional public-health preventive services, in a few "curative" health centers the co-ordination was of clinical practice. More a response to medical specialization, the co-ordination in group or teamwork was to solve the central treatment problem of personal and integrated care of the patient. Pomeroy's "curative" health centers in California, essentially local outpatient clinics, co-ordinated the work of doctors, nurses and social workers in their dealings with a wide range of problems for which people sought medical help. Their scope was treatment rather than the traditional public-health practice of infant feeding, tuberculosis follow-up and screening and venereal-disease treatment.[21] In general, co-ordination of treatment was the exception.

As Candib observed, the efficiency ethic, so powerful in industrial work, became almost a central value of the health-center movement and in the public view of social and medical services in general.[4] Preoccupation with efficiency at the expense of diversity and expanding care at the centers may well have been responsible for their later decline. At least the programs of health centers did not change with changing times and needs.

Preventive Care, Primary or Secondary, Simple or Complex

Most health-center enthusiasts viewed the program of centers as preventive and educational, complementing the curative work of private practice and carefully avoiding competition with it: "no prescription given; no sickness treated."[22] In the United States, where private practice was dominant, only a few centers included curative functions other than those for tuberculosis and venereal disease that were allowed by public statutes. In other countries and rural regions the health centers seldom made distinctions between treatment and prevention.

The centers' preventive program was derived from community problems, which were infectious diseases and poor nutrition. Immunization, vaccination, infant feeding, tuberculosis screening and treatment of venereal disease were the major technics. Similarly, the center's operation was to be responsive to community expectations as a result of district locations and community participation. The program of some centers, however, went far beyond medical and welfare activities to include recreation, day care of children and clubs. Such programs implied a view of health as a way of living, not just freedom from disease. But not everyone saw the program and functions of the health center as deriving from local community needs and expectations or from a social view of health.

The health center implied a relation to other institutions, and it was the "others"—namely, the hospitals—that determined the center's functions and programs. The district described a population, and the center a means for the triage of patients for the hospital. Illness could be sorted by its clinical severity and allocated by its need for technical treatment to the hospital. The center would thus deal with what illness did not get referred; its functions, derived from the internal needs of the hospital, were often viewed as leftovers, chronic illness and disability.

The British plan for health centers was an example of planning implicitly based on the primacy of hospitals and regionalization.[23] The separated duties of the doctor, midwife and nurse were to be administratively joined together in a health center. Like general practitioners, the centers would be linked to hospitals by referrals. Coming shortly after World War I, the plan implied, as did the definition of general practice itself, a regionalization somewhat like that in military medicine, where the wounded were sorted according to severity and allocated for treatment to the front (first-aid stations) or the rear (hospitals). As a hospital outpost or first-aid station, the health center would treat only simple, not complex illness, even though, in actual fact, prevention and chronic illness in the community were exceedingly complex—and are so still today. Perceived as hospital outposts dealing with supposedly simple community-health problems, centers everywhere often had difficulty attracting professional staff and maintaining programs of their own.

Reform Today—Reorganization or Reorientation

The health-center movement developed in many places throughout the world. Centers became a part of governmental systems of health care in such countries as Russia, Yugoslavia and Chile. The English plans were never realized although a flurry of centers was reported after World War II and the famous Peckham experiment.[24] Grant was interested in centers for rural community development first in China and later in Puerto Rico,[25] as was Kark with the Pholela Health Center in South Africa.[26] In the United States the center movement declined in the late 1930's, but it is reappearing today.

The new centers are now being sponsored by hospitals, medical schools, citizen groups, medical societies and, less often, by health departments. Under new sponsorship, these centers are developing at the same time that group practice, a kind of private entrepreneurial health center, receives a stamp of professional and public approval and when another health-center movement in mental health, quite separated from medical practice, has also developed. What has happened to the district idea, community participation, bureaucratic organization and the program itself?

In a new redefinition the district is not only a community but a laboratory, one where the effect of health care as an independent variable may be measured on the "health" of a selected population. This research definition of community reflects a special demand for social accounting and a research interest in the social basis of health and illness. As the costs of services become larger, and the expenditures more public than private, accounting is demanded. Analysis of the impact of health services in the community helps rationalize the public monies spent on centers. Despite its promise of rationalization the research view of community may have limitations. It may arouse community fears of manipulation similar to recently discarded ones of "being a guinea pig" in public hospitals or resentments at being over-researched as compared to suburbia. In the interest of completing evaluation, programs may not change with public needs.

In still another modern view, the district has neither strict nor local geographical boundaries, but is redefined as the clientele of a health center or group practice. Local boundaries may be less important since centers of larger size seem required to deal with the complexity of community health problems and to serve diverse groups. Larger centers can be reached by more efficient transportation; their use can be monitored in community data banks. If boundaries disappear and the centers grow in size and complexity, community participation, traditionally based on small groups, will be more difficult, and some may be left out. If they are sponsored more by hospitals, they may become, as outpatient divisions often have, "colonial" outposts, the major resources held by hospitals.

The idea of community participation is back again. The center's governance and control is democratic by having local residents and consumers represented as advisors, sometimes as the majority of the center's board of directors. The options for community residents to participate also have new meanings of paid work and rehabilitation. The old health center meant only to bring services to the poor. They could become healthy but remain poor just the same. The new center idea offers the poor jobs and training as part of a comprehensive program for their social, economic, educational and medical rehabilitation.[27] The jobs are in and outside the center. Residents may work outside in the neighborhood as aides, helping increase the center's use, or in community "store fronts" as "patient advocates," resolving conflicted encounters with the center or with any community agency. Inside the center, residents may have a real professional job or human-relations work, avoiding depersonalization by guiding patients through the center's services and so removing impediments thought inherent in any bureaucratic treatment.

Quite apart from participation, now meaning paid jobs, training and "having a say" in the agency's goals is the idea of participation in everyday management. If the community outside in the past was excluded from the control of health agencies the professionals inside may have been just as relatively deprived. Today, the center's staff may also take part in the new industrial democracy in management decisions, a movement with roots more in modern psychology than in any political theory of social reform.[28] The advantage, too, may only be psychologic if the staff does not have a voice in the goals of the organization as well.

The bureaucratic idea has returned too with both the new health centers and group practice. Their goals again are efficiency and co-ordination; the reasons are similar too. As the major criticism of medical services is again their economic cost, the major reform is organizational. If arranged to be less costly, health services can be more widely distributed. That bureaucratic goals might be something else besides efficiency alone is rarely discussed, at least not when ultimate reform interests are organizational and the criterion is fiscal. Clinicians may be skeptical of the promise of the efficiency ethic as it reappears in the modern organizational phrase "delivery of medical services." Encounters with patients suggest that neither efficiency nor reorganization alone is the answer to full medical use. Patients may be indecisive about even seeking help, and awkward in coping with illness. The course of their illness itself may be uncertain, and its management and treatment equally so. That bureaucratic arrangements might make best use of the psycho-social treatment of the patient during illness and rehabilitation and these efforts be expansive rather than efficient is another possibility.[29] Fortunately for this possibility, reorientation has been as much a part of the health-center reform as reorganization. The new community-health problems are not, as so commonly perceived, simple but complex, whether they are those of the very young, infant mortality, or those of the old, chronic psychosocial-medical disease and disability. The center's new program, which seeks the prevention of illness and the rehabilitation of residents, promotes a reorientation of medical values, a shift in the goal of care from longevity alone to optimal functioning and achievement, and to a more social view of health.

Whether old efficiency tests, now appearing as cost effectiveness, will brake the expansive social-medical-employment programs of centers is uncertain. In both objective and cost the programs of centers is uncertain. In both objective and cost the programs are quite unlike private-office medical practice, to which they are often compared. The primacy of the center's community programs over the demands of the hospital is also uncertain. Speaking about the Columbia Point Neighborhood Health Center, Gibson expresses the repeated hope that the health center, not the hospital, would be the focus for the organization of care, and that its programs and social orientation would be that of medicine and of medical education.[30] That they are not is no fault of the health center movement. The technologic therapies and orientation of the modern hospital are certainly more impressive and command more resources. For the allocation of more resources to centers more community participation in the hospital than at centers themselves might help. Still, the influence and impact of the hospital's technology is now becoming better understood. As better understanding comes about, change in the hospital's priorities for care may take place. The health center, whether public or private, may then begin to develop the resources to deal with complex problems in the community and become the long idealized center of care, if not a place for the renewal of the community and for the rehabilitation of the poor—or anyone else.

References

1. Davis, M.M., Jr. *Clinics, Hospitals and Health Centers,* New York: Harper, 1927.
2. Hiscock, I.V. Development of neighborhood health services in United States. *Milbank Mem. Fund Quart. 13*:30–51. 1935.
3. Stoeckle, J.D. Future of health care. In *Health and Poverty.* Edited by J. Kosa, A. Antonovsky and I.K. Zola. Cambridge: Harvard University Press, 1969 (in press). Chapter 10.
4. Candib, L.M. *A Social Study of the Health Center Movement: A new approach to public health history.* Cambridge: Harvard University, History of Science Department, 1968. (Honor thesis.)
5. Phillips, W.C. *Adventuring for Democracy.* New York: Social Unit Press. 1940. p. 46.
6. Woods, R.A. *The Neighborhood in Nation-Building: The running comment of thirty years at the South End House.* Boston: Houghton, 1923. p. 279.
7. White, W.C. Official responsibility of state in tuberculosis problem. *J.A.M.A. 65*:512–514, 1915.
8. Stanton, E. Discussion on health center bill. State Sanitary Officers' Convention, Saratoga, New York, September 8, 1920. *New York State J. Med. 20*:359–361, 1920.
9. Burnham, A.C., and Dietrich, A. Forum, "Health Centers." *New York State J. Med. 20*:206–208, 1920.
10. Stoeckle, J.D. "OPD" as ambulatory care at hospital. In *Chronic Disease and Public Health.* Edited by A.M. Lilienfeld and A.J. Gifford. Baltimore: Johns Hopkins Press, 1966. Chapter 4.
11. *The Social Gospel in America 1870–1920 (by) Gladden, Ely (and) Rauschenbusch.* Edited by R.T. Handy. London: Oxford, 1966.
12. Devine, E.T. Social unit in Cincinnati: experiment in organization. *Survey 42*:115–226, November 15, 1919.
13. Alinsky, S.D. *Reveille for Radicals.* Chicago: Univ. of Chicago Press, 1946.
14. Cox, H.G. "New breed" in American churches: sources of social activism in American religion. *Daedalus 96*:135–150. Winter, 1967.
15. Marquette, B. Personal communication.
16. Cabot, R.C. Out-patient work: most important and most neglected part of medical service. *J.A.M.A. 59*:1688, 1912.
17. Wilinsky, C.F. Health center. *Am. J. Pub. Health 17*:677–682, 1927.
18. Terris, M. Herman Biggs' contribution to modern concept of health center. *Bull. Hist. Med. 20*:387–412, 1946.
19. Mountin, J.W., and Hoenack, A. Health center: adaptation of physical plants to service concept. *Pub. Health Rep. 61*:1369–1379, 1946.
20. Haber, S. *Efficiency and Uplift: Scientific management in the progressive era, 1890–1920.* Chicago: Univ. of Chicago Press, 1964.
21. Pomeroy, J.L. Health center development in Los Angeles County. *J.A.M.A. 93*:1546–1550, 1929.

22. *The Health Units of Boston, 1924–1933 and 1924–1944.* City of Boston Printing Department, 1933 and 1945.
23. Great Britain, Consultative Council on Medical and Allied Services. *Interim Report on the Future Provision of Medical and Allied Services.* London: His Majesty's Stationery Office, 1920.
24. Pearse, I.H., and Crocker, L.H. *The Peckham Experiment: A study in the living structure of society.* London: Allen & Unwin, 1943. (Sir Halley Stewart trust publication.)
25. Grant, J.B. *Health Care for the Community: Selected papers.* Edited by C. Seipp. Baltimore: Johns Hopkins Press, 1963. (No. 21, *American Journal of Hygiene Monograph Series.*)
26. Kark, S.L., and Cassel, J. Pholela Health Centre: progress report. *South African M. J. 26*:101–104 and 132–136, 1952.
27. Geiger, H.J. *Tufts Comprehensive Community Health Action Report.* Boston, June 23, 1966. (Memiographed.)
28. Bennis, W.G. *Changing Organizations: Essays on the development and evolution of human organization.* New York: McGraw-Hill, 1966.
29. Anderson, O.W. Health services in land of plenty. In *Environment for Man; The next fifty years.* Edited by W.R. Ewald, Jr. Bloomington: Indiana Univ. Press, 1968. pp. 59–94.
30. Gibson, C. Beyond group practice. Presented at 10th annual family health lecture, Children's Hospital Medical Center, Boston, March 13, 1968.

Part III
Evolution of the Neighborhood
Health Centers of the 1960s

Introduction

Why did the present generation of neighborhood health centers develop when they did, in the late 1960s? Why did the Office of Economic Opportunity get into the health business? What factors lead to the OEO focus on the neighborhood health center as the favored form of intervention? What were the centers initially supposed to accomplish and how were they going to be organized?

The two articles in this section address the questions above from different perspectives and provide additional discussion of issues raised in Chapter 2 "Neighborhood Health Centers as a Social Movement."[1] The chapters by Lisbeth Bamberger Schorr and Joseph T. English and by Sar,A. Levitan provide valuable information on the origins of OEO's involvement in the health area. They outline some of the conflicts of goals, interests, and favored approaches which underlie the development of the OEO program. The Schorr and English article, "Background, Context and Significant Issues in Neighborhood Health Center Programs," contains an extensive listing of the issues which they (both early administrators of OEO's health effort) and their colleagues at OEO, and later HEW, felt were important questions being addressed by the demonstration projects they were supporting. The candid tone of their chapter reveals some of the queries which initiators of the programs felt were most important, and for which they did not claim to have confident answers.

"Healing the Poor in Their Back Yard," by Sar A. Levitan, provides the most detailed published account available of how OEO came to sponsor neighborhood health centers. Levitan highlights the severe problems of coordinating funding and services experienced by the individual centers and by federal departments. He analyzes the surprisingly mild reaction to the centers expressed by the medical establishment.

References

1. Donald L. Madison, "Organized Health Care and the Poor," *Medical Care Review* 26, 8 (August 1969): 783–807, provides additional information with regard to these questions. It places the neighborhood health centers in the context of other health programs for the poor and tries to distinguish different meanings of the elusive concept "comprehensiveness," a watchword of the neighborhood health centers and of many of the other programs as well. Madison's framework helps to address the issue that neighborhood health centers contain elements that can be organized in different forms, that can be implemented by other organizations not necessarily located in neighborhoods.

43

4

Background, Context and Significant Issues in Neighborhood Health Center Programs

Lisbeth Bamberger Schorr and Joseph T. English

When the War on Poverty began, health was not looked upon as one of its major battlefronts. How it came to be just that can be better understood by a look back into the atmosphere in which the early decisions were made.

The passage of the Economic Opportunity Act of 1964, mobilized—in Washington, D.C., and in communities large and small around the nation—a group of dedicated and exuberant men and women from highly diverse backgrounds, who were determined to make real the promise of the new antipoverty legislation. They were young—not necessarily in age, but they had the youth that Senator Robert Kennedy described so eloquently as "not a time of life, but a state of mind, a temper of the will, a quality of imagination, a predominance of courage over timidity, of the appetite for adventure over the love of ease." They were there to implement a piece of legislation that provided an unprecedented opportunity for the federal government to support the development of new ways of dealing with old problems.

In the headquarters of the Community Action Program, we had the task of seeking out and defining some of the ways by which the federal government could most effectively assist local communities in their efforts to eradicate poverty. At the beginning, the number of fronts on which the war on poverty could be waged seemed to be unlimited. The question that occupied us was how could we assure that the money for which we were in some measure responsible would be spent in ways that were to make a real difference, both in the quality of everyday life of individual poor people in this nation, as well as for the future of poverty as a brutal fact of life in America?

The question of health first arose quite incidentally, as communities found that job training for a worker who would be ultimately refused employment because of a physical disability made no sense, that educational improvements meant nothing to children whose physical impairments made learning impossible and that lack of prenatal care could cause harm that no later intervention could reverse.

Proposals came in from around the country, requesting funds to purchase certain categories of health care and services that had been most notably inade-

Reprinted from *Milbank Memorial Fund Quarterly* 66, 3 Part I (July 1968): 289-296.

quate for the poor. Simultaneously, task forces in other governmental agencies were encouraging the Office of Economic Opportunity (OEO) to act in the field of health by making funds available to plug specific loopholes in existing publicly supported services. Such efforts were undertaken in a large number of communities, with general, unearmarked community action funds.

While this was being done, however, several very practical demonstrations indicated that the basic institutional arrangements—governmental and private—whereby health services were made available to the poor were defective, and that to the extent that health services were relevant to health status, the health of the poor could not be improved without fundamental changes in the arrangements whereby health services were organized and delivered. We were thus highly receptive to the advice from consultants that we should devote at least some research and demonstration funds to projects which would deal with the fundamental problem of the organization of medical care. We then entered enthusiastically into preliminary discussions with individuals whose own studies and experience had led them to similar conclusions and who were thinking of undertaking programs with this end in view.

All analysis of the obstacles that prevented poor people from obtaining the best possible health services that American medicine was capable of providing made apparent that any attempt to deal with fundamental problems must be fairly comprehensive, and would, therefore, be immensely complicated and very expensive. Probably the most difficult and significant decision in the health area made by OEO during its first year of operation was to support programs that were addressed to the fundamental problems, despite the cost and complexity of such programs. A second significant decision was a corollary of the first: that to the fullest extent possible OEO funds would not be used to replace others, but instead would be used to encourage arrangements whereby other funds and services would be integrated as part of one cohesive whole. (Interagency efforts to make this principle a reality have been constantly and strenuously pursued—with frequently slow, but sometimes striking, success—since August, 1965.)

Further discussions, which took place among the staff, with a growing number of thoughtful and wise consultants and with an enormously impressive group of potential project sponsors, produced the basic outlines of a new institutional form for the rendering of medical care, which has since become known as the neighborhood health center.

The basic characteristics of the neighborhood health center were envisaged as follows:

1. Focus on the needs of the poor.
2. A one-door facility, readily accessible in terms of time and place, in which virtually all ambulatory health services are made available.
3. Intensive participation by and involvement of the population to be served, both in policy making and as employees.

4. Full integration of and with existing sources of services and funds.
5. Assurance of personalized, high-quality care, and professional staff of the highest caliber.
6. Close coordination with other community resources.
7. Sponsorship by a wide variety of public and private auspices.

Three grants were made by OEO in 1965 for programs designed to incorporate these elements, and, by early 1966, the problems with which these programs were attempting to deal came increasingly to public attention. Alonzo S. Yerby, after describing to the White House Conference on Health the circumstances under which poor people received medical care, called for a national commitment to assure that all Americans, regardless of income, will have "equal access to health services as good as we can make them, and that the poor will no longer be forced to barter their dignity for their health." At the same time, the implementation of both the Medicare and Medicaid legislation provided additional evidence of the difficulties encountered by programs that furnished only money to pay for services and did not afford the opportunity to encourage improved institutional arrangements for providing those services.

In that context, and at that time, therefore, it was not surprising that an immediate response was received from physicians, hospitals, medical schools and health departments who saw in the research and demonstration program the possibility of support for something that had long been urgently needed, and for which federal support in sufficiently flexible form had not earlier been available. (The fact that the early constituency of the neighborhood health center program consisted, by and large, of the providers and not the consumers of service was later to lead to difficulty. We did not fully appreciate that the requirement of full participation by those being served after a proposal had been approved could never make up for the fact that the project had been originated and formulated by the professionals alone.)

By the summer of 1966, eight demonstration neighborhood health center programs had been approved. Enough experience had been amassed to lead Senator Edward Kennedy to formulate an amendment to the Economic Opportunity Act to set aside special funds to support the "development and implementation of comprehensive health services programs focused upon the needs of persons residing in urban or rural areas having high concentrations of poverty and a marked inadequacy of health services." Congress appropriated 50 million dollars for this purpose in 1967, and during that year an additional 33 neighborhood health center projects were approved. As of June, 1968, 30 projects are in operation, and 44 more have been approved.

When all the programs that have been funded to date are fully operational, they will serve nearly one million people and will make available 2,000 jobs for persons living in the neighborhoods served. The currently funded projects utilize 700 physicians on a full- or part-time basis, and involve one-quarter of the nation's medical schools—with another one-quarter indicating intent to participate.

Each of these projects is struggling, in its own way, with issues to which each must develop its own response, reflecting the widely diverse circumstances in which each project has been designed and is operating. Some of these issues are:

1. The development of totally new relationships between the consumers and providers of service, where professionals take responsibility for the professional aspects of the operation, while the new institution (be it a neighborhood health center or other institutional arrangement created to accomplish a similar purpose) becomes truly responsive to and under the control of the people it serves.
2. The development of new kinds of health roles and careers making possible a more effective delivery of services, and methods of training and utilizing new sources of manpower therefor.
3. The extent to which the organization of a neighborhood around one kind of need (health services) can form the basis for successful community action in other substantive areas (e.g., welfare, housing, education).
4. The extent to which an institution created to serve one function (the neighborhood health center) can and should become the physical and organizational focus of other kinds of anti-poverty activities (e.g., legal services, day care).
5. The modification and refinement of institutional and organizational arrangements to assure personalized care, family oriented care, care that will conform to high-quality standards, and be attractive to professional personnel of high caliber.

On the basis of the experience now being accumulated around the country in the 44 different programs, each individual project will become better equipped to fulfill its mission as it evolves its answers to such issues as the above. It should also be possible to shed light on additional questions that must be better answered than they have been in the past, if this nation is going to meet the health needs of all Americans more effectively. For example:

How can the medical care job be divided up in new and better ways, among new kinds of professionals and nonprofessionals, while assuring both quality and acceptability? What kind of education and training is required, and what kinds of institutions are best suited to provide such training?

Will the training and utilization of neighborhood people in ancillary health roles provide the pathway for them or their children into medical, dental, or nursing schools as well?

How many diverse kinds of organizational frameworks can be developed that make possible comprehensiveness and coherence of services, personalized care, the supervision of quality and the opportunity for resident participation?

How can federal agencies be encouraged to work together even when it means giving up a degree of sovereignty here and there, to enable a community institution to deliver a comprehensive package of services that are supported from a variety of sources?

How can the needs of consumers of service for care of high quality, rendered in a setting that is accessible and acceptable to them, be made compatible with a health industry based in large part on individual enterprise, competition and profits? In what circumstances will the public support some supervision over the activities of health professionals?

What is "mainstream" medical care? Do some parts of the medical care system, such as the entry point to the system and the locus of day-to-day (primary) care, require greater adaptation to the needs of various segments of the community (such as the poor) than do the more sophisticated parts of the system, such as hospitals?

Can neighborhood health centers and similar programs be expected to stand in splendid isolation and stark contrast to the more traditional ways of rendering health services in metropolitan areas, or will they begin to tug the rest of the system in their wake?

Can poor people exercise control over institutions that they share with the middle class? Does the inclusion of middle-class persons in the constituency of a service institution increase the chances of its providing high-quality services? How necessary is a degree of control on the part of those being served? What forms of control over what issues are acceptable to the consumers, to the providers? How can the positions of the two groups be brought closer together? What is the future of the nonprofit community health corporation where providers and consumers of service function as peers in meeting the community's needs?

What is the relative importance to the achievement of high-quality care of consumer participation in policy-making and of the caliber of the sponsoring health or medical institution or agency?

What factors will influence maintenance of quality in the provision of services when the program is beyond the excitement and innovative spirit of its early developmental phases?

Regardless of what the answers to these questions will turn out to be, it is clear that the neighborhood health center program provides an excellent example of the kind of federal action that makes possible an effective and flexible response by an enormous variety of local institutions to a set of urgent and complex problems. Of course, important as that fact may be in relation to the future role of the federal government in solving the most pressing social crises, one must go on to note that the aspirations of the thousands of people who are today intimately associated with the program in its many forms surely go further. If these aspirations are realized, the results can be measured in less suffering and enriched lives.

5

Healing the Poor in Their Back Yard

Sar A. Levitan

Behold, I will bring . . . health and cure,
and I will cure them, and will reveal
unto them the abundance of peace and truth.
Jeremiah 33:6

OEO's Medical Program

It was inevitable that the programs initiated under the Economic Opportunity
Act would become involved in the health business. The linkage between poverty
and poor health has long been recognized, and most of the major EOA programs
included a health component. Entry into training and employment programs
normally included at least a diagnostic medical check-up, and frequently
remedial treatment was needed to help the poor bridge the gap from poverty to
gainful employment. Altogether, expenditures on health activities accounted for
about 5 percent of the total OEO budget during its first four years, and 11
percent of CAP funds.

Although medical care as a supportive service for EOA programs was taken
for granted, the extent to which the Community Action Program should fund
health programs became an immediate issue. OEO's policymakers could not
agree whether CAP's limited resources should be allocated to health programs
rather than to housing, education, or other competing needs of the poor. The
case for allocating funds to health programs was weakened by the already
enormous expenditures for health care of the poor. In 1964, federal, state, and
local governments were already spending nearly $8 billion for health and medical
services, and legislation on the drawing board would double these annual outlays
within three years. An estimated $9.7 billion, over half of total health expendi-
tures in 1968, supported programs benefiting poor and low-income persons. On
a per capita basis, medical expenditures for the poor equaled the average annual
U.S. expenditure of $200 per person for the entire population.

Despite these massive public expenditures, the deficit in health care of the

Reprinted from Chapter 7 of Sar A. Levitan, *The Great Society's Poor Law: A New
Approach to Poverty*, Baltimore: Johns Hopkins University Press, 1969, pp. 191-205.

poor was startling, whether measured in terms of life expectancy, infant mortality rate, or incidence of visits to physicians or dentists.[1] In view of these high governmental expenditures, what accounts for the deficiencies in health care? No doubt some of the funds are wasted by inept administration; and, as in other areas, the poor pay more, particularly when the government foots the bill. More importantly, three additional factors help explain the deficiencies.

1. The poor, on the average, need more medical attention, since aged persons are disproportionately represented among the poor, and since physical and mental handicaps are associated with poverty.

2. The poor are offered little preventive medical attention. Moreover, the health care that is available encourages them to ignore correctable health problems or defects until they become major problems.

3. The delivery of existing health services to the poor is inefficient, and community health services are fragmented, disorganized, and often inaccessible. Shortages of medical and allied manpower have added to the difficulties of establishing adequate health services in neighborhoods where economic incentives are limited.

When community action agencies began to submit their plans, a number of them included health components as part of the total package. Most of the funds were for fragmented or specialized services: visual screening, immunization clinics, prenatal care courses, or supplements to existing clinics. Innovative projects were hard to come by, and Head Start accounted for more than half of the funds that were spent in the first two years. In fiscal 1967 neighborhood health centers became the major OEO health program (table 5-1).

Compared with other government contributions to medical services for the poor, the CAP outlay for health and medical services was no more than the proverbial drop in the bucket. Local CAA's could develop neither the planning

Table 5-1
Estimated OEO Allocations for Health, Fiscal 1965-68 (Millions)

Programs	1965	1966	1967	1968
Total	$18.8	$59.0	$117.7	$99.5
Neighborhood health centers	2.0	7.8	50.8	33.2
Family planning	.4	2.4	4.6	8.3
Other research and demonstration projects	1.8	1.0	1.7	1.8
Narcotics programs	—	—	9.4	—
Other community programs	3.4	8.8	7.0	9.5
Head Start health programs	10.3	31.7	31.6	32.9
Job Corps health programs	.5	6.9	11.7	12.8
VISTA health programs	.5	.5	.9	1.0

Note: Details do not necessarily add to totals because of rounding.
Source: Community Action Program, Office of Economic Opportunity.

capability, staffing, nor institutional base for medical care. Obviously, if CAP was to come to grips with these problems with the money available to it, it could fund only demonstration projects. The challenge to OEO was to develop innovative comprehensive health service programs.

The argument for emphasizing comprehensive health services rather than individual and isolated health components was not subscribed to by all concerned at the outset, and the concept remains a matter of controversy to the present time. The great expense and complexity of setting up any sort of comprehensive program were considered important obstacles, as was the anticipated difficulty in enlisting the substantial number of trained professionals that would be required. Simpler programs, which focused on specific health problems such as faulty hearing and vision, or narrow parts of the health care spectrum, such as screening and diagnosis, were seen by many as more practical and feasible. Officials of the U.S. Public Health Service were among those who recommended that if OEO became involved in the health field, it should merely support programs that would fill specific loopholes in existing community services.

On the other hand, the argument was made that while the gaps were substantial, health care for the poor was already so fragmented and disorganized that the addition of a few more unrelated projects would not be particularly helpful. According to this argument, the health needs of the poor would not and could not be adequately met without major changes in the health care system. OEO was the first federal agency to have the flexibility, as well as the mandate, to undertake programs that could have significant influence in changing the health care delivery system.

A Comprehensive Health Care Program

The proposal for developing a health program was made to CAP by professionals rather than by community agencies. Early in 1965, Professors H. Jack Geiger and Count D. Gibson, Jr., of Tufts University's College of Medicine, approached OEO with a plan for comprehensive neighborhood health centers that would be designed specifically to serve the multiple needs of the poor. Their plan was inspired by comprehensive health clinics that were operating in several developing nations. Geiger and Gibson had first presented their idea to the Public Health Service but were referred to the antipoverty agency. Their original proposal, to establish a model center in the Columbia Point public housing development in Boston (which had about 6,000 residents), was expanded to include the operation of two centers—one in Boston and the other in a rural southern area, which turned out to be Mound Bayou, Mississippi. The centers were designed to provide the full range of out-patient services to everyone who lived in the target areas. Particularly appealing to CAP officials was the proposal that the centers use indigenous community residents to perform many functions, and include them in making decisions concerning operation of the centers. In line with OEO goals, Geiger hoped that the neighborhood health centers would stimulate broader social action and institutional changes in other areas.[2] CAP funded the proposed project in June 1965.

The Denver antipoverty board, meanwhile, was having problems assembling a package of proposals. Although some of its members insisted on their own pet projects to the exclusion of others, they all favored inclusion of a health component. With cooperation from the Denver Health Department and guidance from OEO, the Denver community group developed a comprehensive neighborhood health center proposal. CAP funded its application two months after the approval of the Tufts project, and five additional centers during the balance of the fiscal year.

Out of the negotiations over funding these centers, CAP developed a four-point model for comprehensive neighborhood health centers: (1) a full range of ambulatory health services; (2) close liaison with other community services, which implied referrals and exchanges of services; (3) close working relationships with a hospital, preferably one with a medical school affiliation; and (4) participation of the indigenous population in decision-making that affected the center and, whenever feasible, their employment in subprofessional and other positions.[3]

The comprehensive health centers gained a devoted and valuable ally in Senator Edward Kennedy of Massachusetts. Concerned over the health deficiencies and needs of children enrolled in Head Start projects and of adults in training programs, Kennedy first explored the possibility of adding various health services provisions to each of these programs. After extensive discussion, Kennedy concluded that the simple addition of new funds for the purchase of services would not effectively meet the need and that a profound change in the organization of health services for the poor was needed. He was impressed with the potential of the embryonic neighborhood health center program, which he thought might be able to accomplish this. Cognizant that myriad other demands would be competing for the meager resources, in 1966 he proposed a neighborhood health center program with earmarked funds. Fifty-one million dollars was allocated to the program, a sixfold increase over the previous year, but during the following year the amount allocated to one-stop neighborhood health centers declined to $33 million.

The reduced allocation did not, however, reflect a decline in the popularity of the program. During fiscal 1968 CAP funded six additional health centers while most other CAP programs remained at their previous levels or were reduced. The launching of new health centers during fiscal 1968 with reduced funds was made possible by the fact that the operations of most projects that were funded in fiscal 1967 were delayed and consequently did not require refunding during 1968. The Senate Appropriations Subcommittee indicated its enthusiasm for comprehensive health centers by insisting that the $90 million requested for them not be affected despite a recommendation that total OEO appropriations for 1969 be reduced to $1,873 million, or $337 million below the Administration's request.[4]

Earmarking the funds induced some communities which had previously proposed fragmented health programs to apply for comprehensive projects. Thirty-two centers were in operation by August 1968, and an additional 16 were funded and in various stages of planning. Three of every four projects were located in urban areas. The 12 rural centers included a project on an Indian reservation in Minnesota; another rural center served an area in California where migratory labor is concentrated. The projects were designed to serve one million people, assuming they are funded to reach full operating capacity. At the 1968 funding level, neighborhood health centers would provide medical services to about one of every 25 people eligible to receive assistance, including some who qualify as medically indigent even though their income exceeds OEO's poverty criteria.

As with most CAP activities, applications for neighborhood health centers exceeded the available resources; moreover, OEO's criteria were too general to indicate priorities for funding the proposed centers.[5] A number of factors presumably were used to determine whether a community "deserved" to receive support for a center: the extent to which the community had received CAP funds for other purposes; the availability of health and medical services to the indigent of the community; the degree of community support (or pressure), including cooperation from pertinent state and local organizations; and the innovative elements of the proposal. It is not clear what weight these considerations actually carried in the approval of projects, for CAP developed no indices of need for health services, and even with the best intentions, subjective judgments had to enter into the final selection. It appears that "first-come first-served" was a controlling criterion, and the committing of available resources on this basis made more refined standards superfluous. Inasmuch as additional funds were not forthcoming, once CAP had committed itself to a project it was difficult to terminate funding in favor of another proposal, even if the latter seemed more desirable.

A "Typical" Center

Wherever feasible, the neighborhood health centers took over available facilities and used the new funds to expand their services. In the majority of cases, however, facilities were inadequate or altogether lacking, which required the establishment of a new center by renovating an existing building or constructing a new one. The intent was to use indigenous labor for this work, but the practices of the building trades made this hard to achieve. OEO also tried to encourage

the use of local contractors and labor, but for obvious political reasons it failed
to include utilization of local labor in the official guidelines. The Watts center
was built by local contractors who employed low-income residents to put up
the structural modules. Although neighborhood people were employed in the
construction and renovation of other projects as well, it may be significant that
Watts had a riot prior to the approval of its neighborhood health center; in other
cities local labor was not so "lucky," and construction or renovation was done
by outsiders.

Professional staff were recruited from diverse sources, including returning
Peace Corps personnel and recent medical or dental school graduates. Though
salaries were competitive with those of other publicly supported institutions,
they were too low to attract already established and more experienced personnel,
particularly full-time physicians and dentists. Program standards called for one
physician for every 1,500 people served and one dentist for every 2,500 people.
In addition, centers employed medical technicians, social workers, and other
technical personnel. To complement the trained personnel, neighborhood aides
were hired for subprofessional roles. These low-income workers were to be
trained either in the centers or in existing training programs in hospitals, local
health departments, or federally supported programs. On-the-job training at the
neighborhood health centers attempted not only to fill the needs of the facility
but also to increase the future employability of the trainees in the competitive
labor market.[6] It is hoped that the centers will provide the setting in which a
variety of health roles can be restructured to enable the training of persons with
a limited formal education to perform functions previously performed by persons
with much more training and education. The extent to which these goals are
being achieved is not known because CAP has not yet collected hard data on the
operation of the centers. OEO's Health Service Office estimated that about a
thousand local residents were employed in the summer of 1968 by the centers
then in operation, citing this as evidence that the training goals of the program
were being achieved. However, OEO could not supply information on the occu-
pational distribution or the wage or salary rates of the neighborhood employees.
Given the general shortage of personnel in medical occupations, trainees should
have little difficulty in finding jobs in other institutions, provided they receive
meaningful training.

As in other CAP programs, indigenous residents served on the policymaking
bodies of the health centers and were included in decisions on staffing, hours of
operation, development of community support, organization of school health
screening clinics, and other nontechnical problems.

Eligibility Criteria and Funding

Initially, all residents of a poor neighborhood were eligible to receive health center services. This standard was criticized by practicing physicians in the neighborhoods and by others who argued that benefits ought to be limited to the poor. In countering these criticisms, OEO spokesmen pointed out that the broad eligibility criterion was being applied in areas where 80 percent of the population qualified under the official poverty indices.[7] OEO did not identify the data it had utilized to determine the income level of all the residents in a designated area. Certainly the 1960 census data were obsolete by the time the centers were established. Moreover, many Negro and other minority-group families were forced to reside in slum areas even when they had an income that would have enabled them to move out. To overcome criticisms that the OEO-funded health centers were serving the nonpoor, Congress in 1967 limited eligibility to low-income families. Accordingly, the 1968 guidelines specified that the standards of "closely related programs" would control eligibility, in effect making the clientele of neighborhood centers consistent with Medicaid standards, which vary from state to state, or with OEO poverty standards, whichever is higher.

OEO grants for operating centers have varied considerably, depending upon location, population served, facilities needed, and the supportive services offered. Thus the size of grants has ranged from about $300,000 to $3.5 million. Little data is available on the actual utilization of funds, but OEO's Health Affairs Office has estimated that the grants, exclusive of construction and renovation costs, were expended as follows:

	Percent
Medical care	60
Dental care	10
Social services, training, community organization	10
Evaluation	5
Administration	15

To conserve its limited funds, CAP arranged with FHA to assist applicants for neighborhood health centers to secure, whenever feasible, loan guarantees for the renovation or construction of facilities.

In 1967 OEO's Office of Health Affairs assumed (for planning purposes) that the annual cost of care would amount to $125 per person, excluding reimbursement or contributions from other government programs. The actual costs ranged from about $85 per person in Denver, with its target population of 20,000, to double that amount in Boston's Columbia Point. Costs varied with the range of services offered by the centers, the relatively high cost at Columbia Point being attributable to the "highly innovative" approaches and to the small number served. Based on these data, it is estimated that comprehensive medical services for the 22 million poor in the United States would cost about $2.7

billion. If the services could be extended to all the medically indigent, the cost would rise by 30 to 40 percent. However, since OEO's neighborhood health centers are suitable primarily in areas where poor people are concentrated, Dr. Ruth Covell and her associates in HEW have estimated that only about a third of the poor could be served by comprehensive health centers at a total annual cost of $1.3 billion—assuming that adequate personnel and facilities could be secured. Overall public outlays for health services would not necessarily increase by that amount because comprehensive health centers would absorb part of the current expenditures. The savings would be achieved by reducing the duration of hospitalization and by preventive measures that would decrease the need for costly hospitalization. Also, a network of comprehensive health centers would supplant some of the existing health facilities and services.[8]

Further insights concerning the true costs of delivering health and medical services to the poor may come from a special project OEO is funding in Portland, Oregon, where prepaid medical services are being purchased from the Kaiser Health Plan for 1,200 poor families (selected from four neighborhoods by the local community action agencies). The Kaiser organization, under a grant from the Public Health Service, is attempting to compare utilization and the expenses incurred by the OEO-supported group with the experience of its regular participants. On the assumption that the poor will need more health services because of previous neglect, the Kaiser Health Plan initially charged OEO about 30 percent above its normal rates for OEO's participants. This rate will be adjusted on the basis of actual utilization, and the experiment should help fix the true costs for providing comprehensive health and medical services for the poor.[9]

Coordination of Funding and Services

Granted the soundness of the neighborhood health center approach, OEO could hardly have been expected to bring about major changes in the delivery of health services to the poor; and the agency's officials recognized that OEO could not compete with the billions of dollars available for that purpose to the Department of Health, Education, and Welfare. OEO hoped rather to serve as a catalytic agent in bringing about changes in the health care delivery system and in pooling the funds received from scattered sources. Thus it has used its resources to fund a few demonstration projects. To avoid duplication and to maximize the impact of the demonstrations, OEO entered into an "agreement" with HEW. The role of the centers was spelled out in a joint statement by the two agencies:

> OEO is undertaking the program . . . to make possible the pulling to-
> gether of disparate sources of funds and services into a coherent whole,
> by (1) providing the needed 'seed money' and (2) by paying directly

for services which cannot be supported by other sources or services to
poor persons who may not be eligible under other programs.[10]

Since HEW grants were normally designed to serve a target area larger than
the neighborhood health centers funded by OEO, the larger programs were encouraged to contract with the neighborhood center to provide services offered
by the grantee, to assign personnel and/or equipment to the neighborhood
center, or to provide specialized services to the neighborhood health center
population (for example, mental health clinics).

Neighborhood health center clients are often eligible for medical assistance
from Medicaid and federally supported public assistance programs; and when a
center offers medical services, it is entitled to reimbursement. Since public funds
are used in either case, it might appear that there would be no point in the health
centers' collecting these fees. But if the centers are to exploit their innovative
features and prove the claim that they deliver a "bigger bang for the buck," then
a case can be made for the vigorous collection of "debts" from other programs.
However, the necessary arrangements have often been difficult to conclude, and
considerably less money has come into the centers from other sources than had
been anticipated. If it is assumed that the centers will remain part of CAP and
not be transferred to HEW, OEO may intensify its attempts to collect reimburs-
able outlays in order to maximize the funds available for the operation of
comprehensive health centers and to demonstrate its claims about the superiority
of the centers in delivering health services to the poor.

The Denver Health Center provides an illustration of the coordination
envisioned. Before OEO initiated the neighborhood health center program, the
Denver Health Department was planning, together with the Children's Bureau
of HEW, to establish a children's center in a poverty neighborhood. OEO proposed to cooperate with the Children's Bureau so that the Denver Health
Department could establish a neighborhood health center that would serve the
entire family. Instead of one center, two centers were established under one
roof, with OEO providing funds for the adult services and the Children's Bureau
supporting the pediatric services. Additional funds were provided by the Public
Health Service to operate activities within its domain.[11]

Generally, however, agreement on cooperation and coordination at high
levels does not necessarily extend to the administration of the program. The
agreement reached by HEW and OEO has not permeated the lower levels of
their own agencies, let alone the state and local officials responsible for the
administration of health progarms. The HEW official who distributes federal
health funds on the basis of formulas prescribed by Congress may find it difficult
to adjust his funding practices to the special needs of a neighborhood health
center. Similarly, even a well-intentioned state official may find that allocating
federal resources to neighborhood centers that serve a select few in a predeter-
mined area does not fit in with his over-all program for the distribution of funds

in the state. Local health officials may also find it difficult to adjust their programs for aiding the poor to a restricted project that has regulations and rules that are different from those to which they have been accustomed. The difficulties are not insurmountable, but change requires time, and the health service bureaucrats, like most other humans, do not take kindly to change.

Relations with the Medical Establishment

Either the American Medical Association has mellowed or the fight has been taken out of it by the series of defeats that culminated in the congressional approval of Medicare. The AMA had cried wolf too frequently and too shrilly to raise again the specter of "socialized medicine" when OEO proposed the establishment of neighborhood health centers. Also, the AMA had in the past been tolerant of legislation on behalf of the poor who could not pay "standard" fees. Although its president, Dr. Charles Hudson, formally endorsed the concept on behalf of AMA the day after OEO published its initial guidelines, the AMA's position on neighborhood health centers can best be described as schizophrenic. Dr. Hudson's views were reinforced in June 1966 by an official of AMA's Division of Socio-Economic Activities, who commented that "this is something that the AMA looks to with great warmth, to which the AMA is pledging full cooperation, and for which we think there is a very good future."[12] But Dr. Milford O. Rouse, Hudson's successor as AMA president, "viewed with alarm" the establishment of neighborhood health centers, and upon taking office warned the assembled physicians that "we are faced with the concept of health care as a right rather than a privilege." He failed to explain why physicians should not welcome a positive attitude on the part of the American public toward medical services. The AMA's House of Delegates gave OEO an unsolicited warning to stop meddling in health affairs and to leave medical services for the poor under the auspices of Title XIX (Medicaid) of the Social Security Act. Some 18 months later, in December 1967, the AMA held its first conference on health care for the poor. One of the discussion groups at this conference rejected the House of Delegates' position and voted unanimously that health care should be regarded as a human right rather than a privilege. With regard to neighborhood health centers, the conferees acknowledged that local hospitals are frequently "unable to adapt themselves to pockets of poverty," and stated that slum residents should be given opportunities to help plan neighborhood health centers.[13] Other medical groups—the Medical Committee on Human Rights, the Physicians' Forum, the American Dental Association, the National Dental Association, and the National Medical Association (the latter two composed mostly of Negro physicians and dentists)—have had consistent supporters of the neighborhood health center concept.

At the local level, OEO's health centers have had remarkably little opposition, and OEO has been careful to court the cooperation of local medical groups. According to a CAP memorandum:

> Interested professional associations *must* be consulted, and every effort must be made to establish a close working relationship with professional health personnel who are or will be serving the target neighborhood.[14]

Aside from their concern for the health of indigents, local medical and dental associations were led to cooperate with the health program as a matter of simple economics: far from robbing doctors and dentists of their bread and butter, the centers promised to free them of unpaying patients. Where funds were already available for indigent health care, OEO was careful to advise the health centers that patients eligible to receive care under Title XIX "are free to obtain any of these services where they see fit."[15] Physicians and dentists could find little to complain about in the administration of the neighborhood health centers. Two of every three grants for health centers were made to community action agencies, which in all but two cases delegated their administration to the local medical institutions (table 5-2). These institutions—hospitals, medical schools, city health departments—had formerly provided out-patient and clinic services to the poor and continued to do so under the neighborhood health centers. Thus medical personnel were apt to regard the new centers as a modification in the delivery of charitable services rather than as a threat to existing medical institutions.

Pharmacists, however, presented a problem, since the health centers normally included a pharmacy which competed with private drugstores in the neighbor-

Table 5-2
Grantees and Administering Agencies of Neighborhood Health Centers, July 1968

	Grantees	Administering Agencies
Total	48	49[a]
Community action agencies	32	2
Hospitals	4	13
Medical schools	3	10
Health departments	0	7
Medical societies	1	2
Group practice	1	3
New Health Corporation	1	8
Other nonprofit agencies	6	4

[a]Includes one instance of joint administration.

Source: Community Action Program, Office of Economic Opportunity.

hoods. Again, OEO instructed the neighborhood center officials to inform Title XIX patients of their right to fill prescriptions at the local pharmacies, but the immediate accessibility of clinic dispensaries makes this a continuing issue. There are, however, signs that pharmacists and OEO are seeking a rapprochement. According to a spokesman for the registered pharmacists, "The profession's best interest will be served by pharmacists getting active in these community antipoverty programs which are going to roll on, with or without us."[16] But spokesmen for the National Association of Retail Druggists prefer that the health centers be transferred to HEW, anticipating that under HEW the centers would abandon the operation of pharmacies. The druggists apparently feared that the neighborhood health centers would be successful and that this would lead to the establishment of more such facilities.[17]

Is There a Future for the Centers?

In mid-1968 the neighborhood centers were of too recent origin and limited scope to permit evaluation: only 32 centers were actually in operation and the oldest had been in existence for only about two years. It will be some time before definitive judgments can be made about the centers' impact in improving the quality and accessibility of medical services to the poor. Nor is there sufficient evidence that the neighborhood health centers are attractive to professionals, or that they can provide the setting for training the poor to perform subprofessional functions to meet continued manpower shortages. More crucial to the future of the centers is whether separate health care centers for the poor—compounded in many instances by racial or ethnic segregation—can remain viable institutions. And it is not at all clear whether these centers will be more successful than earlier efforts in involving clients in planning and administration and in training indigenous populations to assume subprofessional roles. In these aspects, the health centers share the difficulties and problems of other CAP efforts.

Nonetheless, the concept of one-stop health centers for the poor has already won many adherents. A recent presidential commission on health manpower and its utilization addressed itself to the problem of quality and delivery of medical services to the poor. While concluding that "no clear-cut solution for care of the disadvantaged in our country has been developed," the commission singled out the neighborhood health centers as promising and urged that "such experimentation be markedly expanded."[18] The American Public Health Association and the U.S. Public Health Service have also gone on record in favor of the comprehensive health service approach; and the PHS has pledged that it will "encourage and promote the concept of comprehensive health services through the use of its own resources and its own consultation and assistance activities." The Surgeon General has assigned "high priority for funding of those programs aimed primarily at improvement of the health status of the indigent" and has urged his field staff, in its work with state health planning agencies, to emphasize the need for delivering comprehensive health services to the poor.[19] The emphasis by the Surgeon General on the needs of the poor is a departure from the traditional approach and activities of his agency.

Such examples of support were duplicated many times, but the testimonials have not resulted in any significant funding priority for the program. Although more neighborhood health centers will probably be added to the program, this will not be done at the rate initially envisioned. The ability to recoup current expenditures from Title XIX or from other government sources will be a telling factor. OEO's health officials have estimated that more than half of the current expenditures of neighborhood health centers might be reimbursed from other governmental programs. Therefore, if the claims of neighborhood health service proponents prove correct, even the present allocation of public funds to provide medical services to the poor could result in improving quality and quantity of health services, as these funds are increasingly spent within the framework of a more effective organization and delivery system.

References

1. U.S. Department of Health, Education and Welfare, *Delivery of Health Services for the Poor* (Washington: The Department, December 1967).
2. H. Jack Geiger, "The Neighborhood Health Center," *Archives of Environmental Health* (June 1967), pp. 912–16.
3. Lisbeth Bamberger (Schorr), "Health Care and Poverty," *Bulletin of the New York Academy of Medicine* (December 1966), pp. 1140–49.
4. U.S. Congress, Senate Committee on Appropriations, *Departments of Labor and HEW and Related Agencies Appropriation Bill, 1969*, 90th Cong., 2d sess., Rept. No. 1484 (Washington: Government Printing Office, 1968), p. 86.
5. OEO, Community Action Program, *Guidelines [to] Healthright Programs* (Washington: Government Printing Office, 1968), pp. 3–4.
6. OEO, Community Action Program, "Manpower Development in Comprehensive Health Services Programs" (December 1967) (mimeographed).
7. U.S. Congress, House Committee on Education and Labor, *Hearings on Economic Opportunity Act of 1967*, 90th Cong., 1st sess. (Washington: Government Printing Office, 1967), part 4, p. 3488.
8. U.S. Department of Health, Education, and Welfare, *Delivery of Health Services for the Poor*, pp. 49–66.
9. U.S. Congress, House Committee on Education and Labor, *Hearings on 1967 Amendments to the Economic Opportunity Act*, 90th Cong., 1st sess. (Washington: Government Printing Office, 1967), part 2, p. 873.

10. A joint statement of the Department of Health, Education, and Welfare and the Office of Economic Opportunity, *Coordinated Funding of Health Services* (Washington: Government Printing Office, May 2, 1967), p. 2.
11. U.S. Congress, Senate Committee on Labor and Public Welfare, *Examination of the War on Poverty*, 90th Cong., 1st sess. (Washington: Government Printing Office, 1967), part 9, p. 2893.
12. Dick Kirschten, "AMA Shuns Realities of Slum Health Programs," *Chicago Sun Times*, July 2, 1967.
13. Donald Ganson, "Doctors Bid AMA Push Aid in Slums," *New York Times,* December 16, 1967.
14. OEO, Community Action Program, Health Services Office, Memorandum to Project Directors of Comprehensive Health Services, October 25, 1967.
15. *Ibid.*
16. "OEO Is Here to Stay, So—," *Pharmacy News* (April-May 1968); reprinted in *Congressional Record* (daily ed.), June 6, 1968, pp. S7805–6.
17. Louise Hutchinson, "OEO Is Urged to Close Its Pharmacies," *Chicago Tribune,* July 10, 1968; and address by Willard B. Simmons, "Pharmacy, Patriotism, Politics, Poverty," in *Congressional Record* (daily ed.), September 26, 1968, pp. S1151–12
18. *Report of the National Advisory Commission on Health Manpower* (Washington: Government Printing Office, November 1967), I, 37.
19. Memorandum of the Surgeon General to the Bureau and regional health directors, November 7, 1967.

**Part IV
Perspectives of Evaluation**

Introduction

The neighborhood health centers were established initially under the research and demonstration provisions of the Economic Opportunity Act. Those funded by HEW under Section 314 (e) of the Partnership for Health Act proceed under a similar demonstration authority. The centers have been set up as demonstration projects for reasons of political expedience as much as any actual commitment to the tenets of the demonstration project approach to testing out new programs. Chapter 1 of this reader has already discussed the demonstration project "scenario."

Formal and explicit evaluations do tell us something about how well the centers are doing, but the larger truth is that these evaluations have been irrelevant to the highly political process of gauging the success of the centers to date. There are definite limits to how much these political facts of life can be changed. This book seeks to organize some of the more useful evaluations and descriptive accounts in an attempt to inject the actual experience of the health centers more effectively into the debates about their future and that of related attempts to improve primary health care in this country.

The chapters in this section present a variety of perspectives on the evaluation of the centers.[1] They stress different functions of the centers, they argue from different theoretical and political vantage points. They suggest different methodologies for examining the centers. These chapters provide alternative frameworks for consuming other materials which explore particular features of the health centers (including those chapters in subsequent sections of this reader) and themselves present broadbrush evaluations of the centers as a group.

"Some Accomplishments and Findings of Neighborhood Health Centers," by Daniel Zwick, is the single most informative article in print about the health centers. The author, for several years an administrator with major responsibility for the development and management of the OEO health centers, presents a very economical accounting of what the centers have achieved and what we have learned from their experience on questions of community participation, health care delivery, staffing and management, and financing. It is a strikingly frank report. The article is especially useful because it includes information on some of the goals of the centers which are often glossed over or have not been the subject of intensive evaluation.

Eugene Feingold's "A Political Scientist's View of the Neighborhood Health Center as a New Social Institution" looks at the health center "from the point of view of power at several different levels of generality." The different levels of generality which Feingold defines and discusses suggest alternative ways of assessing the experience of the centers.

The editorial on neighborhood health centers from the *Health/PAC Bulletin* expresses a radical critique of the centers as being "too little too late," and as failing to be effective catalysts of community change. This chapter suggests the importance of looking at a somewhat different set of questions: Have the centers been an effective focus for change in local poverty communities? Have they "led to significant reform of the university medical schools and big teaching and voluntary hospitals associated with them"?

Reference

1. For a statement of the approach to evaluation of the centers taken by the Program Planning and Evaluation Division, OEO Office of Health Affairs, see: Gerald Sparer and Joyce Johnson, "Evaluation of OEO Neighborhood Health Centers," *American Journal of Public Health 61,* 5 (May 1971): 931–942. It notes the array of objectives held for the centers and discusses dilemmas of evaluating them. The authors advocate "an ideal minimal evaluation effort" to address the questions they deem most important and suggest techniques most appropriate for answering them.

Some Accomplishments and Findings of Neighborhood Health Centers

Daniel I. Zwick

The development of neighborhood health centers in low-income communities throughout the United States in recent years has attracted widespread attention and response. An increasing number of community groups and health institutions have begun to plan and initiate similar activities. Scholars and students of medical care programs have started to devote considerable attention to analyses of the progress and problems of the movement.[1]

Substantial federal financial assistance has been provided since 1966 for planning, organizing and supporting new ambulatory care programs in low-income communities.[2] Grant support was originally provided on a "research and demonstration" basis from the Community Action Program of the Office of Economic Opportunity (OEO) and has expanded to a large-scale nationwide effort aided by both the Office of Health Affairs of OEO and the Health Services and Mental Health Administration of the Department of Health, Education and Welfare (HEW). This paper seeks to review and discuss some of the major accomplishments and findings of these developments from the vantage point of a participant and observer at the national level.

Goals and Guidelines

The goals and aspirations of the organizers of the OEO "Healthrights" program were both high and broad. Their concerns encompassed improvements in access to services, reform in health care delivery, extension of community participation, utilization of new types of health workers, relationships between health care delivery and other forms of community action and economic and social development, medical care quality and financing, transportation and outreach and a host of related problems.[3] The comprehensiveness of the approach was a function of the complexities of the problems being engaged. Their objectives have been characterized as the "positive pursuit of health"—for the individual, family, neighborhood and community.

Each of the goals involved profound difficulties and obstacles to effective action and change. Efforts to deal with so many factors at the same time were destined to encounter much frustration and failure. A later leader pointed out,

Reprinted from Milbank Memorial Fund Quarterly 50, 4 Part I (October 1972): 387–420.

"It has been suggested that the neighborhood health center tries to do too much. This criticism may well be appropriate. But in view of the long history of neglect, dare we try less?"[4]

The initiation of the "War on Poverty" in 1964 and 1965 provided a climate and stimulation for innovation.[5] These conditions encouraged a relatively few to undertake tasks that had disheartened many. Their experience seems to support the observations of an analyst of economic development projects overseas:

> If project planners had known in advance all the difficulties and troubles that were lying in store . . . they probably would never have touched it. . . . Since we necessarily underestimate our creativity, it is desirable that we underestimate to a similar extent the difficulties of the tasks we face so as to be tricked by these two offsetting underestimates into undertaking tasks that we can, but otherwise, would not have tackled. It (the hiding hand) takes up problems it *thinks* it can solve, finds they are really more difficult than expected but then, being stuck with them, attacks willy-nilly the unsuspected difficulties—and sometimes even succeeds.[6]

The challenge inspired the imagination and energies of many local groups as well as numerous health professionals and political leaders. Strong feelings focused on the need for greater attention to the serious health problems and related unmet needs in poverty areas.[7] Because the breadth of the attack appeared potentially responsive to the dimensions of the needs, the initiative appeared serious and realistic. High risks, though, were inherent in the mission.

The Congressional mandate in November, 1966 for the OEO Comprehensive Health Services Program set the purpose with comparable scope:

> . . . to assure that (health) services are made readily accessible to residents of such areas (of concentrated poverty), are furnished in a manner most responsive to their needs and with their participation, and whenever possible are combined with . . . arrangements for providing employment, education, social or other assistance needed by the families and individuals served. . .[8]

The statutory provisions received operational interpretation in the OEO "Program Guidelines" in February, 1967.[9] The document sought to set procedures toward the broad concepts and purposes. In practice, the formal provisions were to be viewed as too rigid by some and too ambiguous by others.

An HEW program analysis issued in December, 1967 identified comprehensive health centers to serve the outpatient health care needs of low-income areas, along with proposed changes in outpatient clinics and health manpower and financing programs, as principle means to improve the delivery of health services to the poor. The report pointed out that up to 1,000 such centers or similar projects might be needed.[10] A statement by the Surgeon General of the Public Health Service about the same time committed the resources of that agency to work toward similar objectives.[11]

The principle thrusts of the program were summarized in an OEO staff report:

1. How can consumers and providers of health care work together most effectively in planning and carrying out health services?
2. Can the delivery of health care be organized on a team basis to provide high-quality comprehensive personal health care to poor families in a dignified efficient manner?
3. What kinds of new jobs and new careers can be developed in the health care field for poor persons?
4. What are the best ways of relating these projects to other health and poverty efforts?[12]

Each of the aided projects was expected to engage these issues in its own way.

The aspirations set for the program in its early days resulted in certain misunderstandings in future years. Many viewed them as promises. A few saw them as requirements. Both such views produced disappointment and criticism. As for other OEO programs, cynicism sometimes became the product of expectations that were too simplistic and optimistic.

The tests of accessibility, availability and acceptability set forth in the Program Guidelines, however, have become commonly applied standards for community health services. The bold rhetoric of the 1960's is the common talk of the 1970's.

Resource Development

Between 1965 and 1971, about 100 neighborhood health centers and other comprehensive health services projects were initiated with OEO grant assistance. About 50 additional projects were started with HEW aid. In excess of $400 million was invested in these endeavors (table 6-1). When fully operational, these resources may serve up to three million persons.

Approximately 60 additional comprehensive health care projects for pre-school and school age children living in areas with concentrations of low-income families (Children and Youth Projects) were developed during the same period with HEW financial aid. An amendment to Title V of the Social Security Act in 1965 initiated this program.[13] Over $200 million of federal grant funds have been awarded to assist these efforts (table 6-2).

The new projects are broadly dispersed geographically. They are located in about 120 different communities in 42 states; about three-fourths are in urban

Table 6-1
Amounts of OEO and HEW Grants for Neighborhood Health Centers and Other Local Projects

Fiscal Year	Total[*]	OEO Grants[*]	HEW Grants[*]
1965	$ 2.0	$ 2.0	$ ——
1966	7.8	7.8	——
1967	50.6	50.6	——
1968	39.5	32.8	6.7
1969	64.9	51.1	13.8
1970	98.5	72.3	26.2
1971	155.4	91.6	63.8
Total	$418.7	$308.2	$110.5

[*]In millions of dollars.

Table 6-2
HEW Grants for Local Projects to Develop Comprehensive Health Care of Preschool and School Age Children

Fiscal Year	Amount[*]
1966	$ 13.5
1967	31.7
1968	36.8
1969	39.0
1970	38.8
1971	43.8
Total	$203.6

[*]In millions of dollars.

areas and one-fourth in rural communities. Locations range from northern Maine to the southern border of California to the western coast of Alaska.

This undertaking has been the most extensive concerted public effort in the history of the United States to expand ambulatory health care resources in poverty communities on a nationwide basis. It has built upon and greatly expanded somewhat similar earlier efforts, both in this country and abroad, to make primary health care services more accessible to poor families in organized settings.[14,15] A substantial beginning has been made in overcoming the serious deficiencies that exist with respect to health care services in the nation's low-income communities. Legislative actions in recent years encouraging increased expenditures in poverty by other federal health programs suggest an even broader impact has been made; changes in the "Hill-Burton" health facilities program and the community mental health center program (including more liberal matching provisions, up to 90 per cent and initiation of the National Health Services Corps are examples of such actions.

The scarcity of physical facilities to house high quality health services in poverty areas has been a most serious obstacle to the organization of new programs. Through an extraordinary arrangement involving the cooperation of four federal agencies (OEO, HEW, the Department of Housing and Urban Development, and the Office of Management and Budget) and private mortgage and insurance companies, funds have been made available through FHA-guaranteed loans to build new centers in Chicago, Kansas City, Nashville, Philadelphia, Pittsburgh, Rochester and San Francisco; similar negotiations are underway in other cities. These facilities involved long-term investments of $1.5–2.5 million each. Technical guidelines for planning ambulatory care facilities of these types have been an important by-product.[16] HEW and OEO grant funds have also been used for modular units and trailers and to renovate existing buildings, including former warehouses, stores, apartments and convents.

Although the majority of projects involves the development of new "free-standing" health care centers, support has also been given to the other approaches toward the development of comprehensive ambulatory health care services in low-income areas. Hospital outpatient departments have been restructured, poor families have been enrolled in existing prepaid group practices and new medical groups have been established. More ambitious efforts to organize community health networks to co-ordinate and extend health delivery systems in urban poverty neighborhoods were begun in 1970, by OEO.[17] Table 6-3 indicates the diversity of approaches receiving aid from OEO as of December, 1971.

Attempts to restructure hospital outpatient departments to provide comprehensive family health services have often been found to be the most difficult. Experiments have been started in both large cities (such as Newark, Boston, Cincinnati, Houston and Los Angeles) as well as in smaller cities (such as Dayton, Oklahoma City and Winston-Salem). As might be expected, changes that involve altering long-established institutional relationships and services usually encounter formidable obstacles.

A wide variety of health care agencies has joined in these projects. Commu-

Table 6-3
Projects Receiving OEO Grant Support*

Type of Project	Operational Grants	Planning Grants
Neighborhood health center	19	
Rural services	15	3
Outpatient department	10	5
Group practice	5	1
Community health network	6	6
Total	55	15

*December 31, 1971. Excludes 16 projects transferred to HEW in fiscal year 1971 and 9 projects transferred in fiscal year 1972 (17 of these are N.H.C.-type projects).

nity and teaching hospitals, medical schools, health departments and group practices have been willing to assume new or broader responsibilities along these lines (table 6-4). Over half of the nation's medical schools have been involved, in one way or another. As a result, a broad base of exposure and experience has been established. Many factors appear to have motivated health agencies to undertake these assignments; further study of the specific situations will add to understanding of the forces inducing institutional change in medicine and in the society as a whole during the 1960's and 1970's.

Community Participation

The principle that consumers should participate actively in the development of policies for the centers was a key feature of the original idea and Program Guidelines and has been a major part of the evolving experience. The implications of this requirement were not fully understood by the early planners of OEO.[18] However, the feelings of discrimination and frustration generally present in poverty areas and the lack of responsiveness and sensitivity in health and other community services usually available to them made it urgent to seek substantial changes in methods of doing business. The statutory authorization for the OEO Comprehensive Health Services Program simply stated that services should be designed "in a manner most responsive to their (neighborhood residents) needs and with their participation."

The original OEO Guidelines provided that this goal might be achieved through participation either on an advisory council or a governing board. At least one-half of the former or one-third of the latter were to be neighborhood

Table 6-4
Administering Agencies of Operational Projects Receiving OEO and HEW Financial Assistance, 1965-1971

Type of Administering Agency	OEO-Aided*		HEW-Aided Comprehensive**		Children & Youth	
	No.	%	No.	%	No.	%
New health corporation	30	37	11	35		
Hospital	16	19	7	22	25	37
Medical school	14	17	3	10	22	32
Health department	7	9	4	13	21	31
Group practice	7	9	3	10		
Other	7	9	3	10		
Total	81	100	31	100	68	100

*Excludes 15 planning projects.
**Excludes 2 projects also receiving OEO aid and 25 projects transferred from OEO. Also excludes 19 developmental projects.

residents served by the project. The early and active involvement of other community groups, including health professional associations and official agencies, was also defined as an essential feature.

The participation of consumers in planning health service programs did not seem a radical innovation. Citizen participation on hospital boards and community councils was longstanding. The "Partnership for Health" legislation enacted about the same time required a major consumer role in health planning. The original OEO Program Guidelines drew an analogy to hospital boards of trustees.

Some health professionals recognized that consumer interests could become effective allies in achieving desired changes. An early leader pointed out:

> I believe that one of the mistakes we make in our various professional fields is to feel that we can only make progress by convincing our colleagues through the logic and passion of our approach, that they ought to change. . . . I feel rather that we must look to our allies in the community, because if we examine the history of medicine in terms of organized forms of service, we find that the medical profession reaches to what the community expects. And it is to developing a higher level of community expectation with regard to broad problems and with regard to the best use of resources and programs and institutions that effort must be directed.[19]

The assumption that low-income consumers should participate actively and equally in policy consideration and formulation was a new emphasis, however. This approach called for new attitudes and behavior on the part of not only consumers but also health professionals and program managers. Such changes were not likely to be easily achieved.

The initial projects were generally organized through the efforts of professional staffs of health agencies who were primarily interested in making changes in the methods of delivering health services. The active participation of consumers has increased steadily, often requiring modification in the organization of the health center. As consumers, health professionals and program administrators have assumed new roles with regard to policy formulation and decision-making, many new practices and relationships have had to be learned and tested. Usually adjustments and readjustments have been necessary to find the system and balance that work best in the local situation.

Through participation on advisory and governing boards, consumers have played a major role in the development of almost all centers. In some cases they were the energizing force leading to the planning and development of the programs. In most cases, they have affected the character and concerns of the project in important ways. Their specific activities have most often related to the selection of key staff, service priorities, hours of service, budgets, recruitment of outreach workers and other local personnel and grievances.[20]

The uncertainties and tensions that have often occurred in connection with community participation in health centers have been well reported.[21] Initial analyses of these processes from political and sociological points of view have been published.[22,23] These relationships are likely to be the subject of numerous papers for years to come, thus enriching the discussion of a topic that has received relatively little attention in medical care and public health administration.

Experiences with community participation have indicated the importance of adequate orientation and training if the new roles and authorities are to be handled effectively. HEW grant funds and OEO contract funds were made available for the support of related educational programs early in the development of the health center program. In recent years substantially increased resources have been devoted to such training efforts, especially to prepare boards to handle the duties and obligations that are undertaken in becoming an administering agency and federal grantee.

The experiences of the councils and boards need to be considered in perspective. Many health centers have found themselves involved in basic issues long associated with democratic government. Questions of representation have been essentially the same as those with which western democracy and political science have struggled since the Greek state; it has never been easy to determine who appropriately and legitimately represents others. Voting tallies have often been disappointingly low; as organizers of many other community programs have learned, it is exceedingly difficult to obtain high levels of voter participation in most nonpartisan elections in the United States.[24] It has not been found that these issues are altered substantially when poor people are involved.

Similarly, disagreements between governing boards and program administrators as to appropriate divisions of power and activities have been similar to those often experienced in many other bureaucratic enterprises. In view of the strong interest in jobs, problems of patronage have been encountered; policies on "conflict of interest" have set standards higher than those often applied elsewhere. Internal struggles for influence have been reminiscent of those common in other enterprises where change is occurring that may significantly affect the future well-being and fortune of the participants.

The health center activities with councils and boards have often been more visible and better reported than similar events in other settings. Higher expectations for involvement and effectiveness have frequently been applied than is generally achieved in corporate affairs.[25] Critics have frequently not been as tolerant of error in these cases as in more established institutions.[26] Confrontations have sometimes involved considerable intensity of feeling and differences in styles.[27] Health professionals have seldom been previously prepared to deal with these types of interactions, thus they have been required to deal with new conditions, sometimes under quite uncomfortable pressure. As in other circumstances, the effective resolution of issues has been found to depend largely upon the quality of leadership and the degree of understanding and skills of those present.

Consumer "demands" for health services in neighborhood health centers have been generally in line with comparable expressions among other consumer groups. Usually interest has focused on needs and desires for more comprehensive services. Increased dental care and drug abuse control services, additional hours of service and better arrangements for transportation and child care have been frequent interests. The desires for broader benefits are notably similar to those reported from consumers involved in prepaid group practices.[28] They also appear consistent with the tendency of purchasers of private health insurance to prefer more comprehensive benefits. The common concerns of consumer representatives about the sensitivity and attitudes of physicians and other health care providers attest to the continuing importance assigned to personal care and the doctor-patient relationship.

Experiences in the extension of community participation in the development of health centers bring to mind the observation of Winston Churchill that democracy is the most awkward, the most complex, the most irritating, the clumsiest and the best system yet devised in the mind of man. These developments appear consistent with the Jeffersonian faith that when free citizens have adequate information and opportunity they will act in responsible ways. The incorporation of additional groups within the society's decision-making system can be an important stabilizing action.

The health center program has tended to place increasing control and responsibility in consumers. At noted above, the earlier grants tended to be made to health care institutions who helped organize consumer advisory boards. In recent years much greater emphasis has been given to the support of new neighborhood health corporations that include both consumers and providers on the governing board of directors (table 6-5). In this matter too, bold aspirations have become common standards in less than a decade.

Health Care Delivery

Health centers have sought to organize and provide comprehensive ambulatory health care to individuals and families.[29] Even though this goal has been difficult to achieve, or even to define precisely, it has indicated the scope of concern and ambition of the planners. Primary care practitioners have been general practitioners in some cases, and pediatricians and internists in others. Increasing reliance is being placed on nurse practitioners and other "physician expanders." The centers have a wide range of medical specialists available, either on staff or through consultation. Dental care has generally received substantial attention. Home care services are being increasingly implemented. Counseling and other supporting social services are usually strong. The weakest area is commonly mental health services.

The efforts to develop comprehensive health services at the neighborhood health centers and Children and Youth Projects reflect not only consumer needs and wants but also the broadening professional interest in organizing such programs.[30-34] Trends in medical education and health services delivery have, in turn, been reinforced by these activities. The interactions of these community and professional movements appear to deserve more extensive analyses.

Health care delivery systems in neighborhood health centers usually have employed health care teams. Various patterns of "team care" have been implemented.[35] This focus arises primarily out of the nature of the health and associated problems identified in many poor families; no single discipline or specialty is capable of dealing alone with the complexities of the conditions present. Teams have often encountered the well-known difficulties of altering patterns of behavior and developing new relations among health care professionals and allied workers. Increased attention to these issues appear to be necessary, through both basic and continuing education, if such methods of health care delivery are to be effective.[36,37]

The organization of outreach staffs, commonly called "family health workers" or "community health aides," has been the usual approach to improve communications between the center and residents.[38] The record of relatively low utilization of services by poor families enrolled in a prepaid group practice in New York City has pointed up the importance of this function even when income barriers to health care are removed.[39] Other community action programs serving the poor have demonstrated the contribution of "face to face" approaches involving staff members from the community itself in breaking through long-standing obstacles. These workers provide the personal assistance

Table 6-5
Administering Agencies of Projects Aided by OEO at Time of Initial Grant Award*

Administering Agency	1965-6 %	1967 %	1968 %	1969 %	1970 %	1971 %
New health corp.		24	33	33	52	59
Hospital	50	21	22	67	9	10
Medical school	37	18	11		18	7
Health department	13	18	11			
Group practice		7			9	3
Other		10	22		13	21

*In some cases the administering agency of a project has changed during the life of the project, usually from a medical school to a new health corporation.

often needed by poor families to deal with conditions that make it difficult, or impossible, for them to use health services and to follow through most appropriately. They have often been trained to provide needed home health services.[40] However, as noted above, the integration of outreach staff into health care teams usually requires considerable preparation and continuing effort.

The comprehensive health services concept calls for much greater attention to prevention and early care. The record of missed opportunities, especially among children, indicated this need was an acute one. Most health centers have made substantial progress in this respect, reporting significant improvements in prenatal and child care, immunizations and dental care. Children and Youth Projects have strongly emphasized initial health assessments and continuous supervision of care. However, in this regard also, experience demonstrates again that established patterns of behavior relating to episodic care, on the part of both consumers and practitioners, are not easily altered.[44]

The unification of health services with related social services is another key aspect. The intimate relation of these issues, especially among "hard core families," demands substantial attention and resources.[46] Similarly, many centers have organized programs to deal with closely related community and environmental health issues, such as housing and water supply. Many Children and Youth Projects, as well as health centers, have provided a base for organizing day care services.

Patterns of health care among poor families appear to be a good deal more complex and sophisticated than has been generally recognized, involving a variety of providers to meet different needs and conditions.[41-43] Data from "baseline studies" conducted in eight communities where health centers were later developed indicate that about 90 per cent of those interviewed reported a "usual source of care." A clinic was so identified for about a quarter of the cases in a New York City neighborhood and in two-thirds of the responses in Atlanta.[45] As health centers begin services, they "intervene" into the existing patterns; it appears that, in most cases, they do not deal with nonexisting or wholly disorganized arrangements. Further analysis is needed to understand better how poor families incorporate a health center into their previously established health care patterns.

Families usually "register" for care at the health centers. They have generally not been asked to "enroll" and thereby to accept a commitment to use the health center as their sole, or prime, source of health care. This practice can make it most difficult to achieve continuity of care. An OEO-sponsored evaluation study of 21 health centers found that 72 per cent of the user families considered the health center their "usual source of care," with a range of 48 to 91 per cent.[47] However, among those reporting the center as their "usual source," for most centers, 20 to 30 per cent indicated that their last physician visit was to another facility; reports of the last dental visit are similar. Up to 40 per cent stated that they go to another source for the treatment of their most limiting condition. Although these patterns do not appear dissimilar to practice among other health care delivery systems, they dramatize again the difficulties of achieving centrality and continuity of care.[48]

It has been pointed out that consumer "enrollment" in a health plan is only achieved through the actual behavior of the participants. Many centers are seeking ways of strengthening continuing ties with their registrants and users. The development of such arrangements and commitments will be especially important as health centers seek payment on a prepaid capitation basis.

The development of effective hospital relations has been difficult for many health centers. The problems that some have had in obtaining hospital privileges are somewhat similar to those experienced in the past by physicians in prepaid group practices and by physicians from minority groups. Restrictions of funds that severely limited the dollars available in OEO and HEW grant budgets for inpatient care and that have reduced Medicaid payments for such costs have further complicated this issue. Difficulties of this nature have occurred even in instances when the health center itself is sponsored by a hospital.[49] On the other hand, some centers have systems that insure most effective continuity of care. Strengthening these relations needs the highest priority.

In the past few years special effort has been devoted to the development of projects in rural areas. These projects are focusing on the use of satellite clinics and nurse practitioners and other types of new personnel. One project in Maine is also exploring the use of "interactive television" as a method of long distance communication and supervision.

Efforts to support the enrollment of poor persons in existing prepaid group practices have been aided by both HEW and OEO. These demonstrations have involved plans in Boston, New Haven, Bellaire (Ohio) and Seattle, a HIP group in Suffolk County (New York) and units of the Kaiser-Permanente Medical Care Program in California and Oregon. These approaches have not only proven feasible but also are producing valuable comparative data on utilization and other factors.

The quality of care at the health centers has been found to compare favorably with other providers. An intensive medical audit program, administered by staff of the Department of Community Health at the Albert Einstein College of Medicine, has been part of the OEO grant program from almost the beginning and has also been incorporated into the HEW program.[50] This work appears to be the most ambitious continuing activity of its type in the nation. These reports also indicate that more effort is required to achieve "ideal levels" of preventive health care.

A study of the utilization of services at eight health centers has indicated that "registrants" tend to average from four to five physician encounters a year.[51] Even with complete removal of financial barriers and extensive outreach efforts and transportation services, the use of health care services by poor families did not increase to unusual levels (as compared to the average rate of physician

persons attracted to community health endeavors tend to differ in interest and values from physicians oriented toward hospitals and medical schools.[56] The development of linkages and institutional relations that provide desirable support without imposing unacceptable bonds remains one of the most difficult challenges. The neighborhood health centers and community health networks share this dilemma with regional medical programs and other efforts focused on strengthening community health services.

Nurse practitioners and physician assistants have been utilized by a number of health centers to help meet needs. The settings of health centers, the service demand and their relative flexibility and willingness to explore new patterns of care have encouraged such efforts. These experiences have tended to be favorable and considerable expansion in the use of such personnel is likely.[57]

As discussed above, the employment of family health workers and neighborhood residents in other positions has been a key feature. Over half the staff of the centers are residents of poverty neighborhoods; the income received, as well as other aspects of the center, can have a significant economic effect.[58] However, the traditional obstacles to career advancement in the health field have generally frustrated the development of career ladders. Some health centers have established new supervisory levels and have developed broad educational programs as well as liberal policies on educational leave in efforts to alleviate this problem.

The centers have also shared in the shortages and problems of management personnel that characterize the health field. The scarcity of trained administrators, especially for ambulatory care programs, has been compounded by the need for persons with the additional skills required in community-based projects. Both short- and long-term educational efforts have been initiated to help meet this need, involving a number of schools of public health, hospital administration and public administration.

In view of the sponsorship of many of the initial health centers by medical schools and large hospitals, it was anticipated that greatly needed management resources might be made available by these institutions to aid the fledgling centers. With few exceptions, the record in this regard has been disappointing. Other pressures on established health agencies have appeared to be so acute that, in most cases, they have not been able to make available much of the needed talent. In a few cases, help in planning new programs and services has been provided by staffs of regional medical programs and comprehensive health planning agencies.

As new neighborhood health corporations have assumed increased responsibilities for the operations of the centers, a number have begun to develop contractual arrangements with medical schools for the provision of clinical services. It appears that such approaches may be the soundest method of long-term relations between health centers and medical schools. They serve to define the nature and extent of the commitments that both groups can accept and live with effectively.

Supporters and some critics of OEO have suggested that much of its most important long-term impact may be the result of the opportunities provided leaders from black, Spanish-speaking and other minority groups to assume managerial responsibilities in operating large-scale programs.[59] The health centers have provided many positions for top and middle management personnel in planning and directing local projects with annual budgets usually ranging between $2–8 million. The medical and program managers obtaining experiences in these projects are likely to fill many key positions in the health industry in the future. Similarly, members of governing boards and advisory councils are developing expertise that will be of great value in other settings. Members of these groups are likely to be increasingly active in health planning and other health activities. The acquired knowledge, skills and self-confidence can also have application and impact in other social and economic endeavors.

The National Association of Neighborhood Health Centers may have a significant impact on future health programming. The new national organization of consumers and staffs of health centers provides a forum for the consideration of proposals affecting the future of the health centers, including plans for universal health insurance and health maintenance organizations.

Financing

The initial OEO grant support of health centers assumed that long-term financial support would come largely from Medicaid, Medicare and other financing sources. The organization of the centers, in turn, would make it possible to achieve better use of the increased funds available for heath services.[60] These assumptions appeared reasonable in the mid-1960's; new large-scale federal health financing programs had been enacted about the same time as the first grants were awarded to health centers. The Medicaid program anticipated the development and support of comprehensive health services for the poor in all states by 1975. To help achieve this goal an agreement of mutual support was signed by the Director of OEO and the Secretary of HEW in May 1967.[61] It was estimated that funds from Medicaid and Medicare might finance 70–80 per cent of health center costs.

The nature of the growth of the Medicaid programs has frustrated the achievement of this goal. State programs have been restrictive with respect to both beneficiary eligibility and supported services. Benefits have been reduced rather than expanded. Some state administrators have resisted the completion of procedures to reimburse health centers. Even the most successful efforts by health centers to obtain Medicaid, Medicare and other private third-party funds has resulted in reimbursements for only 50 per cent or so of their budgets; in most cases, such payments have been in the range of 10–20 per cent.

Amendments to the Medicaid program being considered by the Congress in

policies provided that partial-pay plans might include families with incomes up to twice the poverty index—$7,600 per year for a family of four in 1971—with progressive increases in charges. Because HEW grants were not constrained by such statutory provisions, more flexible approaches to this issue were possible. Both OEO and HEW encouraged payment arrangements on a prepaid capitation basis and such plans are being planned and tested at some centers, e.g., Salt Lake City and Louisville.

An amendment to the OEO Act was approved by the Congress in the summer of 1972, and authorized a further liberalization of the policy of that Agency so that grant funds might be used to help centers serve all residents of the low-income neighborhood, either without charge or on a partial- or full-pay basis. To meet the genuine concern of some that "creaming" may occur, as has happened with respect to other public services, it has been proposed that the percentage of registered families below the poverty index be at least equal to the proportion of the poorest families living in the neighborhood.

The development and use of partial- and full-pay private payment plans are essential under present circumstances so that the centers may achieve the goal of becoming neighborhood institutions. Otherwise, they can become divisive forces within the community, marked with derogatory labels. Further, it appears that the health conditions and practices of neighborhood residents tend to be quite similar, regardless of income.[69]

The tortuous history of OEO policies in this regard has been part of the indecision regarding the extent of federal aid to be made available to the "near poor" and the "working poor." Similar issues have been debated in recent years with respect to such other programs as Head Start, Legal Services, Day Care, and Welfare Reform.

It has become widely recognized, however, that public action to develop needed quality health resources and services in low-income neighborhoods must be done in ways that do not perpetuate systems of services for the poor, a condition no longer acceptable to either health professionals or the poor themselves. Additional health care resources are required to serve not the poor alone but all who live in low-income communities.

Growing Taller

Much has been accomplished in five years, but even more remains to be done. No one is likely to suggest that answers have been found to all the major needs and concerns that inspired the effort. Probably the greatest gains have been to increase understanding of the nature and dimensions of the questions. In view of the widespread interest in the health centers their further gains and shortfalls are likely to be well reported and analyzed. One aspect of their development, though, has been perhaps best covered by a speaker at the recent dedication of a center in a rural community in a southern state.[70] The speaker described the project as "a credit to the community" and indicated, "you can't tell us that it isn't going to succeed because we know it is. We're going to make it succeed. We're going to be taller," the speaker concluded, "because we are somebody and we're not afraid."

References

1. *Bibliography on the Comprehensive Health Services Program*, Office of Health Affairs, Office of Economic Opportunity, Washington, United States Government Printing Office, January 1970; addendum dated July, 1970.
2. *History of the OEO Comprehensive Health Services Program*, staff paper, Washington, Office of Health Affairs, Office of Economic Opportunity, January, 1971.
3. Schorr, L.B. and English, J.T., Background, Context and Significant Issues in Neighborhood Health Center Programs, *Milbank Memorial Fund Quarterly, 46*, 289–296, July, 1968.
4. Bryant, T., Goals and Potential of the Neighborhood Health Centers, *Medical Care, 8*, 93–94, March–April, 1970.
5. Levine, R.A., *The Poor Ye Need Not Have With You*, Cambridge, Massachusetts, M.I.T. Press, 1970, pp. 44–90.
6. Hirschman, A.O., *Development Projects Observed*, Washington, The Brookings Institution, 1967, pp. 12–14.
7. Norman, J.C., Medicine in the Ghetto, *New England Journal of Medicine, 281*, 1271–1275, December 4, 1969.
8. Economic Opportunity Act, as amended; 42 USC 2809. The specific authorization for the "Comprehensive Health Services Program" was originally included in 1966 as Section 211–2 and became Section 222(a)(4) through later amendments.
9. *Guidelines for Comprehensive Neighborhood Health Services Programs*, Washington, Office of Economic Opportunity, Guidance No. 6128–1, February, 1967; reissued May, 1968 and March, 1970.
10. *Delivery of Health Services for the Poor*, program analysis, Department of Health, Education and Welfare, Washington, United States Government Printing Office, December, 1967.
11. Stewart, W.H., Priority Statement for the Partnership for Health Program, Washington, Public Health Service, 1967.
12. OEO Activities to Improve Health Care and Health Delivery Systems in Low-Income Areas, Office of Health Affairs, Office of Economic Opportunity, unpublished document, p. 5.
13. Lesser, A.J., Progress in Maternal and Child Health, *Children Today, 1*, 7–12, March–April, 1972.
14. Hiscock, I., The Development of Neighborhood Health Services in the United States, *Milbank Memorial Fund Quarterly, 13*, 30–51, January, 1935.

Services on the Demand for Hospital Beds, *New England Journal of Medicine, 280,* 808–812, April 10, 1969.

54. Colombo, T., Saward, E. and Greenlick, M., The Integration of an OEO Health Program into a Prepaid Comprehensive Group Practice, *American Journal of Public Health, 59,* 641–650, April, 1969.
55. Tilson, H.H., *Stability of Employment of the Physician in Neighborhood Health Services,* Boston, Harvard School of Public Health, January 1972.
56. Richmond, J., *Currents in American Medicine,* Boston, Harvard University Press, 1969, pp. 96–99.
57. Silver, H.K., Ford, L.C. and Lewis, R.D., The Pediatric Nurse-Practitioner Program, *JAMA, 204,* 298–302, April 22, 1968.
58. Ferguson, A., Impact of Health Centers on the Local Economy, Neighborhood Health Center Seminar Program, Series No. 4, Berkeley, University of California Extension, October 1971, unpublished.
59. Moynihan, D.P., *Maximum Feasible Misunderstanding,* New York, The Free Press, 1969, p. 129.
60. Roghmann, K.J., Haggerty, R.J. and Lorenz, R., Anticipated and Actual Effects of Medicaid on the Medical Care Pattern of Children, *New England Journal of Medicine, 285,* 1053–1057, November 4, 1971.
61. Coordinated Funding of Health Services, Joint statement of the Department of Health, Education and Welfare and the Office of Economic Opportunity, Washington, May 2, 1967.
62. 92nd U.S. Congress, H.R. 1, Section 207.
63. Sloane, H.I., Can We Cut the Red Tape? Or Must We Strangle?, *American Journal of Public Health, 61,* 88, May, 1971.
64. Blendon, R.J. and Gaus, C.R., Problems in Developing Health Services in Poverty Areas: The Johns Hopkins Experience, *Journal of Medical Education, 46,* 477–484, June, 1971.
65. *Lengthening Shadows: A Report of the Council on Pediatric Practice on the Delivery of Health Care to Children,* American Academy of Pediatrics, 1971, p. 123.
66. Sparer, G. and Anderson, A., Costs of Services at Neighborhood Health Centers, *New England Journal of Medicine, 286,* 1241–1245, June 8, 1972.
67. *Promoting the Health of Mothers and Children, F.Y. 1971,* Washington, Maternal and Child Health Service, p. 21.
68. *Cost Finding and Reporting System,* Washington, Office of Health Affairs, OEO Manual 6128–1, August, 1971.
69. Richardson, W.C., Measuring the Urban Poor's Use of Physician Services in Response to Illness Episodes, *Medical Care, 8,* 139, March–April, 1970.
70. *Clarion Ledger,* Jackson, Mississippi, December 1, 1971, p. 5.

A Political Scientist's View of the Neighborhood Health Center as a New Social Institution

Eugene Feingold

Reviewing the state of American political science, one commentator has remarked that "political scientists are riding off in many directions evidently on the assumption that if you don't know where you are going, any road will take you there."[1] Political scientists disagree among themselves about just what it is they are (or should be) studying, how to study it, and why it is they are studying it.

From this disarray, I would like to select one of the central concepts of political science, the concept of power, to use as the organizing core for my comments on the neighborhood health center. There has been extensive discussion in the literature of political science about the concept of power, its definition, and its usefulness as a means of understanding and explaining social and political events.[2] I will not discuss these matters here, but rather will speak of power in the way that most people do, as a relationship of influence and control among people and institutions—the ability of a person or a group of persons to affect the behavior of others or the outcome of events.

We can look at the neighborhood health center from the point of view of power at several different levels of generality. These are:

The question of the power of the ordinary man in modern technological society and in the United States in particular;

The relationship between power and poverty;

The power, or, more properly, the lack of power, of minority ethnic groups in American society;

The relationship between the "war on poverty" and the distribution of power in American government;

The relationship between the neighborhood health center and the various constituents of the political community within which it is located;

The relationship between the neighborhood health center and the black community;

The relationships between the community board of the neighborhood health ⟨enter, the center's sponsors, the local community action program, and the Office of Economic Opportunity; and

The power relationships inside neighborhood health centers.

Reprinted from *Medical Care* 8, 2 (March-April 1970): 108-115. Presented at a session sponsored by the Medical Care Section of the 97th Annual Meeting of the American Public Health Association, Philadelphia, November 1969.

preferential treatment. It has been suggested that these tensions can be lessened by "a massive general attack on the outstanding social problems of the society which affect both whites and blacks"—an attack broad enough so that it is not seen as a special effort designed for black people.[14] It was precisely such an effort that the war on poverty and the Economic Opportunity Act represented— an effort to abate the rising tensions within the Democratic party and keep the party in power by turning attention away from problems of "civil rights" to problems of poverty.[15] However, the poverty program has not been able to alleviate racial tensions because the black community has sought participation and power through that program, while urban whites have large ignored it. Thus, the war on poverty is seen by the white community as a progarm designed for blacks, even though the majority of the poor are white. This raises the question of whether an effort to reduce racial tensions by a broad attack on social problems can be successful so long as the black community continues to demand a share in power, as it inevitably will.

This, then, is one aspect of an analysis of the Economic Opportunity Act from the perspective of power—its passage as an effort to re-cement the alliance that had kept the Democratic party our majority party for a generation. The other aspect of the analysis of the poverty program from the perspective of power that I wish to discuss is the role of the Office of Economic Opportunity itself. It was created because neither the Department of Health, Education and Welfare nor the Department of Labor were felt to be appropriate agencies for carrying on the war on poverty. Yet, it has been in competition with the programs of these departments and of other departments, a competition that it has steadily been losing as programs are stripped away from OEO and sent on to other agencies. The Nixon administration has given formal recognition to this in its announced plans for OEO. There have been frequent reports, so far unfulfilled, that the neighborhood health center program, still in OEO, will soon be moved to another agency. One of the reasons for creating a new agency, the OEO, to handle the anti-poverty program was concern over the ability of existing agencies to break away from their usual ways of doing business.[16] It remains to be seen whether the enthusiasm and innovativeness that the OEO staff brought to bear on its problems will continue when programs are put into the older more bureaucratic government agencies. At the same time, the tenuous political position of OEO, a reflection both of its programs and of the antagonism toward the poor in this country, has been one in which its operations have been under hostile scrutiny from the first. It has been forced to back away from its original plans and pronouncements, raising the question of how much support the neighborhood health centers would continue to get as they tried innovating programs for meeting medical care needs even if they remained within OEO's jurisdiction.

I want to turn now from the national scene to the local scene, and look at the power relationships between the neighborhood health center and the local community and the minority group community.

To the extent that the neighborhood health center changes, or has the potential for changing, established relationships, it finds itself the focus of opposition. There are, first of all, the established relationships in the delivery of medical care. Some of the neighborhood health centers have found that local pharmacists and local medical societies have attempted to exercise political influence at both local and national levels to restrict their programs. A study of the neighborhood health center in Watts reported that there was no active recruitment of residents to use the center "out of fear of inciting the wrath of local physicians and dentists."[17]

A particular source of conflict has been the black physician practicing in the ghetto. Such physicians have found themselves antagonistic to proposals for neighborhood health centers for several reasons. They are concerned about losing patients to the centers. As solo fee-for-service practitioners, they are not particularly committed to the idea of comprehensive care in a community-controlled setting, and see the neighborhood health center as simply a competitor. They have been serving the poor free of charge and at reduced fees for many years. Now that some of the poor are able to pay for their care through the Medicaid program, the ghetto-based professionals feel they should get the fees. They see no reason why new government programs for the poor should go to sponsoring agencies, such as medical schools or other white paternalistic institutions, that have discriminated against the black community in admissions and staff appointments and provided poor outpatient care in the past.

In Detroit, the black professionals were able to work together with representatives of the black community to force a change in the plans of the Detroit Health Department for a neighborhood health center. The center presently operates with a staff of black physicians drawn from the ghetto, many or all of them only part-time with the center. This has, of course, created other problems for the center and for the implementation of the ideal of continuity and comprehensive care.

In addition to being a source of competition, the neighborhood health center is also significant in its community because it is a potential source of power. In addition to the services it offers, the center, as a substantial business operation, has jobs, bank deposits, and purchases of goods and services at its command. In the minority community where all of these are scarce, these commodities can serve as a power base within the community, both for the center and for the individuals who control the center. They can be used particularistically, to help specific individuals, in a new version of the nineteenth century political machine. They can also be used for the more universalistic good of the black and poor communities. I am thinking here of at least one neighborhood health center which has tried to use its banking business as a carrot to persuade local financial institutions to modify their lending practices, and its purchases of goods and services as a means of bringing money into the black community.

Moving from the neighborhood health center's relationship with its local community, we come next to relationships between the community board of

sources, local, state, and federal. These funds are not available in a manner that relates to center needs. As a result, center management must spend considerable effort coordinating the various sources of funds and manipulating them so that they fit reality. This is typical of many programs dependent on governmental funds, and points up the need for such funds to be made available in ways that are responsive to actual needs.)

Finally, we move to the question of power relationships within the neighborhood health center itself. First, there is the question of power distribution within the community board. Board members frequently represent different interests, with different values and different outlooks. Both social goals and more particularistic goals of jobs and other patronage for themselves and their friends are pursued by board members in conflict with each other. As a result, many boards have had difficulty in functioning effectively. In one neighborhood multi-service agency incorporating a health center, the stakes were high enough that conflict over them resulted in a death. In other centers, efforts to provide board members with training that would assist them in carrying on their functions faced resistance from some board members who were concerned that such training would change the existing power distribution. Where the health center serves a community that is ethnically mixed (usually black and Hispano-American), struggles for power and rewards are often ethnically-based.

For centers that use the team approach to providing health care, another power relationship is that between the members of the team. Physicians, even those who have accustomed themselves to working with teams, tend to see the team as physician-centered and physician-run. More generally, many of the professional members of the team are threatened by the suggestion that part of their job can be done successfully by someone who does not have their long professional training. Conflict here involves concern about the quality of care offered by the center as well as the more selfish concerns engendered by the self-esteem and ego needs of the professionals who wish to maintain their control and status.

Power struggles of this kind, which might elsewhere be considered labor-management disputes, take on a special character in the neighborhood health center. The paraprofessional, or nonprofessional, members of the health team are usually recruited from and identified with the neighboring community, whereas the professional staff is often identified with the sponsor. The dispute thus takes on the character of, and becomes involved with, the struggle for power between the center's sponsor and the community. Traditional distinctions between an agency's board, its staff, and its clients, and the administrative practices built on these distinctions, need reevaluation in an agency run by a community board and staffed by indigenous workers.[20]

From the perspective of this political scientist, then, neighborhood health centers are characterized by power relationships. These are of varying orders of generality, from power relationships within the center, to those between the center and the community, to the more general social problems of the power-lessness of minority ethnic groups and of the poor. Finally, we have the broad social problem of the power of the average man in modern society. Or, as one "society matron" put it, "What is this nonsense about maximum feasible parti-cipation? Nobody today has any real say in running their lives. We just do what we are told, and try to have fun, to make the best of it. The poor are no better off than the rest of us—where do they get off thinking they should have a say in managing their lives?"[21]

I have talked about politics as a contest for power. Another view of politics stresses "that the full realization of an individual's psychological and moral potential is contingent on participation in political decision-making processes. And the most significant of these decision-making processes for participation are those in which the decisional outcomes directly affect the individual's own life. Political participation contributes to the individual's development because it increases his sense of public and social responsibility, and exposes him to diverse situations and points of view. Exposure facilitates the citizen's under-standing of others in different life situations and thus increases his total range of understanding. Exposure to the decision-making processes themselves pro-vides knowledge about how decisions are made and gives a sense of responsibility for outcomes. Public and social responsibility results from the participant's taking part in the formulation of decisional outcomes and developing a sub-sequent stake in these policies."[22]

We need to have a clearer understanding of the circumstances under which this is likely to be true. Our experiences with neighborhood health centers hopefully will contribute to such an understanding. In the process, they may both provide power to the powerless, and help to make authority legitimate once more. And—who knows? Perhaps they will even provide models for meeting our medical care needs.

Footnotes
(References included)

1. Eulau, H.: Political Science. *In* A Reader's Guide to the Social Sciences, Bert F. Hoselitz, Ed. Glencoe, Ill. The Free Press, 1959; p. 91.
2. March, J. G.: The Power of Power. *In* Varieties of Political Theory, David Easton, Ed. Englewood Cliffs, N. J., Prentice-Hall, Inc., 1966.
3. Wolin, S., and Schaar, J.: Berkely: The Battle of Peoples Park, The New York Review of Books, June 19, 1969.
4. Falkson, J. L., and Grainer, M. A.: Urban Bureaucracy and the Politicization of the Urban Poor. Paper presented at the 1969 meeting of the American Political Science Association.
5. Elden, J. M.: Protest Politics and the New Public Administration. Paper presented at the 1969 meeting of the American Political Science Association.

6. It has been persuasively argued that this is part of a historical cycle which brings to the fore, at different times, one of three values strongly influencing governmental design: representativeness, politically neutral competence, and executive leadership. See Herbert Kaufman's Administrative Decentralization and Political Power, *Public Administration Review 29*:3-15, 1969.

7. Rubin, Lillian: Maximum Feasible Participation: The Origins, Implications, and Present Status. Poverty and Human Resources Abstracts *2*:5-18, 1967. See also Moynihan, notes 9 and 11.

8. Geiger, H. J.: Of the Poor, By the Poor, or For the Poor: The Mental Health Implications of Social Control of Poverty Programs. *In* Poverty and Mental Health, Milton Greenblatt *et al.*, Eds. Washington, American Psychiatric Association, 1967.

9. Moynihan, D. P.: Maximum Feasible Misunderstanding: Community Action in the War on Poverty. New York, Free Press, 1969. Moynihan's point of view has been challenged in reviews of his volume by Naomi Bliven (The New Yorker, June 7, 1969), Joseph Califano (The Washington Post, February 6, 1969), and Robert A. Levine (The Washington Post, January 19, 1969), as well as by Marvin Hoffman in "The Lord, He Works in Mysterious Ways . . . ," *New South 24*:3-37, 1969.

10. A Relevant War Against Poverty: A Study of Community Action Programs and Observable Social Change. New York, Metropolitan Applied Research Center, 1969.

11. Moynihan, D. P., Ed.: On Understanding Poverty: Perspectives from the Social Sciences. New York, Basic Books, 1969, and Sundquist, J. L., Ed.: On Fighting Poverty: Perspectives from Experience. New York, Basic Books, 1969. Discussion of the origins and effects of the community action program run throughout many of the essays in these two volumes.

12. Sundquist, J. L.: The End of the Experiment? *In* Sunquist, Ed., *op. cit.*

13. Breslin, J.: The Political Discovery of the Year. *New York 2*:30-39, 1969.

14. Aberbach, J. D., and Walker, J.L.: Political Trust and Racial Ideology. Paper delivered at the 1969 American Political Science Association meeting.

15. Scoble, H.M.: Interdisciplinary Perspectives on Poverty in America: The View from Political Science. Paper delivered at the Symposium on Interdisciplinary Perspectives on Poverty in America, University of Kentucky, 1967.

16. Levitan, S. A.: The Design of Federal Anti-Poverty Strategy. Ann Arbor, University of Michigan—Wayne State University Institute of Labor and Industrial Relations, 1967. See also Sundquist, ed., *supra*.

17. Davis, M. S., and Tranquada, R. E.: A Sociological Evaluation of the Watts Neighborhood Health Center. *Medical Care 7*:105-117, 1969.

18. Davis and Tranquada, *op. cit.;* Geiger, *op. cit.;* Geiger, H. J.: The Neighborhood Health Center: Education of the Faculty in Preventive Medicine. *Arch. Environ. Health 14*:912-916, 1967; Geiger, H. J.: Community Control—or Community Conflict? *Bull. Nat. Tuber. Resp. Dis. Ass. 10*:4-10, 1969; Goldberg, G. A., Trowbridge, F. L., and Buxbaum, R. C.: Issues in the Development of Neighborhood Health Centers. *Inquiry 6*:37-46, 1969; and

Gordon, J. B.: The Politics of Community Medicine Projects: A Conflict Analysis. *Medical Care* 7:419-428, 1969.
19. Goldberg et al., *op. cit.,* discuss various solutions to this problem.
20. Acosta, R., and Gartner, A.: Lincoln Hospital Mental Health Services: The Politics of Mental Health. New York University New Careers Development Center, 1969.
21. Quoted in Shostak, A. B.: Politics, Poverty, and Problems. Paper delivered at the Eastern Sociological Society 1966 meeting.
22. Hofstetter, C. R.: The Promise of Participation for Learning, Comprehension, and the Acquisition of Democratic Values. Paper presented at the 1969 meeting of the American Political Science Association.

8 Neighborhood Health Centers

Health/PAC Bulletin

The second wave of neighborhood health centers started in the 1960's, took place at a time when hospital outpatient departments (OPDs) were becoming for inner city residents the major source of health care. OPDs were under-financed and organized primarily for the purposes of medical teaching and research, not patient care. OEO reformers decided the new centers were to be placed in poor, mostly Black communities. They hoped to provide neighbor-hood services while promoting structural changes in the health institutions serving the poor. But no serious commitment to do either existed in the major leadership of Congress or the Executive Department. And ironically, most of these health centers in the neighborhoods were actually dependent for sponsor-ship and funding on the very institutions which were to be reformed.

In the upsurge of the health care reform movement, students and profes-sionals in medicine, nursing, dentistry, social work, health care administration and the like, looked to the neighborhood health centers to solve their own dilemmas of personal and professional relevance. Some left the universities and teaching hospitals to work in the ghettoes because they felt alienated from the competitive and hierarchy-bound atmosphere of those institutions. Others left that environment because they thought a decentralized health system based in communities could deliver better care. Many really believed the health care millenium was about to arrive.

What has happened as a result of the neighborhood health center movement? Some 200 centers have come into varying degrees of existence. Most are in urban or rural slums. The early promise that they would spearhead a massive federal commitment for health care reform has turned sour, a victim both of the Viet-nam War and the shuck of the War on Poverty. The neighborhood health centers are but a grain of sand in the sea of effort needed to provide decent health care for poor communities.

Models for Change

There are two ways to assess the health centers' impact. We can look at them as a technical model of health care and consider what they have taught us about the delivery of quality care; how health care team relationships are worked out;

Reprinted from *Health/PAC Bulletin* 42 (June 1972):1-2.

the relation of the center to a backup hospital on the one hand, and to the community served on the other. Questions can be raised about their efficacy as a focus for family health care and community health services, as well as their "cost benefit ratio" when the average visit costs over $30. Neighborhood health centers offer many important lessons. But this should not overshadow the fact that true decentralization of health services was never given a real try.

These technical questions are not our concern at the moment. Rather, our concern is with the health centers as a political model for reform of services in the modern ghettoes. Many in the 1960's thought the centers could become the locus for general community change. Most of those who thought so were white reformers who did not live in the communities concerned. Black and Third World professionals, usually in private practice in these same communities, were almost totally bypassed in the planners' considerations. And by and large, the communities themselves were not consulted.

Too Little Too Late

The general consensus today is that the health centers have not catalyzed community change. They have been too little and too late. As jobs disappear and dope increases in most urban poor communities, the possibility of a health center becoming a major focus for change becomes as grim a joke as phrases like "urban renewal" and "war on poverty."

Another question we can ask is whether the health centers have led to significant reform of the university medical schools and big teaching and voluntary hospitals associated with them. Here again the record is largely negative, but then little effort was ever mounted toward this goal. These institutions have shown themselves far more intractable and resistant than reformers believed six or eight years ago.

Perhaps neighborhood health centers were never designed as models of technical or political change. By dangling federal money on federal strings in front of poor communities, with glib rhetoric of maximum feasible participation of the poor and of community control, a scramble was encouraged which set neighbor against neighbor and community against community. Soon the internal war within communities to secure antipoverty money far eclipsed in zeal the energy of the poverty warriors in Washington. Communities found themselves fragmented and exhausted in the fight over the crumbs. When people were fighting among themselves, they could not see the real enemy.

Today the neighborhood health center is no longer the fashionable rallying cry it once was. The new term is "HMO" or Health Maintenance Organization. Washington is making every effort to sell the notion of HMO's to neighborhood health care centers. It seems likely that the HMO would take away much of the present and potential power of the community. Stripped of its Nixonian public relations cover, the HMO is a vehicle for corporate managers to move into control of health care.

Part V
Consumer Participation and
Community Control

Introduction

OEO and HEW have both required consumer participation in the development and management of the neighborhood health centers which they sponsor. This requirement (and local residents' demands for involvement) have created a great deal of conflict and attracted plenty of public attention. Papers on consumer participation comprise a disproportionately large fraction of the written materials about the centers.

Consumer involvement in the neighborhood health centers has played out many of the same dramas of citizen participation in the larger antipoverty arena. The federal designers of the health centers program admit that the centers acquired more resources because health was a less politically volatile area for federal intervention than was community action, which had stimulated vigorous opposition from local elected officials. As one early OEO administrator put it, "People felt that even the 'undeserving poor' deserved health care."

The articles which follow give a good sense of the wide range of goals maintained in different quarters for consumer participation in the centers. These goals include ways in which participation will contribute directly to improving health services delivered at a center, redistributing political power, reducing alienation, increasing participants' self-respect, encouraging acceptance and use of the center, securing political support useful in conflicts with other agencies and institutions. Jack Elinson and Conrad Herr, in "A Sociomedical View of Neighborhood Health Centers," outline several latent functions of the centers which relate especially to consumer participation in them: (1) Improving the image of the black male in poverty communities; (2) Stimulating and maintaining solidarity; (3) Pacification of hostile communities by colonial powers; (4) Discharging missionary service obligations of the medical-hospital establishment, (5) Filling a political void in social and economic action, and (6) Politicization or radicalization of residents.

It is particularly hard to gauge accurately the extent of accomplishment of the health centers as a group with regard to the broad range of goals expressed for consumer involvement in their planning and operation. Evidence on these points is hard to come by and there is sharp disagreement about what constitutes impressive evidence. Anecdotal evidence is useful and has accumulated in significant amounts. Attempts to develop more systematic quantitative data about the results of participation have been unconvincing. The inherent difficulties of finding and interpreting information about the functioning of consumer participation make it no less important, however. It is our view that public monies invested in the health centers have bought substantial returns, albeit limited ones, with regard to these goals. The gains have been extremely difficult to achieve. They do not add up to a set of readily quantifiable results. They certainly are not a list of achievements which arouse unanimous acceptance or endorsement. We would include as indications of solid accomplishment: (1) the fact of some hundreds of consumer representatives acquiring political skills in the health area, and (2) considerable evidence that participation has provided a route to jobs and career advancement for significant numbers of persons who would otherwise have been denied them.

The accomplishments of consumer participation are an excellent example of the tangible, limited achievements of the health centers which tend to be ignored, downplayed or dismissed today when the objectives attached to participation have less political salience and support.

As a group, the articles that follow offer a series of perspectives on the evolution of consumer participation efforts in different local settings. What emerges is a picture of the simple, but important, general point that the experience of individual centers with consumer involvement has been and will continue to be a dynamic process in which the goals, interests, postures, and behaviors of the different parties involved change over time. The articles offer different conceptions of what this process has been and why.

There have been substantial problems with the model of *representation* in consumer participation. The approach of electing representatives supposed that those persons selected would communicate from and back to constituencies. In practice, they have represented interests, but in very few instances have functioned as representatives in the sense meant by that term in electoral politics. The skepticisms of "Whom do you represent? Are you really representative?" have been used by opponents of consumer representatives as red-herrings. On the other hand, it is important to strip away the romanticism about participation and community. In many centers the vast majority of adult patients served by the health centers do not know or care about the consumer council or board (see Chapter 19).

The conflicts surrounding consumer participation and control have rarely been simply between consumer and provider. The significance of there being several parties with different interests in these disputes is demonstrated in the articles. The role of federal officials is a particularly perplexing one; OEO was "at times an advocate, at other times an inquisitor."

The expectations placed on consumer representative bodies have often been unrealistically high. They have been expected to perform a wide range of difficult tasks and to provide wise counsel with very little training, support or regular information from administrators. The low ratio of eligible participants in the elections to those who voted has been used to discredit their representativeness. Critics pointed to the low level of voter participation in their elections, although it is absurd to expect higher voter participation in a service area to which residents assign a relatively low priority, where there is no tradition of electoral participation, and where the powers of those being elected are usually limited.

Discussions of consumer participation—and this is true of the articles included here—tend to focus on formal structures for, and activities of, participation by consumer representatives. It is essential to note that in many centers consumer participation has occurred at least as significantly, sometimes more so, through the employment of area residents at the centers. The tasks of area residents employed in a variety of paraprofessional and other roles and their influence in these jobs address many of the same goals for participation which are linked most commonly with consumer representation. It is not surprising that many persons have served in both capacities—as representatives and as employees. Centers vary considerably in the extent to which they have stressed participation through mechanisms of representation or through employment. The Martin Luther King, Jr. Health Center in the Bronx is a good example of a center which has eschewed the consumer representatives route, but has pursued vigorously an approach of hiring and training local residents to the point where that center is staffed almost entirely by local persons.

Much of the discussion about consumer participation has been largely polemical—claims and counterclaims about the reputed benefits of, or deficits attributed to, participation. There is a real need for more documentation of the actual accomplishments and problems of consumer involvement in the health centers. What things were different in a center's development and operation as a result of consumer participation or control?

Jeoffry Gordon, in "The Politics of Community Medicine: A Conflict Analysis," argues that medical professionals have tended to deny the political dimensions of health care in the development of the neighborhood health center. He urges medical professionals to stop avoiding conflict, and to see the positive, functional aspects of it. His article offers an unusual perspective for analyzing consumer-provider conflicts as well as a prescription for future behavior.

The case study of the NENA Health Center by Des Callan and Oliver Fein (Chapter 12) presents a vivid picture of the intense and continuing struggles of that center to come into being and to sustain itself. They express a strong argument that the problems of community control are caused by lack of control over basic resources. The NENA case is a significant one, in part because that center was initiated by a committee of residents, not by professionals. It illustrates the importance of a consumer council having its own professional organizer and advisor. The case describes some of the hard obstacles to health center workers who are residents of the area served becoming an organized force within the center with influence over its policies and operations.[1]

H. Jack Geiger's "Community Control—or Community Conflict?" compares consumer involvement in an urban and a rural health center. Geiger concludes with a taking-back of his title, asserting that is is essential and inevitable that there be community control *and* community conflict.[2]

References

1. Other articles which trace the evolution of consumer participation in indi-
    vidual centers include: Milton S. Davis and Robert E. Tranquada, "A
    Sociological Evaluation of the Watts Neighborhood Health Center, *"Medical
    Care* 7, 2 (March–April 1969); 105–117; Kay B. Partridge and Paul E. White,
    "Community and Professional Participation in Decision Making at a Health
    Center," *HSMHA Health Reports* 87, 4 (April 1972); 336–342; Peter
    Kong-Ming New, Richard M. Hessler and Phyllis Bagwell Cater, "Consumer
    Control and Public Accountability," *Anthropological Quarterly* 46, 3 (July
    1973): 196–213.
2. Readers may find it instructive to compare Geiger's account of consumer
    involvement at Columbia Point with Ann Stokes, David Banta, and Samuel
    Putnam, "The Columbia Point Health Association: Evolution of a Com-
    munity Health Board," *American Journal of Public Health* 62, 9 (Sept.
    1972): 1229–1234. Stokes et al. offer the view from the consumers' side of
    the fence.

The Politics of Community Medicine Projects: A Conflict Analysis

Jeoffry B. Gordon

The physicians are the natural attorneys of the poor and social problems fall to a large extent within their jurisdiction. — Virchow, 1848

One of the dramatic activities of the Office of Economic Opportunity (OEO) has been their Healthright program. Created to provide "equal access to health services for the poor . . . so that they do not have to barter their dignity for their health,"[1] these activities met with enthusiastic support from liberal physicians, health workers, and the patient community. As of the end of 1968, OEO had spent $114.5 million to finance 52 neighborhood health centers, of which 42 were already providing services to about 300,000 persons and ten were in the process of being organized.[2] Their scale varied from referral and outreach programs, integrating patients into pre-existing medical activities, to substantial facilities staffed to provide comprehensive health care. Moreover, fundamental to this program was OEO's attempt to insure "maximum feasible participation of residents of the areas and members of the groups served . . .,"[3] i.e., the consumers of health care—in this case, mostly impoverished.

The neighborhood health center was a new institution, created to provide help to people in the context of their environment, primarily insofar as these people are ill, and especially if their environment is disadvantageous. Since the community health center was a strategy for restructuring the medical care system within the broader purpose of reintegrating an alienated population into the political and social fabric of society, the task of establishing and legitimizing this institution has been especially difficult. As innovation evoked resistance (which it always does), the process became politicized. ("Politics" here has the broad connotation of the distribution of power and responsibility among the members of a society, as well as the process of how that distribution is made.) However, those members of the medical professions, among others, involved in this process have tended to deny the political dimensions of health care. It is the thesis of this paper that this has limited their ability to deal with the situation and has hindered the development of the program. Time and again, when opposition arose, conflict was denied, avoided, or squelched as professionals tried to innovate within their usual style of intellectual analysis and imposed technologi-

Reprinted from *Medical Care* 7, 6 (November-December 1969): 419-428.

cal solution. This has been especially handicapping in dealing with consumer involvement. As will be seen, an understanding of political behavior would be of great benefit. In fact, the constructive use of conflict and social dissonance can facilitate the process of social change, if only it is understood, anticipated, and used rather than denied. Furthermore, no comparative analysis of the administrative and political problems involved in establishing a large-scale community health services program *de novo* or integrated within pre-existing services in a deprived neighborhood has been attempted previously. I present here an analysis based upon the meager literature,[4] personal conversations with community medicine organizers,[5] and an informal personal acquaintance with ten health centers[6] established or in creation under federal funding.

The Participants

It is important to review the actors in this drama. As Davis and Tranquada[7] point out, the foci of power "are all separately characterized by conflict." OEO was the funding catalyst. This organization, a compromise coalition of the interests of the Department of Labor, the Department of Health, Education and Welfare, the Council of Economic Advisors, the Bureau of the Budget, and Congress, was created to deal innovatively with problems established governmental agencies had not yet faced, naturally creating jurisdictional jealousy among those Departments. The OEO effort was focused on the "War on Poverty." Although some of its strategies were adopted by other federal agencies: HUD in the Model Cities Program, and PHS in the Partnership for Health Legislation, the new ideas were not really fully accepted in all quarters. Thus, the new Federal agency's capacity for concerted action was diminished.

Consumer participation, the primary technique of the OEO strategy, may or may not be a valid and effective means of political reform.[8,9] On the other hand, this was an ideological commitment recognizing that poverty is the lack of power, influence, and self-respect as well as of funds, and rejecting the once-commonly-held moralistic judgment that poverty is due to personal incompetence and sin.[10] On the other hand, this was a political tactic to insure that these innovative programs would not be wholly controlled by entrenched and unaccountable politicians.[11]

The OEO had many important goals in supporting the Healthright program, including providing health services to the poor, whose medical morbidity is disproportionately high, establishing the comprehensive health center as a model for the medical practice of the future (public or private), and using health concerns as a tactical approach toward interrupting the cycle of poverty. The OEO, as a federal agency, had a responsibility to preserve harmony, but many of the program goals and activities continued to be viewed with suspicion both within and outside the government. Congress had been skeptical about the need for OEO as an administrative strategy for change. The health centers, both as a model for medical practice and in their very provision of services, were liable to antagonize organized medicine as represented by the attitudes of the American Medical Association and many local medical societies.[12] Nonetheless, the OEO worked hard to produce demonstrable results and to avoid controversy, while faced with problems that demanded ingenious innovation and experimentation. The OEO imparted many of its anxieties to its projects. Demonstrations were supervised from Washington with careful guidelines; they were pressured to show rapid improvements in a relatively short time; and they were made very aware of the dangers of controversy locally and of the uncertainty of future funding. Pressures from other quarters sometimes produced guidelines which directly frustrated the program's purpose. Thus, the OEO has not always appeared as a wholly benevolent participant, being at times an advocate, at other times an inquisitor. Now that there is a new presidential administration, OEO faces new uncertainties. Both to resolve jurisdictional disputes and to institutionalize successful projects, some programs will be allocated to the appropriate federal departments. The impact of the possible transfer of the Healthright program to the Public Health Service remains to be seen.

The sponsoring body, insofar as it included medical professionals, was, as well, in turmoil over its involvement. Although some projects, such as those sponsored by OEO community action agencies (8 per cent), new health corporations (17 per cent) and other nonprofit agencies were administered by community organizations, most projects, sponsored by hospitals (23 per cent), medical schools (19 per cent), health departments (13 per cent), group practices (6 per cent), and medical societies (2 per cent), were administered by medical institutions.[13] In addition, as we shall see, many of the community agencies organized around health were fronts for medical institutions. The American medical establishment is a superb example of scientific technological virtuosity, but this may not be the appropriate mode of approach to a slum environment and its problems. The primary emphasis of community medicine is on service, prevention, and rehabilitation, and the total ecology of disease, and not upon research and education, acute disease, and the individual patient. The "ivory tower" attitude of academia combined with the professionalism of the physician produces a tactical style which conflicts with the needs of the ghetto and may adversely confront those members of the medical profession concerned with an emphasis on community service.

Considering the broader definition of health as "complete physical, mental, and social well-being, not merely the absence of disease or infirmity,"[14] health involves the whole context upon which a person's life, productivity, and satisfaction are based. It is simple to appreciate this, but this global recognition does not have immediate motivational effects. For the presence of diagnostic instruments and curative therapies does not insure their use; the desire for comprehensive, and especially preventive and family-centered, medicine, does not insure its development. Health is of relatively little concern to most people while they are well.[15] Even more so, in deprived areas the peri-medical concerns, food, clothing, housing, and employment, have higher priorities than health maintenance (narrowly defined).[16] Meanwhile, science has overcome many of the problems of treatment of acute medical crises and some health professions are beginning to face up to the broader mandate. Both because of a renewal of concern with preventive medicine and environmental problems and because of an increasing responsibility to maintain chronically-ill people at minimal levels of disability, the physician has become more interested in obtaining the active cooperation of the patient. Many of the outstanding problems in medical practice today (*e.g.,* limiting alcohol, nicotine, and drug abuse; nutrition; family planning) revolve around effectively motivating the patient and the prospective patient to be concerned with his health. This is especially true in a deprived environment. The community health center with its technique of consumer participation may be a way to create this cooperation effectively. Consumer participation is the *sine qua non* of the successful approach to the broad problems of disease. Many health professionals, including some of those presently involved in neighborhood health centers, do not accept this approach. Further dissension is created by other characteristics of some neighborhood health centers, *e.g.,* prepayment, salaried physicians, and expanded roles for medical assistants. Many physicians reject these innovations, opposing the health center concept altogether. Thus, there is a great deal of conflict within the medical community.

Finally, the clientele itself, impoverished but proud, frustrated and angry, is no longer a quiet submerged subculture. Propaganda, actual economic improvements, and the phenomena of relative deprivation and rising expectations have created, for some at least, a new identity. The most vocal, the militants, are now very dissatisfied with the *status quo* and are as impatient with their peers as they are with the establishment. The poor, especially in urban areas, are likely to be Negro or Spanish-speaking as well, and the added dimension of racial and ethnic concerns is ubiquitous. Frustration, confrontation, and overt conflict are more and more becoming the modes of problem-centered action by those interested enough to get involved. In the past, service projects were not cooperative ventures; they were imposed—albeit in a charitable way—from the one side, and the clients were at least expected to be happy with what they got. Today that is impossible. The new identity and increased self-esteem of the "other America" has rejected the supplicant's role and demands more than charity.

The Process

What then happens when a health service facility is created? Dr. H. Jack Geiger, one of the original OEO consultants on health and general director of two community health centers,[17] divides the process up into four phases which transpire over several years. Only the satisfactory resolution of all of these stages will permit valid community participation and, therefore, allow success of the project. It is evident that the process is one of confrontation, conflict, compromise and accommodation, of disequilibriums striving to be resolved. It is an illusion to think that the medical and social goals of community health projects can or should be achieved without controversies.

Instant Community

The sponsoring agency, suppressing its internal conflicts between research and service, has decided to make its work relevant and to minister to the needy community. The motivation is not without its romantic aspects. In the professional intellectual tradition, needs are specified and a rational plan of attack is devised which is submitted to the OEO. Community participation is one of the requirements of funding. The community itself rarely initiates the project.[18] Thus, during the planning stages, or worse, shortly thereafter, the sponsor goes looking for community representatives. There is a readily available group of indigenous, important people (*e.g.*, ministers, teachers, active parents or tenants) who have internalized the community and who stand up and say, "Here I am," when the physicians start to search for "the community." Although it is not readily apparent, these pepole generally, in fact, have only a small constituency, but their feeling of self-importance obliges them to assume the leadership role.[19] Their real qualification is that they have some sophistication in the institutions of the wider policy and have identified with it, even though previously they had not been accepted by it. These attitudes at the same time facilitate their acceptance by the professional reformers. Happy with the status their association with the sponsor provides, perhaps conversant in administrative style, but ignorant of the specifics of medical care, and impressed by the wealth and power of the sponsor, these people become the passive Community Board and a symbiosis develops. The sponsor proceeds as planned.

Insight

Invariably the innovating medical center must, in the process of concretizing its plans, examine its motivation. Real community concern, represented by an unselfish dedication to patient service as determined by their own perception of need, is rare. Often the health project is the manifestation of a new focus of academic research and education promoted by the availability of federal funds and articulated by liberal professionals developing their own identity. This insight is made explicit only by the participation of the community. The Community Board by now has discovered it is a rubber stamp and has little power over finances, personnel, or general policy. Their ego is no longer inflated by the mere illusion of power and they begin actively to challenge the establishment for what they thought was their due. Both the Board and the professionals are soon confronted by other angry community voices, from the Mission Rebels (San Francisco) to Mothers for Adequate Welfare (Boston). Each vocally and critically represents aspects of the neighborhood, at least wanting a piece of the action and at most articulating the new self-esteem of the "other America." Except under unusual circumstances (*e.g.*, Newark),[20] the vast majority of the community remains unconcerned and alienated from this whole process. Nonetheless, the confrontation between the sponsor and the self-chosen community representatives over power initiates the real process of community organization for health.

Disintegration and Cooperation

During this period of strife, angers flare and threats are made. The responsible community representatives demanding real responsibilities and power and the young militants demanding recognition threaten to sabotage the project through boycott or even violence. The liberal professional sponsors, encouraged by the OEO, on their own behalf, or representing the community's desires, carry the challenge to their fiscal agent. The committee of the medical school or the board of the hospital or university, neither wholly convinced of the virtues of the experiment nor in this respect altruistically motivated, and never before asked to share their governing control in this fashion, are understandably reluctant to cooperate. The relatively insignificant project suddenly appears to become a threat to their own autonomy. Meanwhile everyone's attention is diverted from patient care. After a longer or shorter period of arbitration, if the project survives, a new order can evolve. The sponsor and the community work together, not out of love for each other, but with an orientation toward the task at hand. This then becomes a very constructive period of mutual education. The medical professionals are introduced to the needs and desires of the community and the lay community is tutored in the problems and techniques of both health maintenance and administrative organization. Slowly mutual respect develops and, hopefully, broadened support evolves on both sides.

Constituency and Service

While the preceding evolution has been taking place, hopefully, actual creation of some medical service facility has also occurred. This may now begin to function in a favorable environment to solve the problems at hand. Further problems will continue to arise, but the project and its participants have reached maturity and are capable of dealing with them without threatening the project's existence. The purpose of the OEO demonstration has been fulfilled and the medical professionals and their constituency can now concentrate on the quality of service and contemplate mechanisms capable of rendering the project financially sound and independent. The real task of creating a facility which promotes and provides compassionate, comprehensive, family-centered care can now be explored. It should be noted that no project has yet evolved into the last stage.

Sources of Conflict

March and Simon[21] have observed three important conditions which explain interorganizational conflict: 1) the existence of a felt need for joint decision-making, 2) a difference in goals, and/or 3) a difference in perception of reality among the parties. The first condition posits that the parties to the conflict are in the same action system. The problem is relevant and cannot be abandoned. In addition, in this case, both the community and the OEO demand a joint-decision process where none existed before; the medical profession must acquiesce. The second and third differences are inherent in serious intercourse between professionals and lay people, especially the so-called "culturally deprived" subculture. As Wilson explains,

> low income . . . people are more likely to have limited time perspective, a greater difficulty in abstracting from concrete experience, an unfamiliarity with and lack of confidence in city-wide institutions, a preoccupation with the personal and immediate. . . . Lacking experience in and the skills for participation in organized endeavors, they are likely to have a low sense of personal efficacy in organizational situations. By necessity as well as by inclination, such people are likely to have what one might call a "private-regarding" political ethos. They are intimately bound up in the day-to-day struggle to sustain themselves and their families.[22]

The professional, especially the physician, on the other hand, is not only "public-regarding," *i.e.*, benevolent and civic-minded, but is used to having his opinion respected and instituted with minimal opposition, since he often considers his self-interest synonymous with the community good. His very cognitive style,[23] intellectual, abstract, deductive, introspective, task-oriented, comprehending wide horizons and long time spans, and operating in a well-structured administrative environment, is in marked contrast to the style of the low-income culture. Racial prejudices only add to this polarization. Thus, conflict is inevitable; goals and realities naturally are perceived differently.

Let us now look at what happens once the process is initiated. Although the health center remains a service project and the people involved in sponsoring and staffing it are concerned primarily with health services, the project has become a political issue, and the sides are joined. Among the six modes of influence—inducement, coercion, rational persuasion, selling, friendship, and authority—relevant to the political process of arbitration,[24] the professionals are likely to rely on two: rational persuasion and authority, while the community tends to rely on coercion.[25] Thus, the sponsor's tactics appear irrelevant to the community and the community's tactic appears outrightly dangerous to the establishment. Thus, conflict is not only a result of a system in disequilibrium, it is introduced purposefully as a variable in that system by one of the parties.

Inferences

If this analysis is correct, it provides a constructive insight; for the first step toward improvement is correct perception of the situation. The service professionals' commitment to "constructive social harmony" has, in the past, allowed him to ignore, deny, or suppress the actual meanings of many types of events which produce disequilibrium and disharmony. Such is the case here. However, viewed as a political process, these circumstances are not so unusual or threatening. They consist of the normal progression of disequilibrium, arbitration, and compromise basic to the political mechanism. As one observer put it:

> Democratic government is the greatest single instrument for the socialization of conflict in the American community. . . . conflicts open up questions for public intervention. Out of conflict the alternatives of public policy arise. Conflict is the occasion for political organization and leadership. . . . Democracy is a competitive political system in which competing leaders and organizations define the alternatives of public policy in such a way that the public can participate in the decision making process.[26]

This controversy has analogies in past community controversies over education, labor relations, urban renewal, taxation, and so forth. Elected officials and lobbyists thrive in this atmosphere of conflicting interests and competition. Accepting the process for what it is, they use it to advantage. Health professionals and others tend to dismiss participation in controversy as "professionally improper," and they have tried to ignore the political dimensions of health care. This attitude should be changed. Once the true nature and importance of the political process is recognized, sophisticated participation will be advantageous.

It is necessary that the organizers of innovative community service projects should be sophisticated not only in their profession, but also in the techniques of political science and sociology insofar as they deal with these situations.

Especially significant and relevant are Louis Coser's *The Functions of Social Conflict*[27] and James Coleman's *Community Conflict*.[28] Although written with different emphases, these treatises succinctly present analyses which encourage a new constructive attitude toward the problem of conflict. Using these references as sources, let us examine a few of the consequences of the process of controversy in order to illustrate how a knowledgeable approach can be beneficial.

While provision of medical care is the most important goal of the Healthright program, it must be remembered that health is generally a low-priority concern in deprived neighborhoods. In addition, lower-class areas have very little intrinsic organization for civic purposes. One of the primary problems of the Healthright program is the development of concern for health and a constituent community to express that concern. Conflict creates communities and makes concerns vivid. As Coser puts it:

> Conflict with another group leads to the mobilization of energies of group members and hence to increased cohesion of the group. . . . Conflict acts as a stimulus for establishing new rules, norms, and institutions, thus serving as an agent of socialization (for both contending parties).[29]

Thus, realizing that their innovative attempts are bound to create a certain amount of disequilibrium, the organizers of the service can use themselves as a "straw horse," so to speak, focusing the conflict constructively, first upon themselves to create the community of concern, then transforming the emphasis on opposition into a concern for the problem itself—in this case health—by a sincere and serious appeal (and proof thereof) to common interests.

> Conflicts may serve to remove dissociating elements in a relationship and to reestablish unity. Insofar as conflict is the resolution of tension between antagonists, it has stabilizing functions and becomes an integrating component of the relationship.[30]

Thus, Coser, while exploring the ramifications of antagonism and confrontation and delving into the distruptive aspects of conflict, emphasizes what positive functions it can fulfill. These should be sought after and made to predominate.

Coleman's exploration of community is an excellent guide to the pitfalls of the normative political process of dissent over social and civic goals. For instance, in order to make constructive use of the conflict situation one must be aware that certain tendencies are likely to be manifest, *e.g.:*

> A dispute which began dispassionately in a disagreement over issues, is characterized suddenly by personal slander, by rumor, by the focusing of direct hostility.[31]

In other words, one's vanity should not be disturbed by personal attacks in the midst of a controversy. One should be even more guarded against this in conflicts with a lower-class community where less distinction is likely to be made between the character of a man and his activities than other groups may make.

One must be aware of new demagogic and irresponsible leaders in opposition.

> New leaders tend to take over the dispute; often they are men who have not been community leaders in the past, men who face none of the constraints of maintaining a previous community position. . . . The new leaders . . . are seldom moderate; the situation itself calls for extremists.[32]

The militant Black Nationalists are a present example of this phenomenon. A practical implication of expecting their rise to power would, for example, have been to promote more moderate, but nontheless sincere, opponents to one's own programs.

Coleman observes that the structure of authority may affect the course of conflict. The device of a community advisory or policy board is an approach to this realization. Nonetheless, anticipation would insure that these channels of power and communication were real in order to better structure the conflict and its results. Mention must also be made of the technique of cooptation (bringing the opposition inside to voice its criticism with or without real influence on the course of events) in order to warn against its premature use. True community support does not grow from cooptation of its leaders; it is preferable to maintain the confrontation until accord is reached through mutual concern.

Finally, Coleman mentions the importance of the mass media of communication, although with a slightly different emphasis. Nonetheless, it becomes important to remember the value of propaganda and the right publicity in shaping the course of events to advantage, remembering that the ghetto dweller has different exposure habits, including a very active word-of-mouth grapevine for important events.

The aforementioned considerations are just a few examples of how political sophistication can be brought to bear on a problem to good advantage. These approaches are not panaceas, nor formulas for success; rather, they illustrate the kinds of concerns which have been ignored in the past, thus mitigating against the success of socially-innovative community service projects.

Conclusion

Although there has been considerable local and national publicity about the OEO Healthright program, it has tended to overlook the considerable difficulties being encountered in the creation of these innovative services. Until now, no comprehensive perspective of the problems has been undertaken by any of the parties involved. The unofficial impression is that many obstacles have prevented the fulfillment of many of the program goals. Although some people have been provided with medical care that is of better quality or would not have been available otherwise, in many health centers services are underutilized; community participation is not powerful; the support of the medical establishment is tenuous; social innovation is minimal or inefficacious. One aspect of this failure has been the inability of the programs to face up to the political problems involved. This paper has been an attempt to define the nature of those problems and to illustrate how their comprehension may be used to advantage. Obviously, some of the suggestions posed demand very skillful and nimble political maneuvering and some risks of failure. However, in view of the many barriers to social change, the situation demands these skills and risks if any lasting improvements are to come from these innovative projects.

Footnotes
(references included)

1. Yerby, A.: Health departments, hospitals, and health services. *Medical Care* 5:70, 1967.
2. OEO: Report On The OEO Comprehensive Health Services Program. Washington, D.C., U.S. Government Printing Office, March, 1969.
3. Economic Opportunity Act of 1964, PL88–452, title II, Part A, sec. 202(a) (3).
4. *E.g.*, Davis, M., and Tranquada, R.: A sociological evaluation of the Watts neighborhood health center, *Medical Care, 7*:105, 1969; also, although not directly related to a health center, see Rothstein, P.: The closing of St. Francis Hospital: A case study in the politics of health planning (mimeo). New York, Health Policy Advisory Center of the Institute for Policy Studies, 1968.
5. Dr. Paul O'Rourke, Director, East Palo Alto Health Center (August, 1968: April, 1969); Dr. Rodney Powell (November, 1968).
6. Columbia Point and Roxbury in Boston, St. Luke's Riverside in New York City, Mission District and Hunter's Point in San Francisco and East Palo Alto, West Oakland, King City, and Watts in California, and Mound Bayou in Mississippi.
7. Davis and Tranquada, *op. cit.*
8. *Cf.* Spiegel, H. (ed.): Citizen Participation in Urban Development. Vol. I. Washington, NTL Institute for Applied Behavioral Science, National Education Association, 1968.
9. Also see Moynihan, D.: Maximum Feasible Misunderstanding. New York, Free Press, 1968.
10. This impression was reinforced by Max Weber's classic analysis, The Pro-

testant Ethic and The Spirit Of Capitalism, (New York, Charles Scribner's Sons, 1930): "[Protestant] asceticism looked upon the pursuit of wealth as an end in itself as highly reprehensible; but the attainment of it as a fruit of labour in a calling was a sign of God's blessing. . . . The religious valuation of restless, continuous, systematic work in a worldly calling . . . [was] the surest and most evident proof of rebirth and genuine faith." Conversely, poverty was the stigma of personal incompetence and sin.

11. Cf. Moynihan, op. cit.
12. The recent acceptance of the neighborhood health center concept by the AMA and the sponsorship of several projects by local Medical Societies is a definite change in attitude and thus is one indication that this process has had some success.
13. OEO, op. cit.
14. Preamble to Constitution of World Health Organization, July 22, 1946.
15. Conant, R.: The Politics of Community Health. Washington, D.C. Public Affairs Press, 1968.
16. Haughton, J.: Can the poor use the present health care system? Inquiry, 5:31, March 1968.
17. Professor of Community Medicine and Public Health, Tufts University School of Medicine; Director, Tufts Delta Health Center and Columbia Point Center.
18. For an important exception see the experience of the West Oakland Health Council, a spontaneous indigenous organization.
19. Wilson, J.: Planning and politics: Citizen participation in urban renewal. J. American Institute of Planners 29:(November), 1963.
20. Cf. Duhl, L. and Steele, N.J.: Newark: Community or chaos, a case study of the medical school controversy. Mimeo, 1968. It is commonly said that the planning of a medical center which totally ignored community concerns in Newark was an important cause of the riot there in 1967.
21. March, J. and Simon, H.: Conflict in organizations, Chapter 5 in their book, Organization. New York, J. Wiley & Sons, Inc., 1958. Quoted by Davis and Tranquada, op. cit.
22. Wilson, op. cit.
23. Wilson, op. cit.
24. Binstock, R.: Effective planning through political influence. A.J.P.H. 59:808, 1969.
25. Wilson, op. cit.
26. Schattschneider, E.E.: The Semisovereign People. New York, Holt, Rinehart & Winston, 1960.
27. Coser, L.: The Functions of Social Conflict. New York, Free Press, 1956.
28. Coleman, J.: Community Conflict. New York, The Free Press, 1957.
29. Coser, op. cit., pp. 95, 128.
30. Coser, op. cit., p. 80.
31. Coleman, op. cit., p. 10.
32. Coleman, op. cit., p. 12.

10

A Sociomedical View of Neighborhood Health Centers

Jack Elinson and Conrad E.A. Herr

We shall not review in any detail the *manifest* purposes of neighborhood health centers. These have been set forth in the specific amendment to the legislative act authorizing the Office of Economic Opportunity. They have, moreover, been explicated in numerous talks and articles by employees of that agency, notably Lisbeth Bamberger and Gerald Sparer; by the co-directors of the first Neighborhood Health Center, under the OEO act, at Columbia Point, Count Gibson and Jack Geiger; and by others such as Joyce Lashof in Chicago. For example, Gerald Sparer has recently noted that objectives attributed to neighborhood health centers "range from eliminating poverty, improving health status, changing the medical care delivery system to providing jobs and access to services for low income persons."[19] Lisbeth Bamberger has pointed out that the objectives of neighborhood health centers are to be accomplished by providing "a one-door facility, in which virtually all ambulatory health services are available; close coordination with other community resources; professional staff of high quality; and intensive participation by and involvement of the population to be served."[3]

These general objectives and essential elements of the *current wave* of neighborhood health centers are now quite well known to all who have taken the trouble to look at them, and, in any case, are sufficiently global to encompass narrower sets of objectives that might be conceived of for *any* ambulatory care health facility. We refer to the *current wave* of neighborhood health centers because, despite an enthusiastic tendency to regard them as "a new institutional form,"[3] the neighborhood health center movement began in this country in the early 1900's. (See Stoeckle and Candib[21] and Rosen[14] on the history of this movement in the United States and other countries.) The health problems of the poor which the earlier centers—some sponsored by the Milbank Memorial Fund—proposed to solve were undernutrition and infectious disease prevalent in the slums, and they were to do that by neighborhood location, community participation, bureaucratic organization, and preventive care. In the modern scene, perhaps there is no more elaborate a program of neighborhood health

Reprinted from *Medical Care* 8, 2 (March-April 1970): 97-103. Presented at a session sponsored by the Medical Care Section of the 97th Annual Meeting of the American Public Health Association, Philadelphia, November 1969.

centers than in Puerto Rico, which has had for some years now in actual operation more health centers as part of a regionalization of health services for fewer than three million people than the OEO has in preparation or demonstration for more than 200 million people.[16]

What we shall try to do here is to make much more explicit some of the *latent, non-manifest,* or *not-so-manifest* functions of neighborhood health centers, or the neighborhood health center *movement*, as it is sometimes called. These functions are never found described in legislative language, and are hardly ever made explicit by the principal proponents of the neighborhood health center idea, or for that matter by its opponents. These latent functions are no secret; they are frequently discussed outside of convention halls and formal meeting rooms. What we shall try to do is take some of the interesting talk heard in less formal social settings—in hotel rooms and bars, in university seminars, at lunches and in living rooms—and give it a hearing at this professional meeting.

What are some of the latent functions of neighborhood health centers? No one has yet made a systematic survey to answer this question. A few which have come to our attention and which are readily identifiable are:

1. Improving the image of the black male in poverty communities.
2. Stimulating and maintaining solidarity among migrant Chicano farm workers.
3. Pacification of hostile communities by colonial powers.
4. Discharging missionary service obligations of the medical-hospital establishment.
5. Filling a political void in social and economic action.
6. Politicization or radicalization of youth.

Improving the Image of the Black Male in Poverty Communities

This may be illustrated by a quotation from a report of the South Central Multipurpose Health Services Center, University of Southern California, in which a recommendation for the organization of a health council for a neighborhood health center is made.

It is of emergent necessity that emphasis be put on establishing a male achievement model in community action programs because, in many cases, the Community Action Council will become the focal point of that poverty community. It has been through my experience that if you

have 50 per cent male and 50 per cent female, the women will dominate the Community Health Council. . . .

It is my recommendation that two-thirds of the Community Health
Council be mandatorily male—even though they may appear in many
poverty neighborhoods to strangle the effectiveness of a Community
Health Council. I feel it is necessary to do this so we can start moving
in a positive direction in poverty communities and begin to establish
meaningful male models where families can identify with positive
images of the Negro male.

The traditional structure and traditional community [power] in black
communities has [been rested] with the clergy or the Negro woman—
which suggests a passive or matriarchal family structure, as she is leading
the family and making all the decisions. You have too many situations
where the Negro male plays no role in meaningful affairs.

If tradition prevails and Community Health Councils are set up equally
male and female, there will always be a tendency for traditional administration to communicate with the woman because it is the easiest
and because it is less threatening.[2]

Stimulating and Maintaining Solidarity among Chicano Farm Workers

Alviso, California is home for the families of a group of Mexican-American
migrant farm workers. A young Anglo labor organizer was working with the
men of this community—literally working with them, for his budget did not
seem to be any larger than his personal earnings from farm labor. He had a cadre
of strong and committed converts, but the cause seemed to lack sufficient
intrinsic appeal to weld the community into an action-oriented whole. The
young Anglo leader was casting about for an appealing adhesive force, an *action*
that would not bring down any further negative pressure from the establishment
and one that could be successful largely through the group's own efforts. The
leader and two of his strongest followers arrived at the door of OEO ready to do
the agency a favor. Alviso offered to fulfill OEO's major mandate. With a relatively small grant they would demonstrate that a community in action could
create social and economic change leading to improved health. Individually, the
staff of OEO were intrigued; but as an agency they were somewhat taken back
by the concept of a neighborhood health center without credentialed health
professionals. "Who did you say would be the medical director?" "No one?"
"But you are going to have a staff nurse?" "No?" "A social worker?" "A health
educator?" "You're not ready for any of those?" "Then who will plan the programs? And the buildings?" "The community!" "Oh!" The grant was made.
Within a year, this community had built, equipped, staffed, and opened a
neighborhood health center.

Pacification of Hostile Communities by
Colonial Powers

One rather gloomy evening, the upper middle class trustees of a large Northern urban Jewish hospital looked out and found their hospital surrounded by deteriorating housing, the streets filled with angry people, and the stores of some of their best contributors to the last building fund drive (1965–1966) in flames. These same angry people were dissatisfied with Mt. Sinai's emergency room and outpatient clinics. The trustees finally realized that this situation had not developed suddenly. The original clientele of the hospital had long ago retreated to suburban Skokie before the Southern black migration. The original clientele, to a large extent, still used Mt. Sinai for their in-hospital care, for Mt. Sinai continued to be the workshop of their private physicians. The surrounding community, to a large extent, used Mt. Sinai for *all* its care because there was no place else to go. The hospital found itself serving two quite different populations, neither of which was satisfied because of the concessions made to the other. If the hospital was not to lose all its support from the well-to-do Jewish community, the black community would have to be pacified. The vehicle for this pacification program appeared in the shape of an OEO funded neighborhood health center. Here the community could safely be "involved." Interestingly, another arm of the establishment was having some difficulty with this community, because it replaced housing much needed by the people, with parking facilities much needed by the company. Sears, Roebuck came forward with an offer to design the neighborhood health center building and to lend the money for its construction.

Another example of pacification has to do with Temple University in Philadelphia, a white lower middle class "streetcar college." When Russell Conwell was, in the early 1800's, barnstorming the country repeating his "Acres of Diamonds" address, North Philadelphia was a white blue-collar eastern European enclave housing many "able and deserving students of limited means," the group Temple was specifically founded to serve. As in the case of Chicago's Mt. Sinai, the character of the surrounding neighborhood changed. Much later, two major events occurred in rapid succession in 1964 and 1965 which tended to bring Temple to the attention of its black neighbors. The first was a major civil disturbance which erupted on the doorstep of the main campus at Columbus Avenue. The campus and its communications facilities were appropriated by the police as a command post for its anti-riot activities. The choice was logical because it contained the only non-hospital phone switchboard large enough to meet the needs of the police force. However, in the mind's eye of some community people, Temple had chosen to serve the enemy. Secondly, in November 1965, by act of the legislature of the Commonwealth of Pennsylvania, Temple University became a state-related institution in the Commonwealth system of higher education. With the resources thus made available, Temple immediately began to expand its physical plant. Like Chicago's Sears, Roebuck, Temple's priorities for space utliization were not compatible with those of the community. Temple's growing pains were being felt by the community not only in the area surrounding the main campus, but also one mile farther north around the Health Sciences Center campus. Here, too, angry people who had no other place to go, were beginning to complain about the service in the emergency room, in the out-patient clinics and on the wards of Temple University Hospital. There was a growing anxious wish among the leaders of the Health Sciences Center that something could be done to cool the community and to provide an acceptable outlet for the community's pent-up energies. Along came OEO, and to retell the story would be unnecessarily repetitous.

Data regarding the effectiveness of the pacification programs—or, for that matter, the effectiveness of the communities' exploitation efforts—are scant and conflicting: North Philadelphia has not seen a repetition of its civil disturbance, but there has been burning in North Lawndale in Chicago.

Discharging Missionary Service Obligations of the Medical-Hospital Establishment

According to Marion Sanders in a recent article in *Harpers Magazine*,[15] Bathgate Avenue in the Morrisania section of the Bronx gives the appearance of foreign soil. The establishment in this case is Montefiore Hospital, one of New York City's large and most respected nonprofit teaching hospitals. The chief of the missionary service is Dr. Harold Wise, imported from Canada. Like all missionaries, use is made of indigenous personnel: there are communication problems with alien cultures. Wise regards the activity as that of "an imperial power, preparing the underprivileged for self-government." He is quoted as hating to be in the foreign service. One of the public health nurses is quoted by Marion Sanders as saying, "There was no question about it when I was offered this job," her startling large eyes gleaming with missionary zeal, "this—this is where the action is."

Filling a Political Void in Social and Economic Action

In the 1960's there was essentially no likelihood that the established political structure—black or white—in Mound Bayou, Mississippi, would encourage sufficient activity to overcome the problems of malnutrition and inadequate housing. While the nutrition of an individual patient is often the concern of a physician and while the housing of a specific family is frequently the concern of a social worker, starvation and widespread housing inadequacies are generally considered political problems. How could these problems be approached? Under what rubric could community organization proceed without mobilizing the total resistance of the establishment? A labor union? A new political party? How about a neighborhood health center? Neighborhood health center it was, and there was considerable resistance. The total available resistance was never mobilized, however, because it was nearly impossible to launch an all-out assault on an agency organized solely for the purpose of improving people's health. For two years it would have been difficult using the OEO's definitions— upon which, incidentally, Dr. Morehead's assessment schedules are based—to recognize the Mound Bayou actively as a neighborhood health center. Instead of personalized preventive services, energies were being expended testing and closing contaminated water wells and drilling new ones in significant numbers. Instead of family-oriented social casework, energies were directed to building houses. Instead of diagnostic and curative services, energies were channeled into the organization of a farm cooperative and a food-processing plant. The very broad definition of "health services" used by the Tufts Comprehensive Community Health Action Program and its basic goals were never covert. The order and magnitude of the priorities in the rural south were, however, not actively proclaimed. Even in this forum when difficulties of evaluation have been discussed, we have tended to talk around this problem of priorities.

Politicization (or Radicalization) of Youth

There is a mobile adolescent health unit in the Lower East Side of Manhattan affiliated with the Judson Memorial Church in Greenwich Village. The health unit is at present privately financed. The unit consists of a 50 by 10 foot construction trailer divided into three rooms containing all the items of a doctor's office, including a small laboratory. The staff consists of an internist, a psychiatrist, a nurse, a technician, a night watchman, and a medical assistant. The services offered include: short-term care for acute and semiacute illnesses; treatment of minor injuries; diagnosis and treatment of venereal disease; counseling and referral for housing, welfare, and legal problems; updating of immunizations; evaluation and prescription for family planning; education in health, illness, and preventive medicine; evaluation of psychiatric problems; short-term psychotherapy on an individual basis; and group psychotherapy. In addition to these more or less conventional health services, the staff distributes a leaflet entitled a "10 Point Program of Health Revolutionary Unity Movement."[22]

Point 5 reads:
We want free, publicly supported health care for treatment and prevention. We want an end to *all* fees. We want an end to the exploitation of

the sick and suffering of our people by avaricious greedy professionals and institutions.

Point 6 reads, in part:
We want complete decentralization of Health Services and their control to meet the needs of our local communities. This should be based on block health officers.

Point 8 is:
We want education programs for all the people to expose all the leading health problems—unemployment, poor housing, racism, malnutrition, police brutality, and all other forms of exploitation.

Point 9:
Any individual, workers' organization or community organization must support all the points of this political program or be seen as an enemy of the workers and the community.

And Point 10:
Our point of departure is to serve the people wholeheartedly, and never for a moment divorce ourselves from the masses, to proceed in all cases from the interests of the people and not from one's self-interest or from the interests of a small group, and to identify our responsibility to the people with our responsibility to the community of workers and residents who must unite in solidarity to achieve victory. Power to the workers! Power to the community! All power to the people!

The political platform of this health unit would appear to go well with Desmond Callan's vivid categorization of another health center on New York's Lower East Side as an "Island of struggle with social reality in alliance with popular forces."

It should be clear from these few illustrations that all of these neighborhood health centers, whether government supported or not at any moment of time, operate in a broader social and political arena than just the health arena. Neighborhood health centers serve as legitimized access to distressed populations and as politically acceptable conduits for funds, especially federal, to be used for purposes far beyond the mere provision of health services.

In identifying functions served by neighborhood health centers other than the improvement of health services, we do not imply rejection or acceptance. When federal money is running to health, it is difficult for social and economic reformers to resist the temptation of placing their efforts in a health context. Noncategorical requests for federal support are not likely to be funded. It is rare to find a frank multipurpose, noncategorical community service center, such as, for example, the Hunt's Point Multiservice Center in the Bronx. That they do exist, however, suggests that from time to time the federal government *is* capable of putting its money where the hungry mouths are, without subterfuge, without equivocation, and without hiding behind the safe facade of health.

References

1. Arbona, G., and Trussell, R.E.: Medical and Hospital Care in Puerto Rico. School of Public Health and Administrative Medicine, Columbia University and the Department of Health of Puerto Rico, 1962.
2. Bates, J.E.: Demonstration Outline of the South Central Multipurpose Community Health Council, South Central Multipurpose Health Services Center, University of Southern California (mimeo).
3. Bamberger, Lisbeth: Health Care and Poverty: What Are the Dimensions of the Problem from the Community's Point of View? *Bull. N.Y. Acad. Med. 42*:1140, 1966.
4. Bellin, S.S., Geiger, H.J., and Gibson, C.D.: Impact of Ambulatory-Health-Care Services on the Demand for Hospital Beds. *New Eng. J. Med. 280*:808, 1969.
5. Community Medicine, *Massachusetts Physician 545*, 1967.
6. Elinson, J.: Effectiveness of Social Action Programs in Health and Welfare. *In* Assessing the Effectiveness of Child Health Services: Report of the Fifty-sixth Ross Conference on Pediatric Research. Ross Laboratories, Columbus, Ohio, 1967.
7. Finer, June: East Side-Village Youth Project. Judson Memorial Church, 1969 (mimeo).
8. Geiger, H.J.: The Poor and the Professional: Who Takes the Handle Off the Broad Street Pump? Presented at the 94th Annual Meeting, American Public Health Association, San Francisco, 1966 (mimeo).
9. Kelman, H.R., and Elinson, J.: Strategy and Tactics of Evaluating a Large-scale Medical Care Program. *Medical Care 7*:79, 1969.
10. Miller, J.I.: Summation of Discussion Group Reports and Concluding Remarks. Presented at the National Conference on Health Care for the Poor, December 1967 (mimeo).
11. Parker, A.W.: Training the Consumer Who Is Serving on Health Center Advisory or Policy-Making Boards. Presented at Conference on Health Consumer Training, June 1969, Washington, D.C. (mimeo).
12. Reader, G.G.: Health Care and Poverty: What Are the Dimensions of the Problem from the Clinician's Point of View? *Bull. N.Y. Acad. Med. 42*:1126, 1966.
13. Robertson, L.S., Kosa, J., Alpert, J.J., and Heagarty, M.C.: Anticipated Acceptance of Neighborhood Health Clinics by the Urban Poor. Medical Care Research Unit, Family Health Care Program, Harvard Medical School and Children's Hospital Medical Center (mimeo).
14. Rosen, G.: A History of Public Health. MD Publications, New York, 1958; pp. 470–478.
15. Sanders, M.K.: The Doctors Meet the People. *Harpers Magazine,* January 1968.
16. Seipp, C., Ed.: Health Care for the Community: Selected Papers of Dr. John B. Grant. The American Journal of Hygiene Monographic Series No. 21, 1963.

17. Sidel, V.W.: Can More Physicians Be Attracted to Ghetto Practice? Presented at the National Conference on Medicine in the Ghettos, Portsmouth, N.H., June 1969 (mimeo).

18. Smith, D.R.: Significant Behavioral Characteristics of Consumer-Health-Advisory Bodies that Are Basic to the Educational Training Process. Presented at the Joint OEO-HEW Consumer Training Conference, Silver Springs, Maryland, June 1969 (mimeo).

19. Sparer, G.: Evaluation of OEO Neighborhood Health Centers. Program Planning and Evaluation Division, Office of Health Affairs, Office of Economic Opportunity (mimeo).

20. Standards for Evaluating the Effectiveness of Community Action Programs. Office of Economic Opportunity, May 1969 (mimeo).

21. Stoeckle, J.D., and Candib, L.M.: The Neighborhood Health Center—Reform Ideas of Yesterday and Today. *New Eng. J. Med. 280*:1385, 1969.

22. Ten Point Program of Health Revolutionary Unity Movement. Lower East Side Health Council, 1969 (mimeo).

11

Community Control—or Community Conflict?

H. Jack Geiger

Community control of the systems that provide basic human services to the communities of the poor is a concept that is here to stay. Community participation is here, more of it is coming, and programs aren't going to work without it.

Application of this concept results in a profound—even revolutionary— change in the systems that professionals (including health professionals) have devised to deliver their services. It calls for profound changes in professional attitudes, orientations, and ways of behaving—changes so fundamental that they are bound to be painful, difficult, and accompanied by conflict.

The collision between community insistence and professional resistance inevitably generates heat. If heat and conflict are not present, usually nothing of importance is happening.

Some of the conflicts with the consumers of health care—particularly where professionals have honestly tried to involve the community in the planning of programs—occurs because there is so little understanding on either side of what "community" means and what "participation" and "control" mean. This is especially true in ghetto communities. There is too little understanding of the basic premises that the professional and the community resident bring to the action and of the reasons for the disagreements that almost inevitably follow.

To cite the most common example, the basic attitude of most health professionals toward the delivery of services is: "We'll run the services, and you can provide the illnesses." When the professional then moves toward community participation, he is really thinking: "How can I get you to participate in what I want to get accomplished?" Or "We'll set the goals, and you can participate in the means." But the community resident wants to know: "When am I going to set the goals? When am I going to manage and plan programs to meet my needs, as I see them? When are you going to go to work to help meet *my* priorities?" When "community participation" has such different meanings to professional and community, conflict is certain.

Reprinted from the November 1969 *ALA Bulletin,* published by the American Lung Association (formerly the National Tuberculosis and Respiratory Disease Association), pp. 4-10.

Two neighborhood centers

During the past five years, the Department of Preventive Medicine of Tufts University Medical School (in Boston) has been deeply involved in the development and operation of two comprehensive neighborhood health centers, one in Boston and one in Mississippi, each heavily committed to the concept of community participation. There are some useful lessons to be learned from that experience, I think, but the translation to your own programs and concerns will have to be your own.

The health centers are in two very different ghettos, one urban and one rural. The Columbia Point Health Center, in urban Boston, serves a large, densely packed public housing project with some 6,000 low-income residents in 26 high-rise buildings on 13 acres. The Tufts-Delta Health Center serves 14,000 people in the 500 square miles of northern Bolivar County in the Mississippi Delta, 100 miles south of Memphis.

The two communities represent contrasting (but linked) styles of poverty.

What happened at Columbia Point

Columbia Point is a kind of San Quentin by the sea: identical brick buildings, concrete, and fences on a peninsula in Boston harbor. The project was built on what used to be a city dump and is cut off from the rest of the city by two expressways and isolated by social and racial discrimination as well.

The housing development is less than four miles from one of the world's best collections of medical centers and teaching hospitals. Despite that fact, most of the people there were cut off from rational, coherent, and accessible health services before the Tufts project began.

North Bolivar County is in the heart of the area where cotton is king and people are surplus, thanks to the introduction 20 years ago of the double-row cotton-picking machine and the chemical herbicide, which destroyed the sharecropper system, itself an almost unchanged remnant of slavery. These two changes in farming techniques ended the need for an intensive labor force for cotton chopping and cotton picking and left more than 60 percent of the work force increasingly unemployed, hungry, and adrift on the land.

Community participation in the two community health centers developed differently in each place. The experience at Columbia Point is, I believe, typical of most such efforts in urban areas.

Four stages in the relationship

In the issue of community involvement, there are, in my experience, four definable stages in the relationship of a professional organization, such as a university sponsor of a neighborhood health center, with the population it serves.

In Stage 1, the university or professional organization–which has usually already drawn up most of its plans for the program, by itself–begins to operate in the community. Most often, the program is worked out without the participation of community representatives before it is funded and initiated. At this point, the professional organization, which may sincerely believe in community participation, wants to create such participation *instantly* to prove its good faith and protect itself from charges of ignoring the community.

And so the professional organization–which usually does not include people professionally trained in community organization–goes the route of "instant community organization." It reaches out as fast as it can to find "community representatives" and create an immediate ad hoc community committee. Without a coherent community organization plan, it runs toward the community.

In so doing, it runs headlong into the arms of people in the community who are racing toward the new institution or agency. These are almost always the existing elite in the community–those community people who are active on other projects already there or who already hold leadership positions in some group or who have strong political or ideological motivations. They have internalized the community; they say, "Looking for the community? Look no further; here we are!" And they believe it.

What the professional organization often really wants is a passive, window-dressing, grateful, powerless advisory committee to give a variety of sanctions to what is already planned by the professionals. And what the existing elite often really wants is the preservation of their relative status–to be "in" on this big new action, regardless of the degree of real power they may have at the start. The community group does very often include some of the most organizationally skilled, most articulate, most verbal people there. They may or may not be leaders of groups with significant community membership. But–most often–their selection and appointment to an ad hoc or advisory or citizens' committee or board *does not involve the great majority of the community's population in any way*. Most of that population, in poor communities at least, is scuffling for survival–struggling with issues like jobs and food and housing–has little interest in organizational structures, and sees little connection between organizational structures and its own needs. The people are often far more concerned with the services to be provided than with the question of who runs them. And so they couldn't care less who makes it onto the citizens' committee or what power the committee has. Elections for such posts often draw less than 10 percent of the community as voters, for just this reason.

Nonetheless, the professional organization goes looking for its instant community board, the existing elite appears, a board or ad hoc committee emerges, and for the rest of Stage 1–which may last six weeks or six months–there is a great honeymoon, because each group has met its immediate needs. The university or professional organization has its relatively powerless advisory committee that it can display to people on the outside, saying, "Look how involved we are in the community; we sit down and talk with the people; we have board meetings and other things; it's just great." The in-group in the community has preserved its relative status; it is where the action and the big new budget and the jobs are; it's at the center of things.

"You're a fake"

But after a time, things begin to change. Both the professional organization and the advisory committee become conscious of the fact that the people in the community don't really control any part of the new program. The advisory committee has the power to decide only the secondary questions, like the color of the paint. It is not doing hiring and firing, it is not setting the program priorities. People in the community start saying to the advisory committee, "What good are you? You aren't doing anything. You aren't increasing the services or getting us more jobs or handling our complaints."

And so, with increasing restlessness and anger on the part of the community, Stage 2 begins. The advisory committee comes to the professional organization and says, "This whole thing is a fake. We don't have any community control. We want to start running things."

At this point in Stage 2, very serious conflict begins. All kinds of buried anger surfaces in the professional organization. It says to the people in the community, "How dare you people demand these things when we are here doing all these things *for* you?" One starts hearing the "you-people" syndrome. And it takes some humility and self-searching for the professionals to admit that they really wanted to run the whole show. It is painful to admit this and then to set such motivations aside and find some alternative basis for response to the community.

The usual response is that the professional organization offers the "community" group a greater share in the formulation of broad, general policy. Most often, the move is regarded by the community group with great suspicion, and properly so. "Broad general policy formulation" sounds like the turf on which people from the community are likely to be out-maneuvered by the professionals, who usually have greater organizational and verbal skills. It doesn't meet the need of the community for real control.

The advisory group then says, "Wait a minute. You make the broad, general policy formulation. We'll control the jobs, the money, and the budget."

The university or professional institution also gets jittery, with some reason. It says, "Wait a minute yourselves. We have professional standards to maintain. There can't be just anybody hired for just any job."

Sometimes, in Stage 2, some concessions are made. But to the university's surprise, this doesn't cool things; it heats them up because the community advisory committee has discovered a system that works. It has gotten some concessions and decides to try to get some more. Furthermore, the expectations of the "community" group were raised. There is a curious thing about the revolution of rising expectations in any community. The more progress you get, the more you got to get, and the more urgent the matter seems to be.

Angry, divisive conflict

And so you come to Stage 3. At this point, there is angry, polarized, divisive conflict between the two groups. There are charges of failure on both sides, lots of yelling, lots of difficulty in maintaining any kind of working relationship, lots of difficulty in conducting any kind of program—which was supposed to be the object of the effort in the first place.

Sometimes the conflict degenerates to a stage where the program is driven out of the community. But other times—and the group from Tufts University went through the process at Columbia Point—it is then possible to sit down and hammer out a sensible relationship issue by issue. At Columbia Point, there emerged a contractual relationship between Tufts University School of Medicine and the Columbia Point Health Association, which is composed of elected representatives from the community.

The two groups have come to an agreement as to how they will share in hiring and firing, how they will conduct regular program reviews, how they will plan and initiate new programs, how they will do this and that, area by area. The new budget and grant renewal proposal—policy by policy and item by item— were developed by the two groups *together.*

Thus, we finally have arrived at Stage 4 in the Columbia Point project. There is now a representative community organization that is not window dressing. *But there is nothing going on in the store.*

Nothing going on?

The problem is that 95 percent of the community itself has no influence on the program or on the community committee. It has nor organized way to indicate its needs and priorities in relation to the services or program operation and no way to exert control over community representatives by making them responsible to local constituencies. Local community organization cannot be accomplished overnight.

"Nothing going on in the store" is probably an overstatement, and so is the 95 percent figure. The Columbia Point Health Association is now reaching out to many more residents to create an active constituency. I believe the effort will succeed, but doing the job from the top down, rather than from the bottom up, is an uncertain process.

Let me add that at the very beginning, before the health center program was under way at Columbia Point, Tufts organized some 40 to 50 living-room meetings, in which small groups of neighbors met to discuss health problems, current patterns of health care, the services they needed, and the things they wanted to see in the health center.

These 40 to 50 groups were not helped to stay functional and active; they fell apart in the rush for an instant ad hoc advisory committee. How much more powerful the community involvement might have been over the next several years if these groups had been further organized—building by building or block by block or stairwell by stairwell—and if their representatives had formed the health association!

I'm sure that, if this had been done, many of the staff members and leaders in the present health association would be the same as they are now—but they would have a more active constituency to work with.

What happened in the Mississippi Delta

Let me turn now to the development of community involvement in the Mississippi Delta. That effort has particular significance when you know something about the history of the area.

Until about 20 years ago, there had been no substantial changes in the basic social order since Abe Lincoln. The name had been changed from "slave" to "tenant farmer" or "sharecropper," but people still lived without the opportunity to manage their own affairs.

In other parts of the country at the time of the Civil War, even the poorest Americans hunted for their own food or raised their own crops. In the plantation economy, you don't do that. You buy your food at the plantation store. They give you a certain amount, and you buy on account. You never see that account; it's not explained to you. If you need medical care, it's arranged through the system. You don't have any choice in it; you don't arrange it.

The kinds of techniques we associate with the self-sufficiency of rural folk in America were not possible under the plantation system. People who are products of that system have very limited organizational experience, restricted decision-making experience, almost no experience with many of the basic things—like voting—taken for granted as part of adult status in the United States.

About two decades ago, a combination of developments began to change things radically in the Mississippi Delta. The chief one was the introduction of the double-row cotton-picking machine. A single machine can replace 70 to 140 workers. In addition, chemical herbicides came into use about 20 years ago to replace the cotton chopping, or weeding.

With these developments, most of the black workers living in the area became surplus. The unemployment rate reached 75 percent, and people began to migrate to the northern and western cities.

As a result, living conditions for black citizens in the Delta became very poor, and they still are. Reported black infant mortality rose to 60 per 1,000 live births—that's 6 out of every 100 babies. For blacks, the chronic disease rate, including tuberculosis, was much higher than in many other rural sections of the country.

Ninety percent of the black rural people lived in housing unfit (by contemporary standards) for human habitation; 70 percent were without a protected or reasonable kind of water supply; the majority of them were hungry. The median annual income was less than $1,000 a year *per family.*

Development of the health center

This was the turf upon which Tufts University, with Office of Economic Opportunity funds, started to develop a comprehensive neighborhood health center.

There was a difference this time. As one of its first acts, the Health Center planners—long before services began—launched a full-scale community organization effort, using local people as organizers under the guidance of a professional.

The community action staff spent a great deal of time at the beginning— almost a year—meeting with people in their homes, in churches, in schools, and on the plantations in the area. This staff literally knocked on the door of every house in northern Bolivar County inhabited by a black family. As a result, ten separate local health associations were formed within the 500-square-mile area. I want to emphasize that community organization of this kind is effective only if it's *local*. Whether it's formed around a stairwell at Columbia Point or around a cluster of rural homes, it must be local.

Each of the ten health associations in the Bolivar County area had its own priorities. In one town, people had to go three miles to haul water to drink. The alternative was to drink out of the drainage ditch. In that community, the main push was for drinkable water. In another community, care of children was the main need. In another one it was care of the elderly.

But can you share some food?

But almost everywhere it wasn't health services that were most important to the community. People said, "Health services are fine, and what you talk about sounds good, and we're happy to share in it, but for the love of God can you share some food?"

There were two or three other priorities that came ahead of health as we ordinarily define it. These were food, jobs, housing, and then maybe education. Health was fourth or fifth on the list. It happens to be a good point of entry for the other things.

What people were telling us was, "We have a somewhat different set of priorities; what are you going to do about it?" The Tufts group was fortunate enough to be able to respond to those sets of priorities.

Once we had the health center going, we started stocking food in the health center pharmacy and distributing food—like drugs—to the people. A variety of officials got very nervous and said, "You can't do that." We said, "Why not?" They said, "It's a health center pharmacy, and it's supposed to carry drugs for the treatment of disease." And we said, "The last time we looked in the book, the specific therapy for malnutrition was food." There was nothing that anybody could find in the regulations that said otherwise, so we continued to do it.

But it was a clumsy mechanism. So we began writing prescriptions for food that could be filled at some local grocery stores, and we paid for them out of our drug budget. That worked somewhat better, but it was still a clumsy mechanism. So we backed off and took a longer look. What we saw were people with agricultural skills, displaced by mechanization, sitting on the richest land in the United States, with nothing to do, and hungry.

We started talking about garden clubs, and 1,200 families said they wanted to belong. But then something else happened. The people, in response to their own need, invented something I believe to be unique in the United States: the first cooperative composed of landless people, the first farm co-op of people who didn't own any farms.

What they said was, "We'll pool all our labor from this 500 square miles. Let the poorest families join the farm co-op. We'll rent or borrow or get land somehow all in one place. The people will work it, for $4 a day cash, plus $6 a day shares in what we grow. We'll grow vegetables, not cotton, so we'll get something to eat."

The OEO innovatively agreed to give such a farm co-op a start, funding it as an emergency food demonstration program. The demonstration cost was about $120,000 to start. The farm co-op got off the ground very late last year, yet in a little over seven months, the people of northern Bolivar County were able to grow a million pounds of food—enough to end hunger and have some food left over.

7,000 people now involved

The black people in Bolivar County have gained a lot of ideas through the development of the ten local health associations and the overall health council which represents them all. The people are looking into the development of rural co-op-owned homes. Although there is no federal housing program that will do anything for families with an annual income of $900 a year, it may be possible for the co-op members or the Health Council members to pool their limited resources and develop housing practical for people in this income bracket.

The council has come to the Tufts group and said, "We want to start a public transportation system." It has come and said, "We want a budget for legal services, not only for ourselves but for help in going to federal agencies to get the water systems, the sewer systems, the food stamp programs, and other things we need." It has come to us and said, "We want to develop youth guidance in health careers because we are very worried about what's happening to the young people; they're leaving home because there are no jobs."

Today, some 7,000 black people in northern Bolivar County–most of them rural, poor, non-elite, and not previously involved–are actively working to redevelop their area. These people are going to council meetings and subcommittee meetings, planning their own programs, working on the farm co-op, and seeking help in obtaining an investment of some $900,000 for a cannery on the farm co-op that could be a basic industry for the area. And all of these things, of course, affect health.

The development process took two years, but the route was not easy. As I said earlier, if you're going to go the community involvement route, you're going to catch some heat from the existing elite. A resident may come to you and say, "You lousy neo-colonial so-and-so, how come you are coming in here and picking your leaders? Clearly, I am the leader of this community. Here I am."

It is very difficult to explain that, if they really are the leaders, they have nothing to worry about, and that *you* are not choosing the leadership; you are just insisting that the mass of the local people have the chance to identify and choose their leadership. You will catch heat from all kinds of groups who are pursuing their own interests, and strange pairings may develop to try to run you out.

There is another kind of heat that you must stand up to. You shouldn't go into the business unless you are prepared to suffer some conflict and get some scars. Nobody is going to tell you, "You are wonderful for doing this." The message is, "Where have you been all these years, and how come you invented the lousy economic (or health or educational) system in the first place?"

Lessons for health organizations

One of the main lessons in the Tufts University experience for TB and RD associations and similar organizations in the health field is that your priorities may not be those of the people you are concerned with and that you had better learn to start modifying, changing, or even giving up some of them. People who are concerned with survival are going to be worried about that before they are concerned with tuberculosis. They are going to be concerned with housing, jobs, food, their kids, and some other things before they are concerned with categorical disease or categorical disease programs.

The second and only other message I have is this: You will have to consider some major structural changes in your organization if you are going to give people a significant say in the provision of basic human services for their families and their communities. The day is gone when a health or welfare organization can impose a program on the community. If you try it, you'll find to your shock and surprise that the "apathetic, uncooperative poor" have a different set of priorities. You may end up with very different program committees than the ones you have now. I don't know a thing about your boards or your program committees, but if they work much the same as they did five years ago, you're in trouble.

One last thing: I regard what I have outlined for you as a process that's going to be full of cofnlict. I don't think the question is "Community Control— or Community Conflict?" It's community control *and* community conflict. I don't think "control" develops instantly. But if you don't go the community control route in providing health services to economically disadvantaged groups, you are going to have even more conflict, and—what is more important—you won't get anywhere at all.

12

NENA: Community Control in a Bind

Des Callan and Oliver Fein

NENA, short for North East Neighborhoods Association, in the northeast corner of New York's Lower East Side, runs one of the few, if not the only community initiated, community controlled neighborhood health centers in the United States that has received major federal financing. Now rounding out its third year of operation, NENA illustrates some of the strengths and limitations of the neighborhood health center movement of the 1960's, and of the community control impetus within it.

NENA has been caught in a series of binds, basically not of its own making, that have often set one sector of the Health Center against another. The Center has been unable so far to wrest from Washington and the outside health establishment the resources needed to do the job NENA promised its community when it set out in 1968. Instead, the NENA story is primarily one of the heavy expenditure of energy keeping the Health Center afloat while trying to deliver even a portion of the services its patients require.

Situated on East Third Street near Avenue C, the Center is open to all persons, regardless of income, who live in its designated district. Once an immigrant slum ghetto of Jews, Italians, Ukrainians and Russians, in the last generation NENA's area has become primarily Puerto Rican, with a sizable number of Blacks and a small minority of whites, mostly elderly Jews and a scattering of hippies and ex-hippies. A small number of businessmen, artists and teachers live in renovated brownstones or the one middle income housing project amid the mass of decaying tenements and low income projects.

Community Struggle for a Health Center

NENA's Health Center developed as a result of several bitter "learning experiences" of Lower East Side residents in the middle 1960's. The first of these occured in the winter of 1966 during the transit workers' strike. Normal bus service in the Lower East Side is very poor, and cabs are vitually unavailable. But with the transit strike, "Lower East Side residents found themselves cut off

---

Reprinted from *Health/PAC Bulletin* 42 (June 1972): 3-12.

from medical care," said Ms. Wanda Moore, present co-chairwoman of the Health Committee of the NENA community board. "Bellevue was the only source of general medical care. But with city buses shut down by the strike, Bellevue was truly unaccessible." Under these conditions, ordinarily treatable illnesses become life-threatening emergencies.

One snowy evening, a child on Sixth Street developed an acute asthmatic attack. Treatment was delayed and the child developed more and more difficulty breathing. Several hours and many frantic phone calls later, the critically-ill child was finally brought in a neighbor's car to Bellevue, the huge city hospital two miles away.

"People were really angry," said Ms. Moore. This experience of near-death because of lack of transportation was not an isolated incident. The problem oppressed everyone. "They wanted a health center right in the neighborhood. So they turned to NENA for help." In particular, the Sixth Street Mothers, a neighborhood block group, turned their attention to health and to NENA.

NENA was established to coordinate groups around community issues. In 1966, NENA had committees to deal with housing, education, narcotics addiction, law enforcement and transportation. But it was not until the Sixth Street Mothers presented their case to NENA that a committee on health was formed. And, in truth, it was health that put NENA on the map.

At the same time, independent of the community's activities, medical students, interns and residents at Bellevue became disgruntled with the health care offered there. They petitioned New York University Medical School, which provides the professional services to Bellevue, to create satellite health centers in the surrounding community.

In the spring of 1966, the Health Committee and the dissident doctors met together and planned a strategy to encourage the medical school to establish a health center in the NENA area. First the Health Committee met to begin planning for a proposed health center in the Lower East Side community. Then these plans were presented to Dean Lewis Thomas of NYU. He assigned faculty members to help refine the Health Committee's plan into a formal planning proposal. Over the next year the Health Committee consulted with many community groups, storefront agencies and service workers to draw up its component of the plan. In March, the plan was handed over to the medical school for submission to a foundation.

Two months later the Health Committee was shocked to learn that NYU had decided not to submit the proposal, the product of a whole year's work. The Health Committee charged NYU's medical dean with bad faith, and broke off negotiations with the NYU-Bellevue Medical Center.

The NENA Health Committee found itself back at the beginning, older but wiser. They had learned an important lesson: don't rely on major medical centers for help. And so the Health Committee began to plot a course which would avoid dependence on either Bellevue or Beth Israel Hospital, which together provide a major portion of health care on the Lower East Side.

During the summer of 1967 the Health Committee went to Washington. By judicious use of their Congressman, they got a consultant from the Office of Economic Opportunity (OEO) to advise them on starting a center. Soon thereafter, the group realized it could not live with two restrictions imposed by OEO grants: first, the grant had to be administered by a medical organization such as a medical school or center. The Committee wanted federal money to go directly to their own community organization. Second, OEO grants could only be used to provide care for the poor. The Health Committee did not want to restrict the use of the health center by income. It was to be a neighborhood-wide facility for all to use.

The Health Committee was unclear about what course to take. But whatever the course, it was clear that an arrangement with a back-up hospital was necessary. At the consultant's suggestion, the Health Committee had approached New York Infirmary, a small acute care hospital, in the fall of 1967. The relationship offered important things to both parties. The Infirmary, which was applying for permission to expand, felt that its association with NENA would demonstrate its need for more beds, as well as meet criteria for community service. For NENA, the arrangement would permit future health center doctors to admit individuals to the Infirmary as their private patients, providing continuity of care. Moreover, it set up a relationship of equality with a community hospital which was better adapted to the needs of NENA's future patients.

Realizing the limitations with OEO, the Health Committee sought other alternatives. Another Washington adviser told them of the availability of Public Health Service funds for health centers, under less onerous guidelines.

During the winter and spring of 1968, a flurry of activity ensued to prepare a grant application. Negotiations with the Infirmary were sped up. A core administrative and medical staff was recruited. And a temporary building was acquired to house the center until larger quarters could be built.

By summer, 1968, NENA's health center had been funded. Fifteen months later, in September, 1969, the Center opened its doors in a small renovated building that formerly housed a boys' club and before that a hotel for alcoholics. The structure was but 21 feet wide and five stories tall. It had no elavator.

NENA Today

Today, the NENA Health Center is located in this same tiny building. It has 35,000 registered patients and a staff of about 125; 250 patients walk through its doors each day. Services available include general family care; some medical specialty services including surgical consultation, dermatology, obstetrics and gynecology, ophthalmology and ear, nose and throat; dentistry; pharmacy; laboratory; X-ray; limited social services; and in a separate storefront, a city-sponsored detoxification program for addicts. There is also a child care program for patients waiting to be seen at the center.

NENA offers comprehensive, continuous care, both preventive and curative, to a few thousand enrolled families, who are seen by a health team, primarily by appointment. It also offers drop-in or screening care, including emergencies, available without appointment eleven hours-a-day to all registrants, whether enrolled with a team or not. In fact, because of the demand and the limits of time and space, enrollment with the health care teams is generally not open to new families.

The Center's small building limits NENA's ability to deliver efficient and courteous care. For instance, three family health care teams (each composed of two physicians, a nurse practitioner, medical assistant, community health worker and secretary) use the five rooms on the second floor. The teams have to alternate sessions and reduce office hours because of the lack of space. The result is that the Center can offer the team approach to relatively few families.

Scores of daily drop-in patients who are not enrolled in the teams are seen in three small examining rooms at the back of the long, narrow first floor. These rooms are also used by visiting specialists. On the first floor, there is only one waiting room. Patients waiting for the laboratory, X-ray, the pharmacy and a visit to the specialist must all wait in the same tiny area.

The third floor of the Center contains three modern dental chairs with three full-time dentists and an equal number of dental assistants. The dental unit is not yet integrated into the health team structure.

The Center's fourth floor houses the administrative and personnel offices. The Health Committee of the NENA Board has its offices around the corner from the Health Center in the community organization's headquarters.

Two major groups have shaped NENA's development over the three-year existence of the Health Center: The Health Committee and the staff. Both groups have contributed their share to the accomplishments, problems and contradictions that have emerged over this period.

The Health Committee

By 1969, when NENA opened its doors, the Health Committee had boiled down to twelve active members. Though the Sixth Street Mothers were still represented on the Committee, several other groups had gained prominence. One of the most powerful of these was a small group, mostly white, which was associated with the local Reform Democratic Club. The ascendence of this particular group on the Committee is no surprise, considering the selection process.

The Health Committee maintains that it is open to anyone who lives and works in the community. However, the selection process narrows this down

NENA's Original Goals

1. Good health services should be available to all people regardless of economic or social class.
2. Health Services should be available right in the community where they are needed, so that local people need not have the extra expense and inconvenience of traveling to overcrowded hospitals.
3. A good outpatient clinic should be an integral part of community life to serve the people just as schools, churches, social agencies and settlement houses do.
4. The facility should be community oriented; and neighborhood people should have a voice in the way that it is run, in order that it serves their particular needs, and so that they can feel that it really belongs to them.
5. The facility will be run by a Board of Directors consisting of community representatives which should meet regularly to discuss problems and to consider new ideas that come directly from the community. The Board can also serve as a liaison committee between the community and established city agencies.
6. Clinic facilities should be modern, pleasant and have a cheerful welcoming atmosphere.
7. Only professional staff of high quality should practice in the clinic. All doctors should have finished their residency and be familiar with the type of patient and clinic they will be serving.
8. Utilizing team delivery of health care each family would continually see the same doctor. This will inspire more confidence on the part of the patient and establish better rapport between patient and doctor. This will also enable the doctor to know his patient and the patient's family. It will save unnecessary duplication of tests, repetition of visits, conflicting instructions, time and money. But most important, it will ensure continuity of care.
9. Courtesy and real concern for the patient as a whole person should be a "Must" on the part of the staff.
10. An appointment system should be worked out so that patients do not have long waits to get assistance, and thus large waiting rooms will not be required.
11. Besides professional staff, neighborhood people be hired to work in as many capacities as they can be trained to fill and employment should be based on ability to do the job, and not on educational standards alone.
12. Because of the systematic exclusion of Puerto Ricans and Negroes from the professions, as many of these people as possible should be hired in the Health Center at all levels.

October, 1967

considerably. Health Committee members are selected in a two-stage process: first, prospective members must join a subcommittee. If their work is deemed worthwhile by the subcommittee chair-person, nomination for membership on the Health Committee may be made. Then the entire Health Committee votes on the candidate.

This process was developed to encourage participation by new people who really had an interest in health. As Ms. Bertha Dixon, present co-chairwoman of the Health Committee said: "The problem with community-wide elections is that the same old politicos who have organized their faction get elected. Often they aren't truly representative and aren't really interested in health."

Unwittingly, however, the Health Committee's selection process more closely resembles the trustee model of the private, voluntary hospital than a community-accountable and patient-responsive model. Like a hospital board of trustees, the Health Committee is a self-perpetuating body, which elects its own successors and has, in effect, an unlimited term of office. While a monetary contribution is not a criterion for Health Committee selection, as it is for many hospital boards of trustees, the requirement of a time and effort contribution to a subcommittee may function in similar ways. Once on the Committee, verbal skills and endurance limit effective participation even further. These reasons explain, in part, the former prominence of white, basically middle class, Reform Dems on the Committee.

On the Defense. Until NENA was funded, the Health Committee had actually been on the offensive. The Committee spearheaded plans for a new health center. Thereby it had taken on NYU Bellevue, which lay outside the community.

After being funded in 1968, however, the Health Committee increasingly assumed a defensive posture with respect to the community and even its own hired administrators. Executive sessions of the Health Committee, closed to the community and the Center's administration, began to abound. "It got to a point," said one Committee member, "where we couldn't meet at the Health Center or the NENA offices and had to meet in members' apartments." The Health Committee abandoned its focus on planning for new programs and a new building, while getting caught up in the day-to-day administration of the Center.

Two examples illustrate the destructive tendencies fostered by this defensive posture. The first had to do with building the new Health Center. It was clear from the first day that NENA acquired its temporary quarters on East Third Street, that a new Health Center was imperative. One logical site was a playground that had been purchased with the temporary building. The only difficulty was that the community had recently liberated the playground from its previous owners, who had strictly forbidden local block children from playing there. In other words, the playground had become a cause celebre among block residents, who now feared that NENA would destroy their hard-won victory.

Rather than deal with this challenge head-on, the Health Committee avoided the issue. For some months, many of its members wouldn't even walk down Third Street for fear of meeting the local antagonists. Just this year, the Health Committee's representatives failed to show up at a crucial community meeting that dealt with the site for the new building. The Health Center administrator was left alone to face the opposition. The avoidance of these issues has cost the Center valuable lead time in pursuing plans for a sorely needed new building.

A second example of the problems caused by the Health Committee's defensiveness arose around its assumption of administrative prerogative. At NENA, for instance, not only must the project director and all professional staff (including doctors) be interviewed and approved by the Health Committee, but also all other staff that deal with the public, from security guards to dental assistants. While the administration agreed to this policy, it is clear that it took an enormous effort on the part of the Health Committee to accomplish this task when the Center was being set up. Such effort might have been directed toward evaluation of existing programs, planning new ones, moving on the building or the Health Committee's one-time role of militant spokesman on health affairs for the community at nearby hospitals.

But the Health Committee's inward orientation became clear when several Health Committee members insisted that two employees be fired primarily because they had insulted the Health Committee. The employees had gotten into an altercation with several Health Committee members when they tried to attend a closed executive session of the Health Committee. But, the issue is whether it is wise for the Health Committee to become so entangled in such detailed administrative matters to the neglect of larger policy matters. Ultimately, the case of the two employees was brought to an arbitrator where it presently rests unresolved.

Community Accountability. It is clear that the NENA Health Committee had some real degree of control over the Center. Why did it become defensive?

With respect to the community, such as the residents of East Third Street, the Health Committee had a reason to be defensive. Since its selection process made the Health Committee accountable neither to the patients that used the Center, nor to the larger community, the Health Committee found it difficult to be open with opposition forces within the community.

Had the Health Committee felt confident about a community-accountable base, it could have acted in a much broader role as sponsor of the Health Center. It could have stimulated community dialogue; written reports for all the community to read; published a newsletter and even held public hearings. It could have put the heat on Bellevue, NYU and Beth Israel to improve services to the Lower East Side and to develop mechanisms for accountability to patients.

It seems the Health Committee veered in the direction of administrative decision-making because it felt that administrative control meant real control. It is apparent that the Health Committee had deep suspicions of the professional staff it hired. It felt somewhat insecure about its role. In part, this was unavoidable when the Health Committee, which had previously been a planning body alone, became an employer of a staff assigned with the task of organizing and operating the new Health Center. It thereby created a new center of power and decision making besides the Health Committee itself. And it wasn't certain that the professional staff shared its agenda.

One other element, peculiar to NENA, complicated this chemistry. Since 1965, NENA had a professional community organizer, who had provided expert assistance throughout the struggle to get funding for the Health Center. Shortly after the new professional staff arrived, this organizer left NENA. The effect on the Health Committee was profound. It had lost its trusted counsellor precisely at the time that it needed one. Unfortunately, none of the professional staff could substitute in this role. The result was heightened insecurity on the part of the Health Committee and increased distrust of the professional staff.

Recent Changes.   Over the three years of the Health Center's life, the Health Committee has been challenged only sporadically by community and worker forces. But these struggles have brought about some changes. There has been a marked decrease in secrecy of meetings, with fewer closed executive sessions. The participation of representatives of the Center's staff has been encouraged. In addition, the Health Committee seems to be refocusing its attention on long-term programs rather than on the day-to-day operation of the Center. Such long-term plans include the building of a new center, proposals for a mental health program and the creation of a patient advocacy program responsible to the Health Committee itself. But, not until the Health Committee deals with its lack of accountability to patients who use the Center, will it be able to overcome some of its intrinsic weaknesses.

The NENA Staff

Of the approximately 125 NENA Health Center staff, some three-quarters are nonprofessional. By a strict policy of the Health Committee, enforced by the administration, all these workers must come from the surrounding community. They are primarily Puerto Rican and Black, with a very few whites. Since the Health Center is known as a community institution, it has particularly attracted to its work force persons who are conscious of their place and stake in this community. It is a work force which is tied in a hundred ways to its community, through extended families, gossip, rumor, block loyalties, political and social clubs. Most of the workers are people who would rather not leave the neighborhood to work in the outside economy, but who would prefer to work close to home.

It is not a work force of political activists. One nurse characterized the staff as a whole as "very conservative. Very few are progressive. People are very easily satisfied with a small raise. Most of them don't feel secure." Another nurse said she had often been told by non-professional workers: "Well, you're a nurse. You can work anywhere. But where can I go?" This shows a pervasive fear of job loss among many of the staff. Despite brief periods when fear of dismissal has had some basis in reality, the fact is that turnover among staff, from either firing or quitting, has been exceptionally low.

Administrators claim that it is almost impossible to have someone fired at NENA regardless of the reason. The ostensible reason lies in the existence of an extensive grievance procedure. Behind this lies the reluctance of the administration and Board to stand up to counter-charges of professional and administrative bias against a community resident who can mobilize local and even Board opinion on his or her behalf.

Thus there is felt job insecurity on the one hand and actual, at least short-range, job security on the other. The explanation of this fear would appear to lie in the uncertainty of many staff members about the true permanence of the NENA Health Center. For many, this is their first good job. They fear their experience, skills and educational credentials are too marginal to enable them to find as good a job, if any, in the "outside world."

Training. Because of the Center's need for skilled workers, and the workers' need to make their skills transferable and to acquire upward mobility, training is highly important at NENA. At NENA, this has happened in a rather informal and unplanned manner. Early emphasis went into specific job and task preparation; little went into creating truly transferable credentials. Thus, to prepare the Center for opening day, "instant" clerks, receptionists, stock room attendants, maintenance men, medical assistants and so on were rapidly created. Later substantial effort went into teaching English and Spanish and preparing students to pass the high school equivalency exam. A number now attend community or regular college part time; others are apprenticed in the pharmacy and the laboratory, and one, now a medical emergency technician, has been accepted into medical school for 1974.

The result of all this activity is that the NENA Health Center, set up in opposition to the teaching hospitals, has in some ways become a teaching institution. But it does not prepare an elite at the expense of the community. Rather, it has resulted in the Center's first housekeeper becoming supervisor of dental assistants, a former center clerk becoming its office manager, and a woman medical assistant preparing to graduate from a training course to enter the hitherto all male field of medical emergency technicians who ride the ambulance. All this has been done with virtually no budget, training staff or separate training program.

Workers' Organization. The very insecurity which has sent so many workers into training programs for self-advancement of NENA has not yet led to major steps towards a workers' organization or union. In the beginning, a common sense of loyalty to the Center and to the Lower East Side united all levels of the staff. Later a staff association was formed, exclusive of professionals and administrators, to speak for employee concerns at administration meetings and also to secure passage and then observance of a code of personnel practices. But the association has not captured the allegiance of large numbers of staff members. Nonetheless, the group does have a seat on the Health Committee and is able to voice the concerns of staff members, though it does not enjoy the right to vote or opportunity to appear at closed executive sessions.

More energy within the staff goes, in fact, into an elected grievance committee, which arbitrates individual complaints. Issues arise on a personal basis rather than collectively as might happen through the staff association.

There is no union at NENA. Anti-union thinking for many on the Lower East Side began in 1968 and 1969 following the teachers' union strikes. These strikes appeared to many poor parents to be against their children, their community and their schools, on the part of mostly white teachers led by an ambitious and racist union leadership.

At the same time, many staff workers felt suspicious of the only potential NENA union, Local 1199 of the Drug and Hospital Workers' Union. The union opposed various community control struggles at Gouverneur Clinic and Beth Israel Hospital, both in the NENA neighborhood, in 1968, 1969 and 1970 (See *Bulletin*, July-August 1969, February 1970). As a result, many on the staff view unionism as being opposed to community interests. And since NENA is above all a community institution, under a fair measure of community control, union sentiment has not developed.

The professional, technical and administrative staff at NENA are a varied group, ethnically, politically, and in terms of dedication to the Center. Interviews for attitude acceptability with the Health Committee have made little difference. One reason, of course, is that the extreme shortage of interested, available and qualified professionals, particularly physicians, makes such activity more ritual than meaningful. In any event, the professional staff do not act as a unified influence at the Health Center.

NENA's Accomplishments

NENA's accomplishments are many:

• Increase in Services—NENA receives many thousands of visits per year. It reaches more people in its district than any other health service, yet it has never recruited patients. Almost one hundred percent of the children in the surrounding tenement blocks are registered at the Center.

• A Neighborhood Atmosphere—NENA is truly a neighborhood center. Spanish is heard in the hallways, children are always present, many of the workers are patients' neighbors. Little wonder a Puerto Rican mother can say: "NENA is like a clinic, but not like a clinic. If I come here, and my daughter needs me, everyone knows where to find me." NENA belongs to the people.

• A Proud Center Staff—Most workers are intensely proud of NENA. They speak of serving their community. A medical assistant will search throughout the building to find an answer to a patient's question. A medical emergency technician boasts of the efficiency of his ambulance shift. Many staff members make it a point "to take care of business"—that means breaking through red tape to get something done for a patient. Even former staff respect NENA: "People who have left work at NENA never talk about it as 'they.' They still say 'we.' We still feel part of it."

• Community Initiated and Community Controlled—NENA was started by community people, and even though its Health Committee is not perfect, it is still controlled by people who live in the community served by the Center. Most of the board and staff obtain their health care from the Center. NENA is one of the very few examples of a health service sponsored and controlled by a non-establishment community body in a big city slum.

• An Independent Health Service—NENA is independent of the major medical centers that dominate the Lower East Side. Through its relationship to the New York Infirmary for inpatient care, NENA has broken away from complete dependence for back-up services on a medical school or large teaching center. NENA is also independent of these major centers by virtue of its funding, which comes directly from the federal government to its own community organization. Two-thirds of NENA's $2 million budget comes from the U.S. Public Health Service, the rest from Medicaid.

Contradictions

But NENA is a bundle of contradictions. For each accomplishment the Center faces a bind:

• Quantity vs. Quality—Though NENA has vastly increased the quantity of health services on the Lower East Side, its major quality service—the comprehensive, family care program run by health teams—has had virtually closed enrollment for over two years.

• Neighborhood vs. OPD Atmosphere—Like its neighborhood, NENA is overcrowded and teeming with people. One mother describes the screening area: "I never know what's going on there. People are rough and don't care. You spend hours waiting when you are sick. The staff are rapping when people sit and wait. There is no explanation why you are waiting. It is just horrible, like a hospital emergency room. Patients are just numbers: Go here! Go there! I don't know what people would do in a real emergency. I once saw a person with a real emergency refused care by a receptionist because he wasn't registered."

• Staff Pride vs. Low Staff Morale—Though most of NENA's staff is proud to work there, staff morale has been sagging. As the Center becomes more bureaucratized, the workers feel a corresponding increase in alienation. "You can't run this place like a business. It is all going on computers. People have a number instead of a name. So does the job. Time cards are like a god. It resembles the Board of Education. The next thing a patient will come in, they'll hook him onto a computer and they'll find out what's wrong with him." Another worker declared: "There are no overall staff meetings to explain what's going on. People are very discouraged."

• Health Committee Control vs. Patient Accountability—At NENA there certainly is a significant degree of control by people who live near and use the Center. But there are no mechanisms, beyond a suggestion box, for patients to play a role in formulating the policies of the Center. No meetings of patients are held. No patient advocate system exists. And the Health Committee has been reluctant to establish a community outreach program that might combine health education and political education.

• Independence vs. Federal Controls—With all the mechanisms that NENA has devised to keep it independent of the medical establishment, it is still captive to the federal government. Each year the whole Center comes up for review, including its pattern of services, table of organization, salary levels, future plans and so on. Renewal of the grant is contingent on Public Health Service approval of all these matters, as well as its own availability of funds. NENA's demonstration grant expires next year. While the Public Health Service will hopefully grant some kind of extension, there is no guarantee how long federal subsidy will continue. With repeated cuts in Medicaid, the prospect of making the Center self-supporting is dismal. Ultimately, NENA has no independence.

Everyone agrees that the NENA Health Center faces manifold and serious problems. More serious, however, is the fact that even a tentative approach to a solution is unclear.

No agent for potential change is evident with the Health Committee or the NENA staff. Most of the nonprofessional workers who have attempted to bring changes to NENA have left the staff or are now absorbed in school. The remaining nonprofessionals are discouraged by staff divisions. They point out that "everyone seems to be out for himself."

Among professionals similar discouragement exists. One Black nurse said: "NENA has helped me to be less idealistic, more pragmatic and unfortunately more apathetic." This nurse was upset with the lack of staff response to a far smaller than expected wage increase. "I can see now how people can be done in," she said.

White professionals have always been in an ambivalent position at NENA. They were recruited because of their professional or administrative skills. But because they felt that political initiative should lie in the hands of community residents, most of whom are Puerto Rican or Black nonprofessionals, they have been unable to break out of their constricted professional roles.

The NENA administration, rather than being a force for change, today appears to be isolated from the basic concerns of the staff and even of the patients. Some do not recognize, or else cannot bring themselves to believe, how discouraged many of NENA's best workers are at all levels, regardless of political persuasion.

The few self-conscious radicals on the staff—professionals and nonprofessionals—have been relatively ineffective. Commented one physician: "Lately the radicals have confronted the administration on specific grievances. They have done almost no educational work to explain their views to the staff as a whole. The effect has been by and large antagonistic. There is sympathy with some of their aims, but a fear of losing one's job if one joins them. There is also skepticism because so few of the radicals truly take care of their work. One is lackadaisical about his work; another is always late, and so on."

Some might view patients themselves as a possible political force. But so far there is no evidence of patient organization.

Why is there no evident change agent at NENA? The major reason seems to be a deeply ingrained sense of NENA's marginality. As one Puerto Rican worker summarized it: "People are all into their own thing. They are off at school, or they are lining up second jobs, because they're afraid the Center's deficit is so huge it will have to close at the end of the summer." This feeling of NENA's marginality and lack of permanence extends into the community. People recognize that the locus of power in health on the Lower East Side still resides at NYU-Bellevue and Beth Israel.

These problems all stem from NENA's profound external limitations. Without a massive infusion of resources, it cannot possibly offer quality services to all who need them. Yet, in the competition for federal funds, NENA ($1.4 million a year in federal grants) with all its independence is still far outstripped by NYU and Beth Israel Medical Centers, which garner more than $50 million each year in government grants. So NENA remains a minor irritant to the medical empire. Unless the community, the Health Committee, and the workers see these forces as "the enemy" and focus their energy there, the prognosis for change at NENA is guarded.

Part VI
Administration

Introduction

Administrative skills have proven to be among the scarcest commodities in the working experience of the neighborhood health centers. In retrospect, one would expect any new organization tackling a complicated set of objectives in a chaotic institutional environment to be difficult to manage. There have been a number of generations of managers at the centers as the requirements of successful management have changed along with the development of the individual centers. Many of the initial directors of the centers were liberal medical professionals, strong on commitment and enthusiasm and reforming zeal, but weak on management know-how. The current directors address a somewhat different set of organizational needs: implementation of effective management routines, tightening up personnel policies, effecting greater efficiencies of operation as the federal project grants are phased out, seeking to demonstrate tangible accomplishments. As a result, they tend to be less the crusading reformers, more the hard-nosed businessmen. Depending on one's point of view, their job is to either bail out and put on a surer footing the innovations initiated by their predecessors or to scrap those innovative aspects of the centers for which financial support is not longer available.

Once it became painfully evident that management skills were in short supply and that administrative problems were rampant in the centers, the federal government invested heavily in various efforts to provide technical assistance and training in management techniques. The fact that the centers have had severe administrative difficulties is interpreted by some as evidence of the inherent weaknesses of the model. This attitude toward the problems of the health centers is simply one more instance of the strong American reforming tradition of making a brief stab at improvement, then drawing back from it when the difficulties of following through effectively become apparent and the political rewards of seeming to have done something about the problems have long since been harvested. A fairer assessment of the situation realizes that by virtue of their innovativeness and ambitiousness, the centers are unusually complicated organizations that are hard to run smoothly. It is essential to figure out which problems may in fact be endemic to the centers as they are set up—their organizational structures, set of objectives, scope of services, all other policies and procedures—and which are difficulties that can be overcome by making modifications in the model and by training persons to be more effective staff. In this case, the fact that there have been problems implementing a complicated program signifies that the conditions addressed by the program are big ones more than it indicates that the approach to attacking them is ineffectual.

Although written in 1970, Paul R. Torrens' "Administrative Problems of Neighborhood Health Centers" is a comprehensive discussion of the management difficulties that persist today. His review describes administrative problems in the areas of authority, power and control; finances; personnel and facilities; and organization of health services. Torrens' analysis includes the following: conflicting and unclear goals for the centers, reflected in contradictory and vague guidelines; conflicting rules enforced by different federal agencies; year-to-year uncertainty about levels of funding and rigidities in the budget systems required; overly optimistic projections of the extent to which the centers could secure third-party reimbursements; too high expectations. Problems of recruitment of staff are linked to the location of the centers, their association with poverty programs, and lack of hospital privileges for physicians.[1] An important addition to Torrens' list is the failure to build in any incentives for administrative efficiency. Because they could count on project grants for a few years, the centers felt no pressure to build operations which could eventually be self-sufficient.

It is hard to determine what are the realistic prospects for influencing those factors which cause administrative problems but which are not tied directly to the defining characteristics of the centers themselves. For example, the training and professional background of physicians are obstacles to implementing the team practice approach in the centers. These obstacles can be addressed directly, but even the most forceful, concerted efforts at reform in these areas would take many years to significantly reduce the debilitating results for the functioning of teams in the health centers. In assessing the efficacy of the health center model, then, how much concomitant reform in other parts of the health care system is it reasonable to assume or to expect? This dilemma is particularly acute in light of the U.S. tradition of reform, combined with a demonstration project scenario that mitigates against learning from the actual experience of the demonstrations and incorporating the learnings into the continuing operations of programs.

Reference

1. For detailed analysis of the employment experience of physicians in neighborhood health centers, see: Hugh H. Tilson "Characteristics of Physicians in OEO Neighborhood Health Centers," *Inquiry 10*,2 (June 1973):27–38; and Hugh H. Tilson "Stability of Physician Employment in Neighborhood Health Centers," *Medical Care 11*,5 (September/October 1973):384–400.

13

Administrative Problems of Neighborhood Health Centers

Paul R. Torrens

The purpose here is to review some of the major administrative problems which affect neighborhood health centers once they are established and functioning. The background for this report is my direct involvement over a three-year period with the creation and operation of one neighborhood health center in New York City, and my more indirect involvement (by way of consultations, site visits, professional meetings, and personal communications) with approximately 20 more centers across the country during the same period of time. The actual issues discussed here were suggested during interviews with more than 25 present or former neighborhood health center staff members from urban projects all over the country (outside New York City); most of those interviewed have also reviewed drafts of this paper and suggested various changes and additions.

General Model of the Neighborhood Health Center

Certain general characteristics are present in most of the neighborhood health centers which have been established around the country. The center itself is usually located within the neighborhood to be served (most often a disadvantaged neighborhood), and it is organized to provide services to a clearly defined geographic area and a clearly defined population (usually the poor residents of that area). Although the health center may be established as a self-contained, independently operating unit, more frequently it is sponsored by some organized health or medical agency. Usually, it is affiliated or associated with a hospital (or series of hospitals) for hospitalization of the center's patients and for completion of tests and procedures not available at the center itself.

The financial support for the center is usually provided by a federal government program, most frequently the OEO. Money is usually granted for a three- to five-year period to help the center get organized and established, with the

Reprinted from *Medical Care* 9, 6 (Nov.-Dec. 1971): 487–497. Introductory paragraphs in the original version of this article on other writings on the health centers have been deleted because they duplicate information included elsewhere in this volume. The original list of references has been retained.

161

hope that payments from Title 18, Title 19, and other third-party payers will provide the center's long-term support.

There is usually a neighborhood board, committee, or health council for the center, which is composed of representatives of the poor and the patients. This body is supposed to ensure participation of the poor in the center's decision-making and may serve as the legally-constituted board for the center or as an advisory body to whatever group is the legal board.

The staff for the center is usually recruited from the resident population of the area to be served, particularly the poorest and most disadvantaged elements of the population. The center usually has a training program to enable the poor to participate effectively in the work of the center; coupled with this, there is usually a program of health career advancement to enable center employees to move into better jobs in the health field.

Regarding medical care itself, the centers usually attempt to deliver general family medical care using a multidisciplinary team. That is, the center's program is not broken down into a multitude of specialty clinics, but instead there is one general program for all patients. (Some centers have one general program for children and one for adults.) An attempt is usually made to enroll families as a single unit and to care for that family as a unit, assigning responsibility for the coordination of the entire family's care to a clearly designated worker or team.

There is usually an attempt to gather the professional staff together into functional teams composed of members of different professional disciplines; these teams are assigned responsibility for a specified number of families or a specified geographic area.

The neighborhood health center usually has its own clinical laboratory, pharmacy, and basic x-ray unit. These facilities handle most of the center's ordinary needs, and the affiliated hospital is called into play only when more specialized tests, x-rays, or medications are required.

All of the neighborhood health centers have developed new categories of health workers for the purpose of increasing the centers' effective contact with their patients. These workers are given a variety of different titles, such as "social health technician," "family health worker," "community health advocate," and "neighborhood health aide." They are also given a widely varying set of duties which may range all the way from simple messenger-companion-nurse's aide duties (such as accompanying patients to the hospital, bathing patients, following up on missed appointments, etc.) to duties which are more like those of a hospital corpsman-assistant physician (such as taking blood pressures and blood specimens, listening to heart and lung sounds, and dispensing some medications).

One striking feature of all neighborhood health centers is their strong commitment to and involvement in social change. In almost everything they do, the staff members of the center are not just interested in improving the physical

health of an individual patient, but are also steadfastly committed to the better-
ment of the patient's total world.

Administrative Problem Areas

Authority, Power, and Control

A primary objective of the neighborhood health center program has been the
redistribution of power so that the community can participate in the operation
of the center which provides it with medical care. It is generally agreed that
there has been at least some redistribution of power, but in many of the centers
the new definitions and locations of power have not been completely crystal-
lized yet and are still unclear. This has frequently resulted in administrative
uncertainty on all levels of the organization.

Probably the most important site of confusion has been the role of the
neighborhood health council. On the one hand, the neighborhood health council usually feels that it should have the ultimate control of all aspects of the
program, since it (the council) represents the people directly affected by the
services and since the center is usually funded by tax funds (which are viewed as
"the people's money"); unfortunately, the health council is usually not an
incorporated entity and has been given neither the mandate nor the machinery
to carry out this important function. On the other hand, the official sponsor
(i.e., hospital, medical school, health department, etc.) usually feels that *it*
should have the final control of the program, since it must bear responsibility
for any fiscal or professional mismanagement.

This confusion is actually built into the structure of the neighborhood
health center program, since the funds are usually assigned to the sponsoring
group or institution, yet it is required that representatives of the poor be
involved in a significant way—without any clear definition of what this
involvement should be. As Feingold has said, "Precisely what was meant by
community participation was never clearly defined by OEO, in the traditional
American method of avoiding conflict through ambiguity. The problem with
this technique is that it avoids conflict at one level only to create it at another."[15]

Since this basic question has not been answered in many of the centers, the
real location of final authority has not been determined. In some centers,
neither the council nor the institutional sponsor *really* agree on the other's role,
so that the limits of each party's authority and responsibility are never clearly
defined. As a result, neither party is able to move forward in a decisive manner,
since each knows that the ground rules governing the distribution of power may
change without advance notice, nullifying or modifying policies and procedures
that had previously been in effect.

This situation is made worse by the knowledge (on the part of both health council and sponsoring institution) that the final authority *really* rests with the governmental agency providing the funds for the center. The sponsoring institution and/or the health council may decide that they wish to make certain expenditures or they may wish to change the center's service program in some important way, but they both know that these steps cannot be taken unless (and until) the governmental funding agency approves the move. Since each health center may relate to two or three levels of the antipoverty bureaucracy (federal, state, and local), to the Children's Bureau, to the Title 19 staff, to Model Cities staff (both federal and local), to a health department (either state or local), and possibly to other governmental or nongovernmental agencies, it is sometimes even difficult to determine which body has the authority to make a final judgment that is binding on all the others.

Uncertainty of this kind on the policy- and the decision-making level, obviously has its effects on the administrative and supervisory staff working in the center. In those instances where there is conflict between the health council and the sponsoring institution (or where there is uncertainty about each party's role), the staff may be given conflicting or even contradictory directions to follow. Sometimes the staff may hesitate or spend great amounts of time trying to bring the conflicting opinions together. Other times, the staff may simply follow the directions of one party to the conflict, only to be angrily confronted by the other party whose directions have been ignored. The end result of this situation is frequently an administrative and supervisory staff that is uncertain of its own position, overly cautious in the exercise of initiative, and quietly resentful of always being "caught in the middle."

In the area of personnel management, this administrative uncertainty is particularly critical. Since the neighborhood health centers attempt to make all employees feel equally important to the success of the program and attempt to encourage free expression of opinions among the center personnel, there will frequently be questions and challenges addressed to the administrative and supervisory staff concerning actions that they have taken or decisions that they have made. If the administrative and supervisory staff are secure in their relations with the health council and the sponsoring institutions, these questions and challenges can be used as an opportunity for positive and constructive action, and can lead to a better and stronger relationship with the center's personnel. On the other hand, if relationships with the council and the sponsoring institution are uncertain or confused, these questions and challenges may simply further emphasize the weakness of the supervisory staff's position, and may further erode their ability to manage their personnel's activities.

Gordon has noted that the presence of conflict within the neighborhood health center provides the skillful administrator with an opportunity for creative activity.[19] While this is undoubtedly true, it should also be noted that many of the sources of conflict are quite beyond the administrator's power to solve, and he is forced to live with the byproducts of conflict without being able to influence their origins.

Financial Problems

Like all other medical care institutions in the United States today, most neighborhood health centers have problems with money. However, many of their problems are unique, arising from the structure and the purposes of the centers themselves.

For one thing, the manner in which the money is made available to the centers causes administrative problems. Most of the neighborhood health centers are supported by granting agencies on a yearly basis. This means that even though funds are tentatively assured for a period of three to five years, the budgets must be resubmitted, defended, and reapproved each year. Obviously, with each resubmission and approval, there is always the possibility of major revisions in the original plan and budget.

With this arrangement, the administrative staff never *really* know how much money they will have to use in the future. This uncertainty serves to discourage the development of any detailed or concrete long-range plans. It also makes it difficult to guarantee professional job candidates that their jobs are secure for several years, when they (and the administrative staff) know that the budget must be reviewed and approved each year; the effect on recruitment and retentions of key staff is obvious.

Another administrative problem with the financing for neighborhood health centers is the relative rigidity and inappropriateness of the line-item budget system in a program that is supposed to be innovative, aggressive, and sensitive to local opportunities for change. Once the yearly budget is approved, it is sometimes not an easy matter for changes in salary or equipment be to made— even minor changes. Indeed, a frequent procedure involves formal application for change that must be approved by the health council, the sponsoring institution, the local representative of the funding agency, and the national office of the funding agency. In the same manner, it is not unusual that all purchases over a certain small amount (sometimes as low as one hundred dollars) must be approved in advance by the funding agency before the purchase can be completed.

The approval procedures can take weeks to complete and can absorb a tremendous amount of administrative time and energy which could be better utilized elsewhere. The system makes sense if it is presumed that the administrators of neighborhood health centers have little experience and need to be controlled by strong guidelines. On the other hand, if the hope is to attract (and retain) competent administrators to neighborhood health centers, the system is not a good one since it places tight limits on the administrator's professional judgment.

These questions are relatively minor (and mechanical in nature) compared to some of the more important philosophical questions about neighborhood health center finances.

For example, it was mentioned earlier that funds are usually given to the neighborhood health centers for a three- to five-year period to help them get started. After that, it is hoped that the centers will secure other funds from Title 18, Title 19, and other third-party payers. This would then allow the grant support to be withdrawn altogether.

Unfortunately, many of the poor and their families do not qualify for any of the present payment mechanisms as they now exist or as they are now administered in many states. This means that the amount of financial support which is available to the neighborhood health centers from third-party payment mechanisms is much less than was originally estimated. Indeed, at the present time it does not appear that the Title 18 and Title 19 programs now in operation can generate enough financial returns to fully support the neighborhood health centers at their present level of operation.

As a result of this bleak long-term financial picture, some of the neighborhood health centers have started to consider opening up their services to non-poor persons in the area who might be able to pay for their services. This would mean that the centers would then have some added financial input to offset the deficits created by dependence on Title 18 and Title 19.

The trend in this direction is not universal by any means. Indeed, quite a few centers vigorously oppose such steps since they feel that the mixture of non-poor patients (who can afford to pay for services) with poor patients (who cannot) will eventually place the poor right back in the disadvantaged position of second-rate citizens receiving a handout—exactly the situation which prompted the development of neighborhood health centers in the first place. In answer to this, the statement is made that unless the neighborhood health centers do attract and serve paying patients, they run the risk of becoming stigmatized as "ghetto" medical programs providing second-rate "charity medicine."

One of the most interesting long-term developments in the neighborhood health centers throughout the country is an increasing amount of interest in national health insurance. Although the interest is not very vigorous nor very well articulated at present, there is a feeling among many knowledgeable people that a national health insurance program is the only ultimate answer to the financial problems of neighborhood health centers.

Personnel and Facilities

If neighborhood health centers are ever to become more than a temporary fad, they must be able to recruit and retain a well-qualified, career-oriented professional staff. They must be able to provide working conditions which are satisfactory to patients and professionally rewarding to staff. In these matters, neighborhood health centers are experiencing serious problems.

As they attempt to recruit high quality professional staff, neighborhood health centers run into several serious obstacles. First of all, the location of the health centers in the depressed, disadvantaged areas of the cities serve as a deterrent to some potential candidates. Next, the bad publicity that *some* antipoverty programs (not necessarily the health programs) have received casts serious doubts on the stability and the sound management of *all* such programs. Finally, the method of funding neighborhood health centers for only one year at a time and the recurrent rumors of the demise of antipoverty programs, both serve to discourage professional candidates who are interested in long-term commitment.

The recruitment of physicians is particularly difficult, since most neighborhood health centers (even those sponsored by hospitals) cannot guarantee active hospital staff appointments (with admitting privileges) for the physician candidates. The medical staffs of many neighborhood health centers are not able to care for their patients during hospitalization, and when prospective candidates learn of this they lose interest in the centers. Kovner's article[22] and Standard's critique of it[35] cast some interesting insights into this problem.

The great psychologic pressures which are present in neighborhood health centers form an additional barrier to recruitment and retention of professional staff. Since the neighborhood health centers are new and somewhat controversial, there has been great pressure for programs to be developed rapidly and show tangible results as soon as possible. Since the neighborhood health centers have been so anxiously awaited by their host communities, there has been great clamor for the centers to move quickly to solve all the health problems of the area. Finally, since the neighborhood health centers operate right at the center of all the economic, racial, and political controversies which are stirring the country today, the staffs are frequently caught in the turmoil surrounding these controversies, even if the centers themselves are not directly involved. A result of all these pressures has been an extremely high rate of turnover among key staff of the health centers.

The selection of a suitable site for the neighborhood health center is a serious problem for many centers. In many of the ghetto areas in which the health centers are trying to locate, it is difficult to find buildings with 20,000 to 30,000 square feet of space (the average amount required by the centers) which are structurally sound and suitable for ambulatory medical care programs. A wide variety of creative alternatives have been developed by ingenious program directors around the country, which have led to centers being launched in former funeral parlors, dairies, grocery stores, warehouses, schools, and other such quarters, but the location of adequate sites for the centers continues to be a problem. Indeed, in a few situations, the centers have been funded for a year or more without any services being delivered due to the inability of finding suitable sites for center operations.

In the future, it may be that the granting agencies which are providing the support for the operation of the centers will also have to provide funds for the construction and renovation of sites. Without this "brick and mortar" support, grants may be made for the development of neighborhood health centers which cannot find a permanent home.

Organization of Health Services

Colombo et al.,[10] in their report, discussed the integration of an OEO health program into a prepaid comprehensive group practice plan and indirectly suggested that it is easier to add one more element into an already existing program than it is to build an entirely new medical care program from nothing. For the neighborhood health centers, the problem of creating an entirely new program is further complicated by the difficulties of implementing such new concepts as "family medical care," "team medical care," and "family health worker."

In "family medical care," it is usually hoped that entire families can be registered as single units, that every member of the family can be placed under the care of the same physician (who will then be responsible for coordinating their total care), and that all members of the family will be brought in as soon as possible for a complete history and physical exam as a baseline for future care. Also, it is usually hoped that there will be some kind of family medical record, which will bring together all the information concerning the family (whether that information be medical, social, or psychologic).

In practice, the ideal has been difficult to achieve. Families do not come in to be registered as single, intact units and they generally do not come in for baseline exams when they are well; instead, they come in as individuals seeking medical care when they are sick and they do not want to spend time giving background information on other members of the family. The different members of the family frequently have widely varying complaints which makes it difficult to place them all under the care of the same physician, and their individual schedules are usually so varied that it is difficult to find a time when many members of the family can come in to see their physician together. Finally, as was mentioned earlier, the family physician frequently cannot provide total care to the family, since he frequently does not have a hospital staff appointment and cannot care for his own patients when they are hospitalized.

Many of these problems could be overlooked if an effective and easily manageable family medical record could be developed to fill the need for medical care coordination; unfortunately, in most centers it has not been developed. First of all, for a family medical record to be optimally effective, it should accurately depict all aspects of the family's condition at the latest possible time and to do this, a large staff of workers would be necessary just to keep track of changes in family composition, social status, living conditions, and the like. Since most neighborhood health centers don't have the staff to keep up with this huge task, the family medical records frequently do not give a complete and up-to-date picture of the families that are under active medical care (to say nothing of those families which may have registered but never sought treatment).

Also, for a family medical record to be maximally useful, it should be readily available to all staff who need it, whether they be in the hospital, in the center, or in the field. In practice, however, just when one member of the staff needs the family record in the hospital to care for one member of the family, another member of the staff will be using it at the center or in the field to care for another family member. It has been suggested that duplicates be made, but this involves an awesome amount of paper-handling. It has also been suggested that various portions of the family medical record (for example, the records of each individual member) be detachable, but then the family record is no longer a complete picture of the entire family.

Implementation of the "team medical care" concept has proven equally difficult. In the original design, most of the neighborhood health centers allocated their staffs to multidisciplinary teams with a fixed composition of professional and nonprofessional staff in each team. In theory, each team was to have a "team leader" (who could be any member of the team) and a weekly team conference would be held to discuss the cases of the entire team.

In practice, the team concept has run into some significant problems. For one thing, it has been found that the original idea of a number of teams with the same fixed composition serving the same number of patients may not be appropriate to a particular situation. One team may deal with more children and young mothers, for example, and may require more services from a pediatrician and an obstetrician, while another team may deal more with older adults and may need more services from an internist, a physiotherapist, or a public health nurse. In practice, many of the centers seem to be drifting away from teams with rigidly fixed compositions of professional, and non-professional staff; instead, they are developing *ad hoc* teams whose composition and function are governed by the requirements of the particular situation.

Communication within the team is also a problem. Members of the various professional groups (particularly the physicians) frequently feel more comfortable relating to other members of their professional group than they do with other members of their particular team; as a result, communication between members of different teams is sometimes better than communication within the team itself.

Sometimes, also, the team members who have the most pertinent information about a family's condition (i.e., the neighborhood health worker) are also the ones who are the least skilled in verbal or written communications; this frequently means that the impact of their information is markedly diminished or lost entirely. Originally, it was hoped that the weekly team conference would improve communication among members of the team, but this has not been the case; the team conference has proven to be a useful educational and morale-building device, but it is not a very good way to deal with the intricate problems of large numbers of patients or families in any detail. Hopefully, some new means of internal communications will be developed which will allow everyone on the team to be well-informed about the progress of all the team's patients without wasting valuable time in fruitless meetings and discussions of limited numbers of cases.

The "family health worker" (or whatever he may be called in the different programs) constitutes the brightest spot in the operation of most neighborhood health centers. Although there has been considerable variation in the actual role and function of the family health worker from program to program, there is general agreement that this new category of worker is an invaluable asset to medical care. The effective utilization of the family health worker allows the programs to penetrate into their communities in a manner that would otherwise be impossible, find patients who would not otherwise make contact with good medical care, and follow the progress of such patients over a prolonged period of time more effectively than was ever possible before.

However, the creation of this new category of worker is not without its problems either. How should candidates be recruited for this position? What should their training be? What functions should they carry out, alone or with others? When they are ready for promotion or assumption of new responsibilities, what are their opportunities for advancement, for further training, for certification? How do you give a previously untrained member of the poverty population the technical skills he needs to function, without making him so much of a professional that he loses his essential contact with an empathy for the fellow members of his community?

In the implementation of all these new concepts, the administrators of neighborhood health centers are eventually going to have to ask themselves: do these concepts really work? Do they really deliver better medical care than the more traditional approaches, and if they do, how do we measure that difference in terms of results and costs? In the beginning, it was assumed that the neighborhood health centers *should* be established, that they would be expensive to establish and operate, and that their newness prevented any meaningful examination of costs with other medical care mechanisms; as a result, relatively little concrete data are available on the neighborhood health center's effectiveness in relation to costs. Administrators of neighborhood health centers have not yet had to be coldly analytical about the benefits and the costs of their new programs, but someday soon, they will have to begin. Indeed, the future of their centers may depend upon it.

References

1. Abrams, H.K., and Snyder, R.A.: Health center seeks to bridge the gap between hospital and neighborhood. *Mod. Hosp. 110*:324, 1968.

2. Bamburger, L., and English, J.T.: Background, context, and significant issues in neighborhood health center programs. *Milbank Mem. Fund Quart. 46*:289, 1968.
3. Bates, J.E., Lieberman, H.M., and Powell, R.N.: Provision for health care in the ghetto: the family health team. *Amer. J. Public Health 60*:1222, 1970.
4. Bellin, S., Geiger, H.J., and Gibson, C.D.: Impact of ambulatory health care services on the demand for hospital beds. *New Eng. J. Med. 280:*808, 1969.
5. Berry, T.: Recent federal legislation: its meaning for public health. *Amer. J. Public Health 56*:582, 1966.
6. Bishop, E., and Christensen, H.M.: Dentists and the war on poverty: a discussion on neighborhood health centers. *J. Amer. Dent. Ass. 75*:45, 1967.
7. Bograd, H.M.: The role of the lawyer in the neighborhood medical care demonstration. *Milbank Mem. Fund Quart. 46*:334, 1968.
8. Brooke, R.: An audit of the quality of care in social medicine. *Milbank Mem. Fund Quart. 46*:328, 1968.
9. Brown, H.J.: Delivery of personal health services and medical services for the poor. Concessions or prerogatives? *Milbank Mem. Fund Quart. 46*:203, 1968.
10. Columbo, T.J., Saward, E.W., and Greenlick, M.R.: The integration of an OEO health program into a prepaid comprehensive group practice plan. *Amer. J. Public Health 59*:475, 1969.
11. Davis, M., and Tranquada, R.: A sociological evaluation of the Watts neighborhood health center. *Med. Care 7*:105, 1969.
12. Elinson, J., and Herr, C.E.A.: A sociomedical view of neighborhood health centers. *Med. Care 8*:97, 1970.
13. English, J.T.: Office of economic opportunity health programs. *Inquiry 5*:43, 1968.
14. Fein, R.: An economist's view of the neighborhood health center as a social institution. *Med. Care 8*:104, 1970.
15. Feingold, E.: A political scientist's view of the neighborhood health center as a new social institution. *Med. Care 8*:108, 1970.
16. Geiger, H.J.: The neighborhood health center: education of the faculty in preventive medicine. *Arch. Environ. Health 14*:912, 1967.
17. Gibson, C.D.: The neighborhood health center: the primary unit of health care. *Amer. J. Public Health 58*:1188, 1968.
18. Goldberg, G.A., Trowbridge, F.L., and Buxbaum, R.C.: Issues in the development of neighborhood health centers. *Inquiry 6*:37, 1969.
19. Gordon, J.B.: The politics of community medicine projects: a conflict analysis. *Med. Care 7*:419, 1970.
20. Hatch, J.: Community shares in policy decisions for rural health center. *Hospitals 43*:109, 1969.
21. Hope, M.: Building an Environmental Health Component into Community Health Centers. Presented at the session on The Role of the Environmentalist in Building the Urban Community, APHA 97th Annual Meeting, Philadelphia, Pa., Nov. 10, 1969.

22. Kovner, A.R., Katz, G., Kahane, S., and Sheps, C.: Relating a neighborhood health center to a general hospital: a case study. *Med. Care 7*:118, 1969.

23. Lashof, J.: The health care team in the mile square area in Chicago. *Bull. N.Y. Acad. Med. 44*:1363, 1968.

24. ____: Chicago project provides health care and career opportunities. *Hospitals 43*:105, 1969.

25. Lepper, M.H., Lashof, J.C., Pisani, A., and Shannon, I.: An approach to reconciling the poor and the system. *Inquiry 5*:37, 1968.

26. Light, H.: Social work in neighborhood health centers. *Bull. N.Y. Acad. Med. 44*:1378, 1968.

27. Morehead, M.A.: Evaluating quality of medical care in neighborhood health center programs of the office of Economic Opportunity. *Med. Care 8*:118, 1970.

28. Parker, A.W.: Problems Facing Consumers serving on Policy-making Boards of Health Centers. Presented at the Public Health Education Section, Contributed Papers Session, APHA 97th Annual Meeting, Philadelphia, Pa., Nov. 10, 1969.

29. Richardson, W.C.: Measuring the urban poor's use of physician services in response to illness episodes. *Med. Care 8*:132, 1970.

30. Robertson, L.S., Kosa, J., Alpert, J.L., and Heagarty, M.C.: Anticipated acceptance of neighborhood health clinics by the urban poor. *JAMA 205*:815, 1968.

31. Salber, E.J., Feldman, J.J., and Offenbacher, H.G.: Characteristics of Patients Registered for Service in a Neighborhood Health Center. Presented at the Session on Child Health Services, APHA 97th Annual Meeting, Philadelphia, Pa., Nov. 10, 1969.

32. Shannon, I.: Nursing Services at Mile Square Health Center of Presbyterian-St. Luke's Hospital. Presented at the Session on New Community Settings and Approaches to Patient Care, APHA 97th Annual Meeting, Philadelphia, Pa., Nov. 10, 1969.

33. Sparer, R.: Baseline Data for Planning and Implementing Local Neighborhood Health Center Programs. Presented at the session on Local and State Data for Health Planning, APHA 97th Annual Meeting, Philadelphia, Pa., Nov. 10, 1969.

34. Sparer, G., Dines, G.B., and Smith, D.: Consumer participation in OEO-assisted neighborhood health centers. *Amer. J. Public Health 60*:1091, 1970.

35. Standard, S.: Comment on the neighborhood health center and the general hospital. *Med. Care 8*:252, 1970.

36. Stoeckle, J.D., and Candib, L.M.: The neighborhood health centers—reform ideas of yesterday and today. *New Eng. J. Med. 280*:1385, 1969.

37. Tranquada, R.E.: A health center for Watts. *Hospitals 41*:42, 1967.

38. Warner, A.L.: Problems in delivering comprehensive health care to the inner city. *Arch. Environ. Health 17*:383, 1968.

39. Wise, H.B.: Montefiore hospital neighborhood medical care demonstration. *Milbank Mem. Fund Quart. 46*:297, 1968.

40. Wise, H.B., Levin, L.S., and Kurahara, R.T.: Community development and health education—community organization as a health tactic. *Milbank Mem. Fund Quart. 46*:325, 1968.
41. Wise, H.B., Torrey, E.F., McDade, A., Perry, G., and Bograd, H.: The family health worker. *Amer. J. Public Health 58*:1828, 1968.
42. Zahn, S.: Neighborhood medical care demonstration training program. *Milbank Mem. Fund Quart. 46*:344, 1968.

Part VII
Costs and Financing

Introduction

Looking at the performance of the neighborhood health centers in terms of the cost of services which they have achieved is critically important because prime criticisms of the centers have been that they cost too much and are inefficient in their use of resources. It seems obvious and inevitable that health services should cost more for poor persons who are sicker as a group than persons able to obtain care from other sources.

Most observers would agree that the health centers badly need improved management and that they can cut their costs by tightening up their administration. A substantial problem in the financial management of the centers has been that their funding through project grants built in no incentives for efficiency. Some health center administrators looked ahead to the day they knew would come of firm pressures to become more self-sufficient, and they therefore actually turned down money for services they would be unable to sustain a few years later. But this posture was rare. A major focus of the HEW office which has become responsible for all of the OEO centers as well as ones started with HEW money is to encourage better management of their operations. Nonetheless, much of the criticism of the costs performance of the neighborhood centers ignores or denies the fact that high quality health services for the poor are bound to cost somewhat more than they do for persons who are better off. They ignore also the rather impressive costs record of at least some of the centers.

The article below by Gerald Sparer and Arne Anderson, "Cost of Services at Neighborhood Health Centers," is the only systematic study to date of this subject. Their conclusions contradict critics of the costs of the centers. They conclude that the costs of medical care at six of the OEO centers are competitive with other institutional providers, including outpatient departments and clinics of hospitals, and large prepaid group practices.

A major problem in comparing service costs at the neighborhood health centers with the costs of visits to physicians in other contexts is that the neighborhood centers deliver a whole host of services over and above those normally available elsewhere. These supportive services—extensive social services, outreach, training, health education, environmental health units, and so forth—are integral to the purposes and success of the centers. It is also extremely difficult to compute unit costs in an institution like a neighborhood health center. How, for example, does one calculate the portion of costs of the various departments of a health center which should be included in computing an average visit cost?

In "An Economist's View of the Neighborhood Health Center as a New Social Institution," Rashi Fein discusses the difficulties of implementing traditional economists' routes to evaluating the health centers. He looks at the health

177

centers as a financing approach. He points out, "Part of the success of the neighborhood health center can be attributed to the fact that it offers care to those in a specific geographic area who need care and it does so by removing the income barrier." Fein argues for univeral health insurance as a more desirable financing mechanism for the centers. He concludes that the competitive advantage or disadvantage of the centers can only be known once national health insurance is a reality and consumers have the freedom to choose where to go for service.

14 Cost of Services at Neighborhood Health Centers—A Comparative Analysis

Gerald Sparer and Arne Anderson

A major operational objective of the OEO-assisted Neighborhood Health Center Projects is to test and develop a broad-scale, community-based, innovative health-care delivery system, offering employment opportunities for community residents while providing good quality care at a reasonable cost.[1] Articles have appeared suggesting that the cost of care delivered at health centers is high. A recent *New York Times* article[2] reports, ". . . the Martin Luther King Health Center in the Bronx (Montefiore Hospital) spends $75 per patient visit, far more than it would cost to treat a person in a doctor's office." In the January, 1971, issue of Medical Economics, an open letter expressed concern about the apparent plushness of some Neighborhood Health Center facilities in Philadelphia. The article cited the cost of "medical encounters," including medical doctor, nurse, laboratory, pharmacy, x-ray and overhead, ranging from $14 to $28, as evidence of "sky-high costs." The American Medical Association News indicated an approved Medi-Cal rate of $37 for one center, and an annual per person cost of $235.[3,4]

Dr. Mildred Morehead, of the Albert Einstein College of Medicine, recently stated that "a goal of providing care with costs similar to or less than the private practice system is to me totally unrealistic . . . especially when services are delivered to persons previously deprived of medical care and who have been acknowledged as having higher chronic illness rates and other severe morbidity."

Since their inception under OEO sponsorship, there have been many such articles and letters about the operations of the Neighborhood Health Centers. The centers have attracted an unusual amount of attention possibly because of the promise that they hold in the solution of health-care delivery problems of the nation. With the recent national interest in alternative forms of national health-insurance schemes, many proposals place special emphasis on prepaid group practice and care for the low-income population, and attention focuses rather sharply on the Neighborhood Health Center experience. Although early interest in the Neighborhood Health Centers has included the quality of care provided, the use of services and the cost of providing those services, cost of services have recently received considerable attention. Two reasons for this may be the sharply escalating cost of health care in the nation as a whole (an increase

Reprinted from *New England Journal of Medicine* 286, 23 (June 8, 1972): 1241–1245.

of over $28 billion in health-care expenditures in a five-year period) and the increasing share of the health-care dollars assumed by the federal government. The federal share of health expenditures amounted to 13 per cent in 1966; by 1970 this proportion had reached 24 per cent.

Articles previously cited concerning cost of services of health centers can be misleading. Dollar amounts are frequently presented without the benefit of a detailed explanation of the types of services provided by the center and the costs included in the calculation. Generally, the information reported clouds rather than clarifies the issues of cost. The purpose of this article is to present the findings of an intensive two-year cost study conducted at six Neighborhood Health Centers using a uniform cost-finding methodology.[5] The findings presented compare the costs of providing units of services, as well as the cost per person at each center, and relate these findings to policy issues being discussed in connection with national health insurance, Health Maintenance Organization (HMO) development and other areas of health-care organization and financing.

Also suggested are uniform definitions for cost categories, levels of health care and service activities.

Cost-Finding History

A review of the fiscal, accounting and budget operations of the Neighborhood Health Centers during late 1967 and early 1968 indicated that none were routinely collecting cost data that would aid in the setting of a unit or per capita rate for health-care services. Cost-finding methodology for ambulatory health care had not been established, and cost analyses were rarely made. This situation differed sharply from the area of hospital cost finding, in which the American Hospital Association had developed and prepared cost-finding methods for hospitals. Drawing upon these cost-finding methods and adding specific emphasis on determining the cost of ambulatory health-care services at the health centers, the Office of Economic Opportunity invited six health centers to participate in the development, test and installation of cost-finding methods for ambulatory care.[a] A general description of the method was

---

[a]We are indebted to the project directors and fiscal and statistical staffs of the six health centers for co-operation and assistance, particularly, Dr. Joyce Lashoff, Mile Square Health Center (Presbyterian–St. Lukes Hospital, Chicago, Ill.). and Mr. Abraham Miller, Martin Luther King Health Center (Montefiore Hospital, Bronx, N.Y.), for help in developing the cost-finding methodology and in the analysis of data collected. The following staff members through their individual contribution at each project made this development effort meaningful and valuable: Mr. Sorin, Mr. Seacat and Mr. Gutman, of the Gouverneur Health Center Service Program: Mr. Ron Brook of the Martin Luther King Health Center; Mrs. Andrea Henry and Mr. George Hoffberg of Mile Square Health Center; Dr. Roger Cohn and Mr. Alfonso Irving of the Columbia Point Health Center, Boston, Mass.; Mr. Jack McVey, Mrs. Blanche Shrader and Mrs. Margaret Godby, of the Mountaineer Family Health Plan, Beckley, W. Va.; and Dr. Len H. Andrus and Mr. Lee S. Roberts, of King City, Cal.

recently issued as a manual, Cost Finding System for Comprehensive Health Service Projects. Also available for distribution is a detailed instructional manual helpful as a guide to the use of the cost finding and reporting system.[6]

The cost-finding method attempts to define units of care common to ambulatory health services without regard to the type of financing mechanism used for payment or the organizational philosophy and practice and links these units with the appropriate dollar expenses for a designated period of time.

Cost-Finding Methodology

The study was initiated in early 1968. The six centers were selected for study by means of three basic criteria: each center had been visited by a team of specialists and was found to be operating in a manner consistent with program guidelines;[1] the centers had at least several years of operating experience, and the volume of service was already high or building rapidly; the centers selected were a cross-section of a variety of Neighborhood Health Centers, including one large and one small urban center, two rural centers; previously existing institutions and those initiated with OEO assistance (table 14-1).

The cost-finding data used in the study were generated from cost-accounting systems designed and structured to capture the complete cost for each of the functional cost categories analyzed (medical, laboratory, x-ray, pharmacy, etc.). Carefully prepared definitions of functional costs were uniformly applied in collection of the cost data at each of the projects. These costs were then linked to the appropriate unit measure of service (medical encounters, laboratory test, x-ray examination, numbers of patients and persons eligible) to produce the

Table 14-1
General Characteristics of Centers Included in the Study

Center	No. of Clients	Annual Volume of Physician Encounters	Fiscal-Yr 1970 Budget	Urban or Rural
			$X10^6$	
Gouverneur, NY	35,000	155,055	5.3	Urban
Montefiore, NY	30,000	78,526	5.4	Urban
Mile Square, Chicago, Ill	17,000	56,258	3.1	Urban
Columbia Point, Boston, Mass	5,800	26,879	1.5	Urban
Beckley, W Va	6,500	20,500	1.6	Rural & urban
King City, Cal	12,000*	—	1.2	Rural

*Estimated.

unit and per capita costs. The system also suggests grouping the primary functional service categories into five increasingly comprehensive levels of care that help compare services among providers.

Levels of Health Care

The first level—primary clinical medical care—consisted of four basic units of care: medical, x-ray, laboratory and pharmacy. The second—primary medical care—included the preceding (first) level of care, plus home health and mental health. At the third level—primary comprehensive medical care—the preceding (second) level of care was combined with supporting health activities (social and community services, training, transportation, community organization and research and evaluation). The fourth level—primary comprehensive health care—comprised the preceding (third) level of care plus dental care. Finally, comprehensive health care, the fifth level, combined the preceding (fourth) level of care with hospitalization and nursing-home care (Extended Care Facility). These levels of care are additive for analysis of the comprehensive health care provided by neighborhood health centers; they may vary for other providers. For example, many prepaid group-practice plans might only include the first level, primary clinical medical care, and the fifth, hospitalization and nursing-home care.

The levels of care and unit and per capita cost data shown in tables 14-1 to 14-5 include direct costs plus the distribution of two sets of indirect cost, which are important to a complete understanding of the information presented. These indirect costs are as follows: allocable costs, which include such costs as medical records, employee benefits and certain consumable supplies; and general service costs, which include administration, housekeeping and maintenance, space and facilities, overhead charges for administration and other miscellaneous items.

The cost-finding and cost-reporting system is actually reflecting expenses—it measures the costs that are used during the particular period. The term "functional cost" is used as synonymous with a replacement for "expense."

Most of the time, in project operations, the expenditure, cost and expense occur simultaneously and are in effect the same. The major difference between expenditures and cost as reflected by the cost-finding system occur in the reporting of fixed and movable assets and donated services and supplies. In the cost-finding system developed for comprehensive health-services projects, assets are capitalized, and the functional cost represents a portion of the useful life of the asset, with the use of depreciation technics to arrive at this figure. Where services or supplies have been donated the value of these services or supplies is imputed as an estimated dollar amount with the use of fair market guides and is included in the appropriate functional cost category receiving the benefits of the services.

Findings

A review of the dollar expenses of each of the general functional categories indicates that about 45 per cent of the direct costs of the centers went to provide primary clinical medical services, the basic ambulatory health care; about 15 per cent went toward supporting health activities such as transportation, training and social and community activities, and an average 25 per cent was spent for general services and administrative support. The remaining expenses were for dental services along with minor amounts for medical records.

After allocable costs and general-service costs have been distributed to the direct health categories and to all the supporting health activities, a consistent pattern emerges. That is, about 55 per cent of the costs are directed toward primary clinical medical care in both urban and rural settings, whereas supporting health activity services average about 18 per cent in the urban centers and 24 per cent in the rural centers studied (table 14–2).

Average Unit Costs

The average unit costs, a first clue to efficiency and productivity, help answer questions about the relative efficiency of neighborhood health centers.

The average visit cost for primary clinical medical care in 1970 ranges from about $22 at King City to about $37 at Montefiore, with rates showing an upward drift between the two years to between 3 per cent and 15 per cent (table 14–3). Some of this increase is attributed to routine salary increases and other inflationary pressures.

In New York City, the approved rates for Medicaid reimbursement for an

Table 14-2
Percentage Distribution of Costs at Selected Neighborhood Health Centers by Level of Care,* 1970

Center	Percentage Distribution				
	Primary Medical Care	Home Health & Mental Health	Sup- porting Health	Dental	Total
Gouverneur	74.8	8.0	10.2	7.0	100.0
Montefiore	53.1	14.1	21.6	11.2	100.0
Mile Square	52.4	18.3	15.2	14.1	100.0
Columbia Point	56.9	7.2	14.9	21.0	100.0
Beckley	52.3	17.4	23.0	7.3	100.0
King City	66.7	1.4	25.0	6.9	100.0

*Allocable & general-service cost have been distributed.

outpatient visit vary, depending on the hospital, but a frequent range for a voluntary hospital in the downstate area is about \$30 to \$40 per visit.[7] Thus, on an average unit-cost basis, the neighborhood health center is considered competitive on unit costs to other alternative institutional providers. Morehead and Donaldson have shown in their quality-of-care comparison study[8] that the neighborhood health center scores somewhat higher than teaching-hospital outpatient departments, suggesting that the neighborhood health center offers a good product at competitive costs.

Medical Encounters

When the cost of the physician encounter alone is considered (a physician encounter is defined as a face-to-face meeting between a patient and a physician in which some health care is given to the patient), the cost ranges from a low of about \$16 at King City to \$28 at Montefiore, with the average at about \$23 per medical encounter (table 14-3). This figure compares with the \$22 estimated for 1970 by both Kaiser–Portland and Group Health Association, Washington, D.C.

When all professional and medical encounters are used—including physician, nurse practitioner or a nurse acting as a primary provider—the average costs per encounter dropped to a low of \$14.12 at King City and under \$22 at all other centers except Columbia Point (table 14-4). At Columbia Point, a small decrease

Table 14-3
Unit Cost of Services Including General-Services Costs 1970

Center	Annual Average Cost ($)				
	Primary Clinical Medical Care[*†]	Physician[*] Encounters	Laboratory Tests	X-Ray Study	Prescriptions
Gouverneur	25.44	19.36	1.67	9.38	1.34
Montefiore	36.74	28.38	1.27	17.05	§
Mile Square	32.97	22.85	3.71	14.93	2.49
Columbia Point	33.17	25.66	2.83	§	5.74
Beckley	35.66	24.16	1.63	7.70	3.24
King City[‡]	21.56	16.09	5.89	22.56	4.20

[*]Only physician encounters included.

[†]Includes medical, laboratory, x-ray & pharmacy costs; individual items listed for each center do not total to primary clinical medical cost given because a visit may not always include all services or same quantity of each service.

[‡]Data based on reports covering period of 7/1/70 to 12/31/70.

§ Not applicable.

was experienced in the number of services provided in 1970, whereas cost increased.

Volume and services patterns obviously affect unit costs. Gouverneur, with about 155,000 physician medical encounters and 188,000 physician and non-physician medical encounters, more consistently shows low unit costs (table 14-4).

The influence of both volume and service style is best observed at Montefiore, where almost ¼ of medical encounters, 24,000 out of 102,000, are provided by nurses and nurse practitioners. Their cost declines from $28.38 to $21.79 when the influence of these nonphysician medical providers is included. The previous analysis of unit-cost data of medical-care services using the two different denominators (physician encounters and physician and nonphysician encounters) points out the need for additional development of more refined methodology. At present, the use of physician encounters as the divisor or denominator in the calculation of unit costs of medical-care services, which includes all expenses connected with the operating medical-care services, over-states the unit costs of medical care (table 14-3). The use of all medical encounters (physician, nurse and other primary providers) in table 14-4 has a tendency to understate the unit cost.

As analyses of project costs continue, additional efforts are being made to refine the reporting of nonphysician encounters, and attempts are being made to identify and analyze costs associated with physician encounters in a more exacting way.

Limitations and Related Issues

In addition to the issues raised regarding the comparison of the types of services,

Table 14-4
Cost in Dollars per Unit of Medical Service According to Type of Encounters in Neighborhood Health Centers, 1970

Center	Physician Encounters		Physician Encounters & Nonphysician	
	Number	Unit Cost	Number	Unit Cost
Gouverneur	155,055	19.36	188,237	15.95
Montefiore	78,526	28.38	102,241	21.79
Mile Square	56,258	22.85	62,109	20.69
Columbia Point	26,879	25.66	27,578	25.01
Beckley	20,500	24.16	24,589	20.14
King City	36,393	16.09	41,487	14.12

in discussion of costs of health care, other factors must be comparable. These include the quality of care, the utilization rate, which might be affected by the client population characteristics related to age, sex and illness (needs), patient understanding of health care and the system characteristics (accessibility, patient handling, manpower utilization, etc.).

Each of the six centers studied had scores above average for OEO-assisted Neighborhood Health Centers on quality of care as reported by Dr. Morehead in her paper comparing Neighborhood Health Centers to other providers.[8] Utilization data vary from 4.0 to 4.6 physician encounters per year.[9] This cost analysis is limited to ambulatory-care costs, because costs, charges or even utilization data on inpatient hospital services are not available.

Per Capita Costs and Prepaid Group Practice

A frequent question asked regarding provision of health-care services to low-income persons is: "Why not contract with Kaiser, HIP and other existing pre-payment group practices to provide these services?" These groups are nationally recognized as representing an acceptable standard of cost and quality of care, measured most often in terms of premium and utilization rates.

The Office of Economic Opportunity has, in fact, experimented with these providers through awards to four such prepayment group practices, Health Insurance Plan of New York, Kaiser at Fontana and Portland, and Group Health of Puget Sound.

Only at Kaiser Portland are there actual experienced utilization data.[10] Available data from the group-practice plans are based on the negotiated premium rates for primary clinical medical care plus budgeted amounts for additional nursing support, home care, mental health and supporting activities. The negotiated budgets for these prepaid group practices for the three basic services (medical, laboratory and x-ray) range from $74 to $93 per person annually. When pharmacy is added (a benefit not usually fully covered by these plans) the range increases to $83 and $111 for what is equivalent to primary clinical medical care in Neighborhood Health Centers as shown in table 14-5. Addition of other support components brings the project cost level of the primary comprehensive medical-care package for these prepaid group practices to range from $164 to $241 per person per year.

The similar cost data for Neighborhood Health Centers would range from $96 to $153 for primary clinical medical care, with only Columbia Point exceeding $133. The costs of primary comprehensive medical care would range from about $134 to $233—an apparent competitive advantage for the neighborhood health centers (table 14-5).

Table 14-5
Annual Cost per Registered Person at Selected Neighborhood Health Centers According to Level of Care, 1970

Level	Gouver-neur	Monte-fiore	Mile Square	Columbia Point	Beckley
Primary clinical medical care	108	96	106	153	133
+ Home health mental health & other health	11	26	25	19	44
= Primary medical care	$119	$122	$131	$172	$177
+ Supporting health activities	15	39	25	57	56
= Primary comprehensive medical care	$134	$161	$156	$229	$233
+ Dental	10	20	25	40	18
= Primary comprehensive health care	$144	$181	$181	$269	$251

Implications—Are These Costs Replicable?

The study indicates that mature Neighborhood Health Centers of reasonable size can operate complex systems efficiently. Probably, the smaller centers, centers in temporary quarters, and centers struggling with start-up administrative problems cannot become competitive until their population exceeds 10,000 registrants. When the center is serving less than 10,000 people, the administrative support, in addition to the basic facility cost, becomes too heavy a burden to carry if a competitive cost level is to be achieved.

For policy purposes, particularly in view of the rising emphasis on insurance and other prepayment methods of financing health care, it is useful to answer the following questions based on the information available in this comparative analysis:

What does it cost to deliver health care to low-income families? The cost for Neighborhood Health Centers primary comprehensive health care range from $144 to $270 per person per year, with a clear cost advantage to the larger-scale center.

Is the Neighborhood Health Center viable and competitive as a health-care delivery system? From the standpoint of the quality of services, volume and use of services and costs, the Neighborhood Health Center is viable and cost efficient as compared with other providers.

Do the Neighborhood Health Centers' objectives of multiple social and health services interfere with delivery of health care at competitive cost? The great complexity of bringing about a new health-care institution, with broad community service objectives, is apparent, but they have not interfered with the provision of good clinical medical care at costs competitive with established major prepayment groups.

Are the supporting health services provided by Neighborhood Health Centers, which are beyond those usually offered by other institutional health providers, so costly as to make them economically unfeasible for application to a large number of low-income persons? This question is difficult to answer at present. Special studies are needed. The issue here is not whether these items are part of medical care but whether they will be part of medical care to large numbers of persons who have abundant needs for such services.

References

1. Sparer, G., Johnson, J.: Evaluation of OEO Neighborhood Health Centers, *Am. J. Public Health 61*:931–942, 1971.
2. Dilemma in health care: rising cost and demand. *New York Times*, September 13, 1971, pp. 1, 28.
3. OEO Centers' contribution still uncertain. *Am. Med. News*, May 24, 1971, pp. 10–13.
4. Daschbach, R.J.: OEO Neighborhood Center. *Am. Med. News*, June 28, 1971, p. 4.
5. Cost-Finding System for Comprehensive Health Service Projects. Washington, D.C., Office of Economic Opportunity, Office of Health Affairs, January, 1917.
6. Comprehensive Health Services Cost Finding and Reporting System Manual (OEO Manual 6128–1). Washington, D.C., Office of Economic Opportunity, November, 1971.
7. Hospital Rates for Period January 1, 1970–June 30, 1970 (Hospital Memorandum Series 70–4). Albany, New York, State of New York Department of Health, January 26, 1970.
8. Morehead, M.A., Donaldson, R.: Comparisons between OEO Neighborhood Health Centers and other health care providers of rating of the quality of care. Presented before the Medical Care Section, Annual Meeting of the American Public Health Association, Houston, Texas, October 25–29, 1970.
9. Strauss, M., Sparer, G.: Basis utilization experience of OEO Comprehensive Health Services projects—1968 data. Presented before the Research on Health Planning Processes and Techniques Section, Annual Meeting of the American Public Health Association, Houston, Texas, October 25–29, 1970.
10. Colombo, T.J., Saward, E.W., Greenlick, M.R.: The integration of an OEO health program into a prepaid comprehensive group practice plan. *Am. J. Public Health 59*:641–650, 1969.

15

An Economist's View of the Neighborhood Health Center as a New Social Institution

Rashi Fein

Some time ago I was speaking with a friend in the Office of Economic Opportunity in Washington. His responsibilities involve neighborhood health centers. I mentioned to him that I was to appear on this program to speak on something like, "An Economist Looks at Neighborhood Health Centers." He laughed and said, "But no economist has." I rather think that he is right.

It is not my intention to report to you on my thorough examination of neighborhood health centers in general or even of a particular neighborhood health center. I have not undertaken that research. Rather I intend to share with you some views on the possible strengths and weaknesses of such centers as models in the medical care spectrum.

I am certain that an economist's evaluation of neighborhood health centers is generally expected to assess the input and output relationships, what the economist would term "the production function." The evaluation would focus on the delivery of medical care. It would look at the use of personnel and equipment on the one hand, the number of visits (which serve as a proxy for health effect) and other such measures on the other hand. In so doing, the evaluation would follow rather traditional cost effectiveness approaches and might even move to cost benefit analysis. In the latter, the attempt would be made to quantify the inputs and assign dollar values to them and to quantify the benefits and assign dollar values to these outputs. When that is done, the ratio of benefits to costs would be computed and it would be determined whether that ratio was greater than or smaller than 1.0. If the ratio were smaller than 1.0, presumably this project (and similar projects) should not be supported. Alternatively, were the ratio higher than 1.0, the project would be worthwhile. Whether it should be supported, however, would depend on how this project compared with alternative projects, on a priority ranking (determined by the difference between benefits and costs).

I do not propose to spend time on a careful examination of the validity of this kind of evaluation or on the problems that one encounters in undertaking it. Nonetheless, it is useful to remind ourselves that such evaluations are extremely difficult to mount. There are conceptual problems involved in the selection of

Reprinted from *Medical Care* 8, 2 (March-April 1970): 104–107. Presented at a session sponsored by the Medical Care Section of the 97th Annual Meeting of the American Public Health Association, Philadelphia, November 1969.

189

an appropriate discount rate, in the development of adequate proxy measures, etc. There are basic problems connected with the fact that most health measures used in such analysis tend to focus on health conditions that impinge on income and thus ignore the benefits involved in the elimination of pain and of worry. There are extremely difficult problems connected with the fact that we should, at this stage, be much more interested in understanding the differences between centers than in arriving at some national benefit cost ratio (for though this program may be federally funded, it is not a federal program). There are additional problems connected with the fact that the inputs that the economist is likely to examine will overlook such things as community participation, the role of particular individuals, etc., all of which are important in determining the success or failure of a particular center. Indeed, community participation is both an input and an output. There, also, are problems connected with the fact that the economist's measure of output is likely to ignore nonhealth outputs such as the impact on the community, the role the neighborhood health center may play in addressing nonhealth problems, etc. (measures which are important and which, by the way, also inflate costs). Finally, the economist's assessment is not likely to look at the processes at work in a neighborhood health center. In essence, what I am saying, therefore, is that much of what economists are expected to do is far too narrow, and that even within the narrow range of problems that economists are expected to address, conceptual issues remain.

It should be understood that this is not a plea for ignorance or for inactivity on the research side. Rather, it suggests the importance of having various disciplines participate in the evaluation effort. It does attempt to alert all of us, however, to the fact that the economist's evaluation is likely to be given more weight than it deserves if only because it is most often a quantitative evaluation. Some persons are very impressed with quantitative evaluations particularly if the numbers are computed in some esoteric manner and even more so if they involve terms preceded by a dollar sign.

I do not intend to dwell at length on that kind of evaluation. It has its place, and many of you are quite familiar with this type of examination or alternatively with the simpler and perhaps, therefore, less adequate (but also less dangerous) evaluation of the manpower requirements in a neighborhood health center, a subject of some considerable interest because of its possible implications for the total health sector.

It seems to me, however, that the neighborhood health center represents much more than a model of delivery mechanism. I am aware that it is in those terms that it is usually commented upon. There are those who are most excited by the mechanism, there are others who say that it is a very expensive way to deliver care. There are still others who say that while the latter may be true, it at least represents a new departure. Given this approach, some would like to extend the neighborhood health center concept across the land while others are more skeptical. But even to the economist, let alone to other social scientists, the neighborhood health center should represent more than a delivery mechanism. While the issue is often ignored, it also represents a *financing* approach and I should like to speak on that subject. I do so in part because the efficiency of the neighborhood health center as a deliverer of medical care is a subject with which we are all by now familiar (and on which this economist can bring no new results). I also do so because it seems to me that there are important issues on the financing side.

Part of the success of the neighborhood health center can be attributed to the fact that it offers care to those in a specific geographic area who need care and it does so by removing the income barrier. It does not subject those who want to use the center to the investigation indignities of the existing welfare system. This it does most readily if it is located in the heart of a poverty neighborhood where it can assume that almost everyone who enters its doors would be eligible even if income criteria were set and were diligently investigated. If one builds a water fountain in the middle of a desert, one does not have to ask whether each person coming to the fountain really needs to take a drink; one can assume that. So it is with neighborhood health centers in the heart of poverty areas. If, however, one begins to discuss a proliferation of neighborhood health centers, one must recognize that we will enter into difficulties. The more centers there are, the more extended their network, the more they "cover" the poor population, the more likely that eligibility problems will arise. It can be argued that neighborhood health centers could never serve the entire poverty population and yet—because of budget constraints— be limited only to that population unless the centers engaged in that very process that we deplore: investigation, determination of eligibility, periodic checks of income and perhaps even of expenditures. And were the centers to do that, their effectiveness in relating to the poverty population might well be jeopardized. Thus, their success may well be related to the fact that they are few in number. Expansion of the program can surely be undertaken; yet, there may be a point at which success that leads to further expansion may require new features that would jeopardize success itself.

Those remarks are perhaps addressed chiefly to the question: *"Can* the neighborhood health center be expanded to serve all the poor?" But there are other problems with the neighborhood health centers. Let me make clear that I favor such centers but only as a *second* best solution on the financing side. They are second best because while they do provide services to people who need them and, therefore, increase the range of choice and the number of options, they do not offer a full measure of choice. Medicaid aside (and Medicaid presents yet another set of problems), the neighborhood health center says to the poor, "Come get your service from us free. If you do not like us, you are of course free to go elsewhere but elsewhere you must pay." Obviously, even as this increases the range of choice the poor do have, it restricts the choices that they can really make below that, which it seems to me, they and we should desire.

The financing mechanism places the poor at some considerable disadvantage. Free service at the center and fee for service elsewhere is *not* a first best choice. To the economist, the elimination of two classes of medical care does not only mean we move to one class of quality of care—but also that we provide everyone with more choices. I would prefer that we add to the weapons that the poor have with which to influence providers by giving them that most powerful weapon: the power to take their business elsewhere. This cannot be done while the financial cards are stacked in favor of the center. While I would not suggest that the problems of community participation, power, and inputs, have been solved in the business sector, I am nonetheless impressed by how much better the business sector has responded to such issues than have many governmental institutions even when it has not even been consciously trying to respond. The force of competition for the consumer's dollar or good will is not unimportant. A little more of that kind of competition in the health sector might well be useful and might well prevent many of the indignities now inflicted upon people seeking service. In that sense, then, the financing pattern of neighborhood health centers does not provide the full measure of opportunity to the poor, and, therefore, in a sense because the neighborhood health center has a captive clientele, the full measure of performance that one would desire.

Therefore, as I see it, there are at least two important financing problems with the existing pattern of neighborhood health centers: the problem of consumer sovereignty and the problem of replicability. Are there any solutions to these two major problems? Is there a mechanism which could overcome these deficiencies?

Since this is not a paper on universal health insurance, I do not intend to discuss that approach at length or in detail. It should be noted, however, that those who believe in neighborhood health centers as a delivery mechanism should, in my view, favor universal health insurance as the financing mechanism for the neighborhood health center. Were everyone covered by universal health insurance, the problem of eligibility for services in the neighborhood health center would be solved. Anyone, not only the poor, could come to the center. Everyone, not only the poor, would have the financial means to pay for the services provided. Whether one were poor or not would no longer be an issue.

But universal health insurance would do more than that. In addition to saying anyone can come to the neighborhood health center because it is now financed by the consumers rather than through a direct government appropriation, it would also provide the poor with health insurance which they could take anywhere. Thus, anyone can come to the center, and, further, the poor can go anywhere. This means that the center *must* meet the needs of its patients, it no longer has a financial advantage over other providers of care, but it also means that if the center is a better provider of care it can offer its services to the non-poor as well.

Universal health insurance thus converts the neighborhood health center into a delivery mechanism and a delivery mechanism only. I consider it most important to separate, in so far as possible, the delivery mechanism from the financing mechanism so that each can be judged on its own merits. With universal health insurance, this occurs.

And finally, in a political real world, universal health insurance would, it seems to me, permit the neighborhood health center, if it really is a better delivery system, to grow and grow rapidly. No longer would government have to appropriate money to operate centers, money which it feels is so limited that we can never hope to have sufficient funds to cover the entire poverty population. With universal health insurance providing the funds for operation, the problem of budgets is altered. Now government could provide funds for start-up costs, for planning, for stimulating an activity. The costs of operation would come from other pockets. Under such a situation, one could envision substantial and rapid growth of this delivery system.

This, then, is one way that an economist might look at neighborhood health centers. They are providing and paying for services for a part of the population that needs services desperately, but there are better ways of paying for these services. It would be good to turn to them. They would bring more equity into the situation and would provide for more rapid growth of neighborhood health centers, if they indeed are a better way of delivering services.

Part VIII
Patients' Use and Response

Introduction

The main reason for establishing the health centers was to improve the health care available to poor persons. The quality of care provided through the centers is difficult to measure (although one substantial attempt to do so has been undertaken; see Part IX). The patterns of use of the centers are easier to study and give some indication of the level of success of the centers in attracting and serving the poor.

Several key aspects of the centers—their neighborhood location, outreach programs and paraprofessional personnel, family-oriented medicine and team practice of medicine, consumer participation, employment of staff from the areas being served—were included, to varying degrees, because of their hypo-thesized effect on improving the accessibility and quality of health care. A major goal of the centers was to encourage persons not previously receiving adequate care to use the centers.

Do the persons for whom the centers were intended in fact use them? To what extent? Are the patterns of utilization "appropriate," do they jibe with professionals' (and with consumers') notions of when a patient should or should not come in for a visit?

The evidence presented in the chapters which follow is that the centers are being used, and in "appropriate" fashion. Some of them have had to turn patients away, to close their enrollments, because they are unable to serve any more persons; others have not reached the volume of persons which they were originally designed to serve.

The findings with regard to extent of use have significance for proposed future health care reforms. Some maintain, for instance, that co-insurance and deductible provisions are essential in any national health insurance plan to guard against patients using greater amounts of health care than they actually need or than the system is capable of providing. The evidence of the centers is that when the financial and other barriers to care are removed, poor persons do use health services more frequently than do better-off individuals, but that the differences are not particularly great in prepaid group practice settings and after the first six months of use.[1]

In "Actual Public Acceptance of the Neighborhood Health Center by the Urban Poor," Seymour S. Bellin and H. Jack Geiger report a high rate of patient satisfaction at the Columbia Point Health Center, and a high rate of those eligible using the center and comparing it favorably with alternative sources of care. A follow-up study by Bellin and Geiger, "The Impact of a Neighborhood Health Center on Patients' Behavior and Attitudes Relating to Health Care: A Study of a Low-Income Housing Project," documents changes in patients' attitudes since the creation of the Columbia Point center. They document significant changes in attitudes toward health, health care, and sources of care which paralleled changes in utilization of services during the same period.

"Basic Utilization Experience of OEO Comprehensive Health Services Projects," by Mark Strauss and Gerald Sparer, calculates the utilization rates of eight OEO Comprehensive Health Services projects—five neighborhood health centers and three OEO-financed projects within prepaid group practices. The authors' comparison of the utilization rates of project registrants with national survey data indicates that patients use the centers and related projects somewhat more frequently than do various categories of persons in a national sample. They document the existence of an initial, six-month long surge of utilization. The chapter concludes with observations about the implications of these data for planning Health Maintenance Organizations which will serve the poor.

Bruce Hillman and Evan Charney, in "A Neighborhood Health Center: What the Patients Know and Think of Its Operation," write that most patients accept the Rochester Health Center enthusiastically. Their satisfaction is due primarily to the availability and quality of care and the attitudes of health center staff. One-quarter of the patients occasionally use other sources of care. The study documents a very low awareness of, or caring about, issues of community control.

References

1. Constraints of space force us to exclude from this volume articles which report the utilization experience of OEO projects which "buy into" existing prepaid group practices. The comprehensive health services projects differ significantly from neighborhood health centers, but include many similar features as well. Gerald Sparer and Arne Anderson, "Utilization and Cost Experience of Low-Income Families in Four Prepaid Group Practice Plans 1970–1971," *New England Journal of Medicine 282*(July 12, 1973) 67–72, documents basic similarities in patterns of use between regular enrollees in four prepaid group practices and enrollees whose participation was financed by OEO. Merwyn R. Greenlick, Donald K. Freeborn, Theodore J. Colombo, Jeffrey A. Prussin and Ernest W. Saward, in "Comparing The Use of Medical Care Services by a Medically Indigent and a General Membership Population in a Comprehensive Prepaid Group Practice Program," *Medical Care 10*, 3 (May–June 1972): 187–200, report in greater detail the experience of Kaiser–Portland's OEO project.

16

Actual Public Acceptance of the
Neighborhood Health Center by the
Urban Poor

Seymour S. Bellin and H. Jack Geiger

During the past four years, the Office of Economic Opportunity has sponsored a
network of neighborhood health centers as part of the war on poverty. These
centers were designed as an innovation in the system of health care services
which would overcome the many barriers to optimal utilization of preventive and
therapeutic services especially characteristic of low-income populations. Many
health centers also go beyond the more usual limited focus upon the provision
of traditional health services alone, by attempting, in a variety of ways, to intervene in the cycle of ill health and poverty.

Although our health center has these larger objectives, we limit our attention
in this paper to two more traditional questions: (1) Has the Health Center been
widely accepted and intensively used by the low-income community for which it
is specifically intended? (2) Has this new facility led to continuous, co-ordinated
health-care utilization by a population that had previously received episodic,
discontinuous, or fragmented care?

After more than three full years of operation of the Columbia Point Neighborhood Health Center in Boston, we are in a position to examine these issues in
the light of hard data on actual utilization of health care services and the evaluation of these services by the community.

The Columbia Point Health Center, the
Community Setting, and Sources of Data

Health Center. The Tufts-Columbia Point Health Center provides comprehensive ambulatory care, which includes a wide range of preventive and therapeutic
services for the total family. These services are provided in a new way through
three family health care groups (FHCG), each consisting of an internist, a
pediatrician, several community health nurses, social workers, and indigenous
community residents trained as home health aides, social work assistants,
nurses aides, and medical assistants. Each such FHCG offers continuous

Reprinted from *Journal of the American Medical Association* 214, 12 (December 21,
1970): 2147-2153.

The Tufts Comprehensive Community Health Action project reported herein was
performed pursuant to Community Action Program grant CG 8816 from the Office of
Economic Opportunity.

primary health care to a third of the Columbia Point population,
using the Health Center's support services (laboratory, x-ray equipment,
pharmacy, etc.), incorporates part-time but regular specialty services
(eg., obstetrics-gynecology), and takes definitive responsibility for arranging
other specialty services or inpatient care at related hospitals. The goal in organizing these services is to provide continuous, individual, and family-centered
health care along with the advantages of specialization.

The project also seeks to use the delivery of health services as a point of
entry for inducing broader changes in the physical and social milieu that contributes to the cycle of ill health and poverty, including participation of the
residents in the design and operation of their health services through a Community Health Association that shares in a wide variety of policy decisions and
has independent, health-related programs of its own. The goals and programs of
the Tufts Comprehensive Community Health Action Project have been described
more fully elsewhere.[1-9]

The Community Setting. Columbia Point is a low-income public housing
development situated in South Dorchester. It now contains about 5,500 persons
residing in 1,200 households. About two-thirds of the population is under 20
years of age. The community has been geographically isolated from other residential areas and the normal complement of neighborhood-based public and
commercial facilities and services. Until the Health Center was established in
December 1965, health-care facilities were not easily accessible to the great
majority of residents. Aside from a twice-weekly Health Department well-baby
clinic at Columbia Point, the nearest source of health care (except for a few
private practitioners) was the Boston City Hospital, situated about an hour's
trip by public transportation from the housing project.

Family income at Columbia Point is low, about three households in five
have gross weekly incomes of less than $80, or under $4,200 annually. Nearly
two households in three depend for their family income solely on sources other
than earnings, including welfare and social security benefits.[10]

Sources of Data. A health and health-care utilization survey was undertaken of
a random sample of families residing at Columbia Point at two points in time: in
November 1965, just before the Health Center opened its doors, and two years
later.

Before the Health Center opened its doors, one respondent, almost always
the female household head, was interviewed in each of 357 households, consti-
tuting about 26% of all occupied dwelling units in November 1965. Two years
later, in 1967, 260 of these 357 households were still in residence, and another
round of interviews was obtained in 219. In addition, a new sample of 215
households was drawn and interviewed at this time. The 434 households, consisting of the baseline study households still in residence and the new sample,

comprised 35% of all occupied dwelling units in November 1967. A comparison of these samples with respect to such demographic characteristics as age, marital status, family size, and education and such patterns of health behavior as obtaining an annual routine physical examination reveals that they are representative of the total community in residence at the two points in time at which the interviews were conducted.

Furthermore, we performed an internal comparison of those respondents who were interviewed twice (i.e., those of continuous residence from 1965 to 1967) and those who were drawn as an additional sample in 1967. In all major demographic respects except for race and income—age, sex, education, marital status, and family size— differences between the two groups were negligible. Despite the fact that the new sample had a somewhat higher percentage both of black persons and households with higher incomes, the two study populations were similar with respect to key health attitudes and behaviors.

We also examined the possibility that households remaining in residence long enough for the second interview comprised a self-selected group differing from those who had moved either in demographic characteristics or in pattern of health-care utilization (as measured in 1965). There were no major differences along these axes; in other words, self-selection to stay or move out apparently did not involve the health attitudes and behaviors involved in this study.

The household samples were drawn randomly from a listing of dwelling units provided by the public housing authority and contacted in a preliminary census of occupied dwellings. These before-and-after surveys, performed by an independent outside agency, afford data on reported utilization of and attitudes toward the Health Center and its services.

In addition to this questionnaire, data on utilization of the Health Center by residents were obtained from the Center's medical records and its continuous recording system of medical care encounters (all contacts between residents and health professionals, at home or in the Health Center).

The original census of all residents of Columbia Point and the baseline health survey were designed by Daniel Yankelovich, Inc., in cooperation with the staff of the Tufts Department of Community Health and Social Medicine. The firm also assisted in the design of the following health survey and carried out all the data collection and processing. Both surveys were done with full assurance of anonymity, i.e., the respondents knew that their replies were confidential and that no names, household numbers, or individual interviews would be reported to any Health Center or Tufts University personnel.

The Findings

Public Acceptance of the Neighborhood Health Center. Are residents of Columbia Point accepting the of Health Center and do they use its facilities? Evidence of public acceptance is afforded by data from the Health Center's records on actual utilization of its services. The volume of use has been high from the very day that the Health Center opened its doors. During its third full year of operation, 78% of persons in continuous residence at Columbia Point for the full year visited the Health Center at least once (table 16-1). Of those who lived there less than the full year, 64% had had at least one Health Center contact. For the total population, the corresponding figure was 75%.

When the entire population of Columbia Point is taken as the denominator, there was an annual average of 7.3 health professional encounters per resident at the Health Center. When users of the Health Center are taken as the denominator, the equivalent figure is 9.8 health professional encounters annually per user.

Nearly two in every three Health Center encounters involved a physician. The residents had, on the average, 4.6 physician encounters at that facility alone during 1968 (table 16-2). There were, undoubtedly, additional contacts with physicians elsewhere than at the Health Center, particularly for the small minority of persons who did not use the Health Center as their central source of care. The annual average number of encounters with a Health Center physician

Table 16-1
Encounters with All Health Center Professionals in 1968 by Continuity of Residence*

	Throughout 1968	For Only Part of 1968	Total
No. of population in residence category	4,846	1,559	6,405
No. contacting Health Center staff at least once in 1968	3,799	998	4,797
Population contacting Health Center at least once in 1968, %	78.4	64.0	74.9
Annual total No. of Health Center encounters for population	. . .	. . .	46,850
Annual average No. of Health Center encounters for all residents	. . .	. . .	7.3
Annual average No. of Health Center encounters for Center users only	. . .	. . .	9.8

*Columbia Point Population. Data drawn from the Health Center's utilization-recording system, in which every service contact between a professional staff member and a patient is recorded on special form (independent of medical record), key punched, and tabulated each month by computer. Any given visit may result in contact, or "encounter" with more than one health professional, each of which is recorded and counted.

Table 16-2

Average Annual Encounters With Health Center Physicians in 1968*

Total Columbia Point population (in residence at any time during year)	6,405
No. of residents contacting Health Center at least once during year	4,797
Total No. of encounters with Health Center physician during the year, all residents	29,313
Annual average No. of physician encounters at Health Center, all residents	4.6
Annual average No. of physician encounters at Health Center, Center users	6.1

*For all Columbia Point residents and those using the Health Center. Data drawn from the Health Center's utilization-recording system in which every service contact between a professional staff member and a patient is recorded on a special form (independent of the medical record), key punched, and tabulated each month by computer.

for users of that facility was 6.1. These figures compare very favorably not only with other low-income populations, but also with more affluent populations. For example, a national health survey, which included all contacts with a physician or with personnel such as a nurse operating under the supervision of a physician, reveals an annual average of 5.0 physician visits for the total population, 4.6 for the lowest income category, and 5.7 for persons with incomes of $7,000 and above.[11]

The Health Center is the regular or central source of care for about five out of six people in the community, according to our 1967 survey of a random sample of households after two years of Health Center operation. This figure is based on the survey responses of respondents (female heads of household) for themselves and all other family members. The Health Center was the regular source of care for about 97% of the children, according to the respondents. It was, finally, the regular source of care for 71% of the respondents themselves (table 16-3).

As part of the health survey, the respondents were asked what they liked and disliked about the Columbia Point Health Center. Whereas 96% of the sample made one or more favorable comments, only 37% made one or more unfavorable comments. Among favorable features of the Health Center, convenience was mentioned most frequently, closely followed by the personal manner in which care was given and by quality of care. Complaints were not only less frequently mentioned, but tended to be scattered over a wider number of issues. The two most frequent dislikes centered on inconvenience and quality of care. Thus, the very same features which are criticized by some are praised by several times that number of other residents. When the two-year follow-up survey is compared with the baseline, there is a marked increase in overall satis-

Table 16-3
Regular Source of Care*＊

Regular Source of Care	% of Population
None	12
Private physicians	6
Hospital outpatient clinics or emergency rooms	11
Columbia Point Health Center	71
Total	100

*＊Reported by a random sample of 434 household heads at Columbia Point in the 1967 health survey.

faction with medical care, which is attributed to the Health Center.

Does the success of the Health Center in attracting and holding patients merely reflect the lack of adequate standards by which medically disadvantaged persons are able to judge the quality of care offered? Are patients who have previously experienced private medical practice, for example, more critical of neighborhood health center services? Our data dispel such a notion. Before the Health Center opened its doors, nearly 25% relied upon a private physician as their regular source of care. Nearly 50% used a variety of hospital outpatient clinics and emergency rooms, among which Boston City Hospital was the most frequently mentioned. The balance, nearly 30%, disclaimed any regular source of medical care. Of those previously without a regular source of health care, the Health Center was successfully reaching 75% two years later. It also drew clientele in nearly identical proportions from those who had previously used private physicians and those who had used hospital outpatient clinics. To be sure, a minority, 17%, were using other facilities as their regular source of care in 1967. Even these people, however, were also making use of the Health Center services.

At the Health Center, no fees are charged and no means test is used as a barrier to service, since the vast majority of the Columbia Point population has incomes below the poverty guidelines or are eligible for Medicaid or Medicare. Furthermore, the community is geographically isolated from alternative sources of health care. Thus acceptance of the Health Center might be attributed to convenience and, to a lesser extent, to the absence of fees, which may over-shadow other considerations in the choice of health care. This objection can be overcome, however, by examining comparative evaluations of various sources of health care which Columbia Point residents were asked to make in terms of criteria in addition to convenience and cost.

Do residents feel that they must pay a price in (1) quality or care, (2) its comprehensiveness, (3) the personal manner in which it is rendered, or (4) waiting time, in order to enjoy the advantages of cost-free care at their doorstep? In the second health survey, residents were asked to compare their experiences at the Neighborhood Health Center with their experiences with private physicians and the hospital outpatient clinics in each of these aspects of health care delivery. Their responses were analyzed according to their regular source of care previous to the opening of the Health Center. It should be noted that our respondents had personally had experience with at least two of the three sources of health care they were asked to rate, and were therefore making experienced, not hypothetical, judgements.

We compared evaluations by adult residents who now regularly use the

Table 16-4

Evaluations of Different Sources of Health Care in Four Criteria by Regular Source of Care Prior to Advent of Center*

No.	Private Physician 33	Hospital Outpatient Clinics 73	None 50
		Previous Regular Source of Care	
Quality of care is best at, %			
Private physician	6	5	4
Hospital outpatient	0	12	2
Health Center	72	53	70
All are same	13	23	14
Don't know	9	7	10
	X^2 not significant at 0.05 level		
Care is most complete at, %			
Private physician	3	5	10
Hospital outpatient	3	9	2
Health Center	85	58	68
All are same	3	21	10
Don't know	6	7	10
	X^2 not significant at 0.025 level		
Care is most personal at, %			
Private physician	6	14	16
Hospital outpatient	0	7	2
Health Center	82	61	66
All are same	6	11	4
Don't know	6	7	12
	X^2 not significant at 0.05 level		
Waiting time is shortest at, %			
Private physician	3	18	8
Hospital outpatient	0	4	2
Health Center	85	60	66
All are same	9	9	20
Don't know	3	9	4
	X^2 not significant at 0.05 level		

*By Columbia Point residents who presently regularly use the Health Center.

Health Center classified by prior source of care. Regardless of the previous type of health care, there is clear consensus on all four criteria (table 16–4). The Health Center is rated superior to all other sources of care by the great majority of all three groups of residents: those who had regularly patronized a private practitioner previously, those who had previously used a hospital outpatient clinic, and those who had previously used no regular source of health care.

In this connection, it is noteworthy that among current patrons of the Neighborhood Health Center, proportionately more former private patients rate the Health Center as superior on all four questions compared with patients who formerly regularly patronized hospital outpatient clinics or who had no central source of care (table 16-4). Although these differences, with a single exception, are not statistically significant, the consistency of the responses and the fact that they are contrary to popular expectations, lead us to conclude that they are real. While the private practitioner is widely seen as synonymous with high-quality care and the personal manner in which it is rendered, it appears that only a small minority of poor patients have had such a positive experience with private medical practice. This may help to explain why it is that, given the high public expectations of private practice and the disappointing actual experience, the former private patients even more fully appreciated the Health Center advantages than those who had previously patronized other sources of care.

We turn next to compare the evaluation of users of the Health Center with those who, despite the apparent advantages in cost and convenience of the Health Center, continue regularly to make use of other sources of health care. Since those who do not use the Health Center as their central source of care are in a small minority, absolute numbers of such persons in our sample are small and the percentages must be regarded only as suggestive.

It is natural to expect a tendency for patients to favor the source of care which they currently use on a regular basis. This tendency is markedly evident for residents who regularly utilize the Health Center on all four criteria upon which they were asked to rate health care delivery (table 16-5). However, among persons who currently patronize private practice physicians or hospital outpatient clinics, this tendency is much weaker and less consistent. Among both of these groups of patients, a substantial percentage acknowledge either the superiority of the Columbia Point Health Center or its equivalence to the source of health care they regularly use. For example, while current patrons of the private practitioner are more likely to choose this source as offering the highest quality of care (25%, as compared to 12% of regular users of the hospital outpatient clinics, 5% of Health Center users and 3% without a regular source of care), 12% of current users of a private practitioner nevertheless choose the Health Center as offering the highest quality of care, and 38% felt that the quality of care in the several sources was about the same.

Continuous, Coordinated Care. Concern has also been expressed[12] that low-income families would perpetuate a fragmented pattern of utilization of health-

Table 16-5

Evaluation of Different Sources of Health Care in Four Criteria by Current Regular Source of Care*

No.	*Current Regular Source of Care*			
	Private Physician 16	*Hospital Out-patient Clinic* 16	*Health Center* 156	*No Regular Source* 31
Quality of care is best at, %				
Private physician	25	12	5	3
Hospital outpatient	. . .	25	6	16
Health Center	12	25	63	48
All are same	38	25	18	10
Don't know	25	13	8	23
Care is most complete at, %				
Private physician	25	0	7	10
Hospital outpatient	12	25	5	13
Health Center	19	38	67	54
All are same	19	31	13	10
Don't know	25	6	8	13
Care is most personal at, %				
Private physician	43	19	12	16
Hospital outpatient	0	19	4	6
Health Center	19	31	67	59
All are same	19	12	8	6
Don't know	19	19	9	13
Waiting time is shortest at, %				
Private physician	25	19	11	10
Hospital outpatient	0	12	1	0
Health Center	38	50	67	71
All are same	25	19	14	13
Don't know	12	0	7	6

*By a panel of Columbia Point residents interviewed both in the 1965 and the 1967 health surveys.

care facilities by adding the neighborhood health center to a list of facilities to be used in a selective way. Evidence thus far indicates that this fear is groundless. The vast majority of residents obtain all their medical care services, both preventive and curative, from the Health Center; when they used highly specialized services not available at the Health Center, it was on referral by the Center staff. Utilization of all other ambulatory health care facilities in the Boston area by the Columbia Point residents has dropped to a small fraction of the utilization before the Health Center opened in December of 1965. In addition, the overwhelming majority of mothers obtained their health care, as did 97% of their children, at the Health Center. Thus, it is clear that the Health Center is providing primary care for families in the area it serves.

Evidence is also available on patient compliance with medical regimens. Whereas nearly three out of five adult respondents acknowledged failing to follow a physician's instruction at some time in the year before the Health Center opened, this dropped to one out of three two years later. Thus, the pattern of fragmented, discontinuous health care which had been a typical experience at Columbia Point, as in most low-income communities, was markedly reduced with the advent of the Neighborhood Health Center. Our results, in this respect, suggest that many patterns in the use of health-care facilities are susceptible to modification once adequate, convenient, and personalized service is provided.

Comment

Actual experience at Columbia Point reveals that the Health Center has earned the patronage and confidence of the great majority of the community residents it serves. Preliminary impressions from other neighborhood health centers indicate that the Columbia Point experience is not unique.[13] A further indication of the effectiveness of this Health Center and, incidentally, other forms of group health practice as well, is to be found in the success of these programs in reducing the demand for hospital beds.[14,15]

These successes have occurred despite the persistence of certain shortcomings. Apart from the specific dissatisfactions voiced by residents, the staff itself has not been satisfied with its own progress in creating an effective role for paramedical personnel, in the completeness of its outreach to the community, and in developing a systematic approach to community medicine. The fact that some unresolved problems persist in an organization after only a few years of operation should occasion no surprise; indeed, many of the problems result from the overwhelming rate of acceptance and utilization of the Health Center and the heavy service load this caused from the very start of its existence.

These findings, based on actual experience, constitute a documented answer to the critics and skeptics of the neighborhood health center concept. Most recently, for example, Robertson and his colleagues[12] arrived at pessimistic prognostications about public acceptance and effectiveness of neighborhood health centers. The discrepancy between their conclusions and our data may be due to the fact that their conclusions were not based on a study of any population actually using a neighborhood health center, nor were they based on a study of any population that expected the opportunity to use a neighborhood health center in the future. Instead, their conclusions were based on "anticipated" use of a hypothetical neighborhood health center as reported in response to a questionnaire offered to a sample of low-income families who used the medical emergency clinic at the Children's Hospital Medical Center in Boston. It should also be noted that their respondents were asked about neighborhood health centers—with which they had had no experience—at a time when only one was in existence (for which few, if any, of the respondents were eligible) and others were only in the planning stage.

How can we account for the success of the neighborhood health center? We wish to call attention to two major issues: (1) Can service be delivered in a highly personal and continuous fashion? (2) Is decentralization of health services away from hospitals and into neighborhoods really necessary?

Skepticism of the health center often focuses on its alleged inability to provide health care services in the personal and continuous fashion which is widely believed to be essential to patient loyalty and utlimately to an optimal health service delivery system. We believe in the desirability of personalized continuity of care and, as far as we can tell, health services at Columbia Point have been both continuous and personalized. Since we explicitly asked our respondents to evaluate how personal the Health Center's care is, we are on firm ground in concluding that care is experienced in this manner. This is a positive judgement made by the audience that really counts, the recipients of care, not the professional providers at the Health Center, or others.

Although continuous and personal care of patients by one physician seems to be desirable, focus on this single issue overlooks one of the most significant advantages of the FHCG—the fact that it provides a whole set of health professionals and aides, working together, with whom a continuous and personal relationship is maintained. If a change in one professional or one physician does occur (and this has not been an unusually frequent event at the Columbia Point Health Center), the patient still has five or six other familiar sources of care to continue with in the other members of the group. This effect of the FHCG is an important subject for empirical study and verification.

On the second issue, decentralization of health services, questions have been raised on at least two grounds: (1) is convenience of location important, relative to such other qualities as its comprehensiveness of care, in a compact city with a relatively good public transportation system, and (2) does the neighborhood health center ignore advantages of centralization of scarce skills and facilities in existing hospitals?

To begin with, there is always the difficulty of accurately assessing how others see and experience reality.While Boston may seem to some observers to be compact and to have a relatively good public transportation system, 14% of Columbia Point residents spent over five hours from door to door each time they sought medical care before the advent of the Health Center. An additional 70% spent two to five hours in the same quest. It was a major reason given by residents who reported having put off seeking medical attention. Certainly, Columbia Point residents have a different view of public transportation in Boston. While Columbia Point is not typical of all of Boston, neither is it unique.

Second, the either/or formulation that is often implied is false and misleading, that is, *either* convenience of location *or* comprehensiveness of care. The evidence provided by the Columbia Point Health Center, in our view, indicates that both can be done.

Third, it is particularly important to draw a distinction between crisis or emergency care, for which low-income people have traditionally had to pay the price of journeying elsewhere, and continuous coordinated care aside from crisis or emergency. For example, before the advent of the Health Center at Columbia Point virtually all the persons with a chronic ailment had been seen by a physician sometime during the history of the ailment. Only half of these persons, however, were under continuing medical supervision. Furthermore, about 30% of all current acute physical conditions had not been brought to the attention of a physician. For some of these conditions, significant delay occurred before medical attention was obtained. In other instances, medical attention was never sought. Our objective is to encourage people to seek prompt medical attention even for signs and symptoms, like a sore throat, a persistent cough, or recurrent minor joint ache which may appear benign and inconsequential. It is for these problems that distance, accessibility, and cost are such major barriers both for patients and for the health professionals.

In dealing with the second question—does the neighborhood health center ignore the economic advantages of centralization of medical care at the hospital— one must first ask: are we dealing with the interests of the consumers or the providers? If comprehensive family-oriented care as good or better than hospital ambulatory care can be provided in the neighborhood in such a way as to reduce the costs in time and effort to the consumers, why shouldn't it be done? The only countervailing arguments are cost and convenience to the health care personnel and organizations, and the tendency of established institutions, such as hospitals, to maintain the structure and location of services most convenient to its staff and administration. In times of soaring hospital costs and health manpower shortages, these are important considerations, but not the only ones. They should not lead us to lose sight of the real question involved here: is the hub of the health care universe the hospital or the community?

The answer obviously depends in part on who is talking, the professional or the consumer. It is worth pointing out that the hospital-centered plan, located away from the social entity of the neighborhood and community, in a massvie institution with complex funding and elite direction, is most likely to block the new dimension in today's health care that is, effective participation in, and some control over, the provision of basic human services by those served. A health center is a possible vehicle for such consumer participation; as even the middle class knows well, a hospital is an unlikely one.

There now exist or are being organized some 60 neighborhood health centers, differing greatly in objectives, scope of services, organization of services, and in other important ways. There also exists a variety of other forms of group medical practice, in addition to traditional solo practice. This great diversity affords an unparalleled opportunity to learn, on the basis of actual behavior, what are the precise consequences of many innovations and variations in organizing health care. Every effort should be made to encourage rigorous comparative research directed to these fundamental questions.

References

1. *Tufts University Comprehensive Community Health Action Program Report to Office of Economic Opportunity.* Boston, Tufts University School of Medicine, Department of Community Health and Social Medicine, 1966 (mimeographed).
2. Geiger, H.J.: The neighborhood health center: Education of the faculty in preventive medicine. *Arch. Environ. Health 14*:912–916, 1967.
3. Geiger, H.J.: Of the poor, by the poor, or for the poor: The mental health implications of social control of poverty programs. *Psych. Res. Rep. Amer. Psychiat. Assoc. 21*:55–65, 1967.
4. Geiger, H.J.: The poor and the professional: Who takes the handle off the broad street pump? Read before the American Public Health Assoc., San Francisco, 1966.
5. Geiger, H.J.: Health and social change: The urban crisis. *Med. Educ.,* to be published.
6. Geiger, H.J.: Community control or community conflict. *Bull. Nat. Tuberculosis Assoc. 55*:4–11, 1969.
7. Gibson, C.D.: The neighborhood health center—the primary unit of health care. *Amer. J. Public Health 58*:1188–1191, 1968.
8. Hatch, J.: Community shares in policy decision for rural health center. *Hospitals 43*:109–112, 1969.
9. Kelly, C.H.: Fighting poverty with health care. *Amer. J. Nurs. 68:1504–1511,* 1968.
10. *The Columbia Point Housing Project: A Description of a Public Housing Project in the Urban North.* New York, Daniel Yankelovich, Inc. (mimeographed).
11. *Medical Care Financing and Utilization: Source Book of Data Through 1961.* Health Economics Series 1, publication 947, Health Economics Branch, Division of Community Health Services, U.S. Dept. of Health, Education and Welfare, 1962.
12. Robertson, L.S., Kosa, J., Alpert, J.J., et al.: Anticipated acceptance of neighborhood health centers by the urban poor. *JAMA 205*:107–110, 1968.
13. Colombo, T.J., Saward, E.W., Greenlick, M.R.: The integration of an OEO health program into a prepaid comprehensive group practice plan. *Amer. J. Public Health 58*:641–650, 1969.
14. Perrott, G.S.: Utilization of hospital services. *Amer. J. Public Health 56*:1–57, 1966.
15. Bellin, S.S., Geiger, H.J., Gibson, C.D.: The impact of ambulatory health care services on the demand for hospital beds: A study of the Tufts school of medicine, neighborhood health center at Columbia Point in Boston. *New Eng. J. Med. 280*:808–812, 1969.

17

The Impact of a Neighborhood Health
Center on Patients' Behavior and Attitud
Attitudes Relating to Health Care: A
Study of a Low Income Housing Project

Seymour S. Bellin and H. Jack Geiger

Evaluation Criteria

Ultimately, the justification for health services, whether rendered by the traditional solo practitioner, a hospital outpatient clinic, or a neighborhood health center, rests on demonstrating a reduction in death, disease, and discomfort. Modification of death and disease rates is especially difficult to demonstrate over a short period of time in urban, industrial communities, which have controlled infectious disease and eliminated hunger and malnutrition for the great majority of their residents. The problem is compounded when the target community is very small as in the case of Columbia Point. Although an effort is being made to measure death and disease rates, we are also conducting descriptive studies of variables such as utilization of health care services which are more easily measurable in the short run.

Since the Tufts Comprehensive Community Health Action Program's objectives are broad, even with respect to health, a variety of criteria must be employed in its evaluation. As has already been noted, the Health Center not only intends to improve the quality of care given to the residents who find their way to the doors, but to reach those who, until now, have not made use of health care services. Its objective also extends ultimately to a greater emphasis on early detection and primary prevention. The following dimensions of the target population's view of its current health services are reported in this paper, all on the basis of self-reports in response to structured interviews:

1. Promptness in seeking care for health problems.
2. Early case finding; periodic asymptomatic health examinations.
3. Qualities of physicians, e.g., competence, motivation, quality of care rendered.
4. Beliefs about physicians' attitudes towards patients.
5. General evaluation of medical care received.

Reprinted from *Medical Care* 10, 3 (May-June 1972): 224–239. Introductory material about the Columbia Point Health Center and its community setting contained in the original version of this paper has been deleted because comparable information appears at the beginning of the previous article (Chapter 16).

6. Specific evaluation of the Health Center and a comparative assessment with two other major sources of health care on four dimensions.

In addition, the paper directs attention to such situational factors as money, time, effort—costs and resources—involved in obtaining health care. An examination will be made of the reasons people stated for postponing care, barriers acknowledged in the use of emergency health care services, times spent in seeking health care, and indebtedness contracted for medical reasons.

Sources of Data

The data for this evaluation are based on a survey undertaken at two points in time with a representative sample of Columbia Point residents.[a] The initial survey consisted of interviews with 357 household heads and was conducted just prior to the opening of the Health Center in December 1965. It provides a baseline picture of what people at Columbia Point believed, felt, and did about their health problems and the health care facilities available to them before the Health Center was available. Two years later, the survey was repeated with those families who were still in residence in the community. This before and after study makes it possible to assess any changes that may have occurred which might be attributed to the Health Center.

Of the original sample of 357 households, 253 were still in residence 2 years later and, of these, 219 (or 86%) were successfully reinterviewed. At the time of the repeat health survey, this panel sample was supplemented by an additional random sample of 215 households not previously interviewed in the second survey. Thus, a total of 434 households were interviewed in the second survey.

Two major surveys, undertaken 2 years apart, are treated here as if they were independent random samples. A comparison of these samples on major demographic variables reveals that with the exception of race and income, no statistically significant differences exist (table 17-1). Despite the fact that the second survey had a somewhat higher percentage both of black persons and of households with a higher income distribution, the two study populations were similar with respect to key health attitudes and self-reported behaviors.

The health surveys received public endorsement by the Columbia Point Health Association, an elected council of local residents, which speaks for the community in formulating policy and initiating programs on health-related issues. (It also serves as an advisory board to the Health Center on matters

---

[a]The original census of all households in residence in the community from which the subsequent household sample was drawn and the two subsequent health surveys were designed by the firm of Daniel Yankelovich, Inc., in collaboration with the Tufts Department of Community Health and Social Medicine. The first is located at 575 Madison Ave., New York, N.Y.

Table 17-1

Selected Social Characteristics of the Columbia Point Survey Samples:
Wave I Health Survey (November 1965) and Wave II Health Survey
(November 1967)

Social characteristics of respondents	Baseline health survey Nov. 1965 N = (357)* % = 100.0 Per cent	Follow-up health survey Nov. 1967 N = (436)* % = 100.0 Per cent	X^2
1. Age of household heads			
Under 25	14	13	
25-44	49	47	
45-64	15	17	n.s.
65 and over	21	23	
2. Race			
White	66	59	
Non-white	34	41	p $<$ .05
3. Family income			
Under $60/week	55	52	p $<$ .001
$60-$70	30	18	
$80 and over	15	30	
4. Marital status			
Married	41	38	n.s.
Not married (separared, divorced, widowed, single)	59	62	
5. Presence of minor children			
Yes	69	67	n.s.
No	31	33	
6. Health insurance			
Yes	29	25	n.s.
No	71	75	

*Percentages exclude "no answers"

affecting policy and practice.) The actual interviewing was carried out by Daniel
Yankelovich, Inc., which employed nonresident interviewers. The interviews
were conducted in the home and respondents were assured in detail of confi-
dentiality and anonymity. An effort was made to explain to respondents the
purpose of the survey: to find out what the community's health needs and
desires were, how satisfactory and unsatisfactory health services were, and to
find ways of improving them. Evaluations of the Health Center were obtained
in a variety of forms—including both open and structured questions. The critical
incident technique also was used to encourage respondents to cite specific
examples of both good and bad experiences at the Health Center. Such questions minimize the risk of eliciting socially approved responses or "response set"
biases.

Findings

*1. Aspects of Reported Use of
Health Care Services*

Early Detection: Asymptomatic General Health Examinations. Although there is no unanimity of opinion about the value of periodic general physical examinations, a majority of public health authorities favor it. Prior to the Health Center, however, only 28 per cent of the respondents reported that they had *ever* had such an examination for preventive purposes.

Two years after the Health Center opened, the proportion of respondents who in the previous 12 months had received a general health examination in the absence of any known or specific health problem increased dramatically from 17 to 59 per cent $(P = <.001)$.

Preventive Health Measures: Polio Immunization. Success in primary prevention of illness has tended to be uneven where effectiveness depends on the initiative and cooperation of the individual. Polio immunization compaigns, for example, have usually been least effective in low income communities. Columbia Point has been no exception. Before the Health Center opened its doors, only 57 per cent of the adult respondents and 78 per cent of their youngest children had been immunized against poliomyelitis. Eighteen months later, the prevalence of reported polio immunication was virtually unchanged among adults (59 per cent) but increased to 92 per cent among children[b] $(p = .01)$.

Delay in Seeking Care. Twenty-three per cent of the people interviewed before the Health Center opened acknowledged that they or someone in their family had put off seeking medical care in the preceding six months. This figure underestimates the actual prevalence of delay in seeking medical attention, since not all persons had medical problems during that period and individuals differ both in their ability to recognize early signs or symptoms of illness and in their definition of those which merit medical attention. Two years later, the proportion of families who reported that they or someone in their family had postponed medical care in the preceding six months delined from 23 per cent to 10 per cent $(p = <.001)$.

---

[b]A special survey was undertaken of a random sample of households in connection with a Medicaid Sign-up Campaign in which a question was included on poliomyelitis immunization.

A spot check by staff pediatricians, in 1968, revealed that a substantial minority of children had not had their complete series of immunizations, and they pointed up inadequacies in the follow-up procedure in effect at that time.

*2. Beliefs and Sentiments Relevant to
Health Behavior*

Attitudes about illness and sources of health care services are important to the
extent to which they influence actual health behavior and can help to account
for the gains in utilization of health care services previously described. Our
attention will be directed initially to beliefs about when medical attention
should be sought. Two issues are singled out for consideration: a. beliefs about
the importance of asymptomatic physical examinations, and b. beliefs about
what kinds of signs and symptoms of illness should be brought to a physician.

Subsequently, our attention will turn to attitudes that relate to the choice
of health care sources and the kinds and levels of utilization of health care
services. These attitudes include an overall assessment of one's own medical care,
an explicit evaluation of the Health Center, and structured questions evaluating
various aspects of the doctor-patient relationship, including patients' beliefs
about physicians' attitudes toward patients. Next, respondents' comparative
evaluations of and preferences among major alternative sources of health care
will be examined. Our aim is to ascertain to what extent there are correlative
changes in attitudes that might help to explain the changes in levels of utilization based on Health Center records reported in a previous paper, and in self-
reported use of preventive and curative services described earlier here.

Beliefs Regarding When a Physician Should Be Seen: 1. Knowledge of symptoms which merit medical attention. Even prior to the opening of the Health
Center, a relatively high degree of sophistication with respect to signs and
symptoms of illness which should be brought to the attention of a physician
was evident among Columbia Point residents (table 17-2). Agreement was
highest on the most serious signs of illness—for example, severe shortness of
breath (89 per cent), a cough that lasts for several weeks (80 per cent), or an
unexplained loss of 10 pounds (73 per cent). There was also a high degree of
agreement on what appear to be the least serious symptoms: a sore throat (30
per cent), foot corns (21 per cent), and a slight cold (4 per cent).

Two years later, there was a higher proportion of respondents who felt that
medical attention should be sought for every item. Even though the percentages were high in 1965, they were even higher in 1967. The gains were greatest
for upper respiratory infections, i.e., sore throats (from 30 to 50 per cent), and
foot corns (from 21 per cent to 39 per cent), undoubtedly reflecting the attitudes of elderly patients who appreciated the podiatry services made available
to them.

The substantial increase in level of utilization of ambulatory health care
services cannot be attributed to gains in knowledge about signs and symptoms
of a more serious nature that deserve prompt attention. Even before the advent

Table 17-2
Conditions for Which a Doctor Should Be Seen

	Baseline health survey Nov. 1965 N = (357) % = 100.0 Per cent	Follow-up health survey Nov. 1967 N = (436) % = 100.0 Per cent	Improvement or decline	x^2
Serious				
Severe shortness of breath	89	92	+3	n.s.
Lump or discolored patches of skin	88	92	+4	n.s.
Rash or itch for week or more	84	90	+6	.05
Cough for several weeks	80	87	+7	.05
Feeling of dizziness	73	77	+4	n.s.
Unexplained loss of 10 lb.	73	78	+5	n.s.
Mixed				
Frequent headaches	70	80	+10	.01
Feeling tired all the time	69	80	+11	.001
Backaches fairly often	66	78	+12	.001
Diarrhea or constipation	57	65	+8	.05
Minor Conditions				
Sore throat, runny nose	30	50	+20	.001
Foot corns	21	39	+17	.001
Slight cold	4	9	+5	n.s.

of the Health Center, there already was considerable sophistication and consensus with respect to such symptoms, and according to information reported by respondents, serious ailments (e.g., chronic nature) were likely to be brought to a physician's attention sooner or later. This opinion suggests, however, an increasing disposition by Columbia Point residents to bring to the attention of physicians symptoms at an *earlier* stage when they were less painful or disruptive to the daily routine, or of a more minor nature. This interpretation is consistent with the findings cited earlier in this paper that a reduction occurred in the proportion of residents who reported that needed medical attention had been put off.

2. Beliefs in asymptomatic checkups. Perhaps an even more significant index of the disposition of people to seek prompt medical attention (than recognizing the medical significance of particular signs of illnesses) may be the belief about the value of asymptomatic general health examinations. There was a marked increase in the proportion of people who endorsed the utility of such an examination. At the time of the first survey, 47 per cent disagreed with the statement that "there is no need to see a doctor regularly if you are not sick"; in the second survey two years later, the figure was 62 per cent (p = <.001).

Attitudes toward Sources of Ambulatory Health Care: Respondents were asked to rate their current medical care, health care services available to the Columbia

Point community, two open-ended questions about the Health Center, structured questions about physicians and their relationships to patients, and for a
comparative evaluation of major sources of health care.

1. General Evaluations of Medical Care and the Health Center. The proportion of respondents who reported that they were "very satisfied" with their
own health care services increased sharply from 56 to 81 per cent, after the
Health Center was established. It is conceivable, although highly improbable on
the basis of what we know about developments in other ambulatory health care
services for which Columbia Point residents would be eligible, that the gain in
satisfaction of this magnitude would be attributable to sources other than the
Health Center. To minimize the inferential nature of our conclusion, we examined replies to a question in which respondents were asked to rate on a five-point
scale various features of the community including its health care services. This
question provides a more direct assessment of the Health Center as the primary
health resource of the community. The proportion of residents who rated
health facilities in the community as "very good" or "good" was a strikingly low
24 per cent just before the Health Center's doors were opened. Two years later,
this figure increased dramatically to 91 per cent (table 17-3). Only shopping
facilities, after the construction of a nearby major shopping center, and schools,
after a new school was built, showed comparable increases in favorable assessment. Since only 71 per cent of the respondents acknowledged the Health
Center as their regular source of care, a majority of those who claim some other
source, or no source at all, must nonetheless have concurred in the more favorable evaluation of this aspect of Columbia Point.

Table 17-3

Selected Aspects of the Columbia Point Community Which Are Rated "Very Good" or "Good" in the Baseline and Follow-up Surveys

Aspects of Columbia Point	Baseline health survey Nov. 1965 N = (357) % = 100.0* Per cent	Follow-up health survey Nov. 1967 N = (436) % = 100.0* Per cent	Improvement or decline Per cent	x^2
Health facilities	24	91	+67	.001
Police protection	14	16	+2	n.s.
Teenager's behavior	6	12	+6	.05
Shopping facilities	24	92	+68	.001
Upkeep of housing	25	16	−9	.01
Recreation facilities	33	35	+2	n.s.
School facilities	42	72	+30	.001
Helpful neighbors	42	44	+2	n.s.

*Does not add up to 100 per cent since each aspect of Columbia Point was rated by all re-
spondents.

2. Specific Evaluation of the Health Center: What people like and dislike about it. Such global evaluations, of course, offer us no insight as to the bases for the favorable assessment. In view of the geographic isolation of this community from major sources of health care services in the past, sheer convenience may be the decisive consideration in accounting for the shift in overall assessment, assuming that no counterbalancing disadvantages are experienced in other salient aspects of health care delivery, e.g., quality of care, the personal manner in which it is rendered, etc. The Health Center was designed explicitly to do more than simply provide equivalent services at greater convenience; its purpose is to assure good quality, coordinated, continuous, and personal centered care, a new organizational form of health care delivery and a more comprehensive definition of health, as well as accessibility and relevance. It is, therefore, important for both practical and theoretical reasons to understand the actual bases for patronage by residents of this community.

An examination of responses to two sets of open-minded queries makes clear that while convenience in access (e.g., reduction of travel and waiting time) is a highly salient concern to residents in this community, considerations of quality of care and interpersonal relationships are also important. Respondents were asked to specify what they liked and disliked about the Health Center. Responses to this question, previously reported in more general form, are presented here in greater detail. In addition, they were asked to recall at least one experience that had increased confidence in the Health Center and another which undermined their confidence in it. In order to reduce the possibility that respondents would feel inhibited about reporting personal negative experiences at the Health Center, respondents were asked (for both favorable and unfavorable incidents) to report experiences that happened to them *or* to someone else they knew. Ninety-six per cent of the people whom we interviewed mentioned something they liked about the Health Center but only 37 per cent mentioned something they disliked. In response to the "critical incident" questions, similarly, 73 per cent were able to recall an important favorable experience at the Health Center and only 22 per cent an important unfavorable experience.

Three aspects of the Health Center services were favorably mentioned by relatively large numbers of residents. Convenience—that is, proximity of medical services and the reduction of waiting time—received the most frequent mention (60 per cent). Since Columbia Point is so inaccessible to the health services previously used by most residents, and a great majority of residents used hospital outpatient clinics and emergency rooms, the salience of convenience is understandable. Not far behind in frequency of mention was interpersonal relationships with the staff—the personal attention and courteous treatment received (47 per cent). Quality of care was mentioned by 36 per cent and good facilities by 23 per cent (table 17–4).

Although the great majority of community residents are very satisfied with the Health Center, responses to the two open-ended questions disclose a few

Table 17-4

Reasons Given for Liking and Disliking Health Center by Columbia Point Residents, 1967 Survey

A. Reasons for Liking Health Center		
Total Respondents	N = (436)	% = 100.0*
1. Convenience	262	60
2. Personal service, attention	205	47
3. Quality care	156	36
4. Good facilities	99	23
5. Any cost reference	55	13
6. Nothing liked	4	1
7. Don't know, never been there	–	–
B. Reasons for Disliking the Health Center		
Total Respondents	N = 434	% = 100.0*
1. Inconvenience (excludes "insufficient staff")	33	8
2. Lack of personal attention	32	8
3. Poor quality care	44	10
4. Lack of facilities	18	4
5. Any cost reference	0	0
6. Nothing disliked	261	60
7. Don't know, never been there	14	3

*Does not add to 100 per cent since more than one reason may be given by each individual.

focal points of dissatisfaction. Responses to the question, "What do you dislike about the health center?" centered on the same three themes: inconvenience mentioned by 8 per cent, or a maximum of 13 per cent if we include complaints about "insufficient staff," poor quality of care (10 per cent), and unsatisfactory interpersonal relations (8 per cent). Hence, the very same aspects of the Health Center which are the focal points of dissatisfaction by some residents are the source of favorable mention by several times as many others. The "negative incident" question resulted in a similar pattern of responses which differed primarily in that it elicited concrete instances of patient dissatisfaction with the Health Center. While it is probably utopian to expect fully to satisfy everyone in a single facility, it is extremely important for those responsible for any service to consider in detail each grievance or complaint. (The Health Center since its inception has had a joint grievance committee with consumers to deal with patient complaints.)

3. Attitudes about Physicians. In addition to these open-ended questions, several aspects of the health care delivery system were singled out for systematic evaluation and embodied in structured questions. Residents were asked to rate physicians, traditionally the key persons in the health care delivery system, on a number of qualities, including competence, quality of care rendered, communication, personal interest in the patient, and attitudes toward preventive care and minor patient complaints. While a large majority of people credited most

physicians, even before the Health Center was established, with being competent and interested in helping their patients (85 per cent and 91 per cent, respectively), they were somewhat more critical of the quality of care (20 per cent agreed that "doctors don't give you a really good examination"), of the lack of sufficient personal interest in the patient (31 per cent), of their failure to give patients a chance to explain what their trouble was (28 per cent), and most critical of the failure of the physician to explain what their trouble was (43 per cent). In addition, some residents imputed to physicians attitudes which might be expected to discourage patients from seeking asymptomatic checkups or from seeking prompt medical attention for signs or symptoms of illness at an early stage. Twenty-five per cent complained that "doctors only want to see you when you're sick. . ." (i.e., are not interested in preventive care), and a similar percentage maintained that doctors were not interested in hearing about minor complaints (table 17–5).

Two years later, Health Center physicians as a group were favorably rated on virtually all qualities by larger proportions of residents. The proportion of residents who attributed competence and dedication in general remained high (89 per cent and 92 per cent, respectively). The proportions that complained that doctors do not give good examinations dropped from 20 to 11 per cent. Doctor-patient communication as a source of dissatisfaction also declined; the proportion who agreed that "doctors don't explain enough to their patients" decreased from 43 per cent to 14 per cent and that "they don't give patients a chance to tell them exactly what their trouble is" decreased from 20 to 11 per cent. Relatively fewer residents complained about the lack of personal interest by the physician. The percentage was reduced from 31 to 12. Finally, the disinterest in preventive health examinations imputed to physicians also declined; the proportion of residents who agreed that "doctors only want to see you if you're sick—they don't want you to come in just for a checkup" declined from 25 per cent to 8 per cent. The percentage who felt that doctors "are not interested in hearing about minor things" decreased from 26 per cent to 14 per cent.

4. Comparative Evaluation of Major Sources of Care. As has been reported elsewhere, respondents were asked to compare the Health Center, hospital outpatient clinics and emergency room services, and private practitioners on four major dimensions: quality of care, its comprehensiveness, the personal manner in which it is given, and convenience. A majority of respondents chose the Health Center over its nearest rival by a better than 2 to 1 ratio on all four criteria; still others rated the several sources as equivalent on each criterion.[1]

Finally, the residents were asked which source of health care they would prefer if all alternative sources of care were free of charges. Although some who use the Health Center stated they would shift their patronage, the Health Center was preferred over the private practitioner, the next most preferred source of care by more than 3 to 1, even in this hypothetical situation (table 17–6). If all other sources of care were just as accessible as the Health Center,

Table 17-5
Evaluation of Physicians

Attitudes toward doctors*	Baseline health survey Nov. 1965	Follow-up health survey Nov. 1967	x^2
	Per cent who agreed		
	$N = (357)$	(436)	
	$\% = 100.0$	100.0	
Competent, Quality Care			
Doctors are competent and know what they are doing	85	89	n.s.
The doctors don't give you a really good examination	20	11	<0.1
Communication			$<.001$
They don't tell you enough about your condition; they *don't* explain just what the trouble is	43	14	
The doctors *don't* give you a chance to *tell them* exactly what your trouble is	28	11	$<.001$
Rapport, personal interest			
Most doctors are really interested in helping you	91	92	n.s.
They don't take enough personal interest in you	31	12	$<.001$
Doctors don't really know your medical history, the illness you have had, your reactions to medicine	26	15	$<.001$
When to seek medical attention			
Doctors only want to see you if you are sick—they *don't want* you to come in just *for a checkup*	25	8	$<.01$
Doctors *aren't* interested in hearing about *minor* things	26	14	$<.01$

*These questions were asked about doctors *in general* in the Wave I Health Survey. In the second survey, they were asked about Columbia Point physicians.

undoubtedly, still others would shift. Nonetheless, it is clear that a majority of residents now feel they are able to enjoy the benefits of free, convenient care without sacrificing either quality of care or the personal manner in which it is rendered.

3. Situational Determinants

The barriers of time, energy, and cost constitute another important class of determinants of patterns in the utilization of health care services. [c] Access to and use of health care services are affected not only by means tests and fee schedules, location, availability of public transportation, and time when services are available, but also by personal circumstances of the patient. This includes not only his potential resources in money, but also in time, energy, and social credits (e.g., availability of assistance from others), as well as the social claims upon these resources (e.g., responsibility for children, extra-household employment, etc.). The various components of resources and liabilities (or costs) have a limited interchangeability: the time-energy costs of health services which are difficult to reach by public transportation can be reduced by car or taxi. The inflexibility introduced by responsibility for small children can be offset by access to baby-sitters—for hire, in a child care area at a health center, or through other forms of reciprocity. In accounting for underutilization of health care services among the poor and for subsequent improvement in utilization attributable to the Health Center, such situational factors constitute a major alternative (although not necessarily a mutually exclusive) explanation to the frequently cited hypothesis that underutilization reflects learned behavior, a social class subculture, a culture of poverty, or the like.

Our findings confirm the expectation that the potential cost barriers to health care utilization are markedly reduced subsequent to the introduction of the Health Center. This will be documented by an examination of responses to several questions included in the interview schedule: 1. reasons cited by respondents who acknowledged postponing needed health care; 2. reported barriers to the use of emergency health care services; 3. time spent door-to-door, in seeking medical care as estimated by respondents, and 4. reported financial indebtedness for medical reasons.

Table 17-6
Sources of Regular Health Care Which Would Be Chosen if All Sources Were Cost-free

Hypothetical choice of regular source of medical care if all facilities were free	Wave 2 health survey Nov. 1967	
	N	Per cent
Private Doctor	87	20
Columbia Point Health Center	275	63
Hospital Outpatient Department	57	13
Other	17	4
Total	436	100

---

[c]Time and effort are costs typically neglected in accounting for human decision behavior.

Reasons for Postponing Needed Medical Care: We noted earlier that 23 per cent of the respondents, interviewed before the Health Center opened its doors, acknowledged that they or someone in their family had put off medical attention. When respondents were asked about the reasons for the delay, financial cost, and convenience—ie., considerations relating to geographic inaccessibility, hours of service, and waiting time—were identified as major impediments. Forty-five per cent said they were unable to pay for physicians services or for medicine. Seventeen per cent said they could not afford transportation to the sources of care. Twenty per cent complained that it took too long to get there, and 10 per cent felt too ill to travel. Female heads of more than one in five households reported that they were unable to find anyone to take care of children or dependent adults while they sought medical care.

Two years later, among the relatively fewer households that still acknowledged putting off needed medical care, the reasons reported were scattered over a wider variety of categories although considerations relating to money cost (e.g., physicians' fees and medicines) and transportation remain numerically the most significant. Such respondents probably are among the minority ineligible for welfare medical benefits, who continue to patronize other sources of health care services than the Health Center.

Barriers to Use of Emergency Services: Respondents were also asked whether they had actually made use of emergency health services and, if so, whether they had experienced difficulty in using those facilities because of problems in arranging for child care, in reaching emergency room service, or arising from a long wait for treatment. Among persons who had occasion to use a hospital emergency room before the Health Center was established, a maximum of 18 per cent had difficulty in arranging for care of younger children,[d] 27 per cent mentioned trouble with transportation, and 47 per cent mentioned the long waiting time at the emergency room. Two years later, fewer respondents experienced such barriers in access to emergency room service—whether at a hospital or at the Health Center, since the Health Center also provided transportation to nearly all emergency services required by its patients. Among households that made use of emergency health care services subsequent to the inception of the Health Center, the proportions who reported difficulties in arranging for baby-sitters, obtaining transportation, or with long waiting periods for care dropped substantially: the figures are, respectively, 6 per cent, 7 per cent, and 12 per cent.

Time Spent in Obtaining Services: The time spent, door-to-door, in obtaining needed medical care also decreased markedly after the Health Center opened its

---

[d]This figure is not adjusted for childless households.

doors. Previously, 84 per cent of the respondents reported that they spent two hours or more each time they sought care. (Fourteen per cent reported spending five hours and longer per visit.) Two years later, the percentage reporting two or more hours declined to 17 per cent.

Among residents who used the Health Center, 79 per cent reported that they received care within a half hour of their arrival. The proportion who complained about excessive waiting time in the physician's office declined from 56 per cent before the inception of the Health Center to about 20 per cent afterwards.

Financial Considerations: The significance of financial considerations in affecting access to, and utilization of, health care services is underestimated by the data presented thus far. The reader will recall that relatively few respondents, in reply to the open-ended question as to what they liked about the Health Center, made any reference to the absence of fees for comprehensive health care services, including laboratory services and pharmaceutical supplies. Although such considerations are usually prominent among reasons for postponing care, only a fraction of Columbia Point residents are so affected. A major reason for this is that a substantial proportion of Columbia Point residents were eligible for welfare medical benefits. Even before the Health Center opened, residents who were willing to pay a price in inconvenience and accept emergency room and hospital outpatient clinic care were able to obtain some health care services in Boston. This is reflected in the fact that prior to the Health Center, virtually all chronic medical ailments were reported to have been brought to the attention of a physician at some time during the history of the medical ailment. Only half of these chronic conditions, however, were under continuing medical supervision.

It is also likely that financial considerations may have discouraged residents from seeking medical care at earlier stages of illness or taking advantage of preventive health services. Although half of the families made *no* outlays for medical care or related transportation expenditures prior to the inception of the Health Center, the remaining families spent an average of $8.00 monthly for these purposes. (Much of this, it should be kept in mind, was for emergency room and outpatient clinic care.) Fifteen per cent of the respondents reported that medical expenses lead to financial indebtedness, a figure which was reduced to 3 per cent two years later.

4. Summary

This paper is one of a series reporting the results of a comprehensive evaluation of the impact of a neighborhood health center on its target community. Two major sources of data are drawn upon for this evaluation: 1. data on *actual* utilization based on medical records, and 2. attitudes toward, and reported use of, health care services based on a survey of a random sample of households interviewed at two points in time—just before the inception of a neighborhood health center and two years later.

A previous report, based on actual utilization, showed high levels of utilization of Health Center services by this low income community, approximating comparable figures for more affluent populations. We noted further a shift in actual utilization from such major sources of ambulatory health care services as Boston City Hospital (outpatient department and emergency room), heavily used by Columbia Point residents in the past, to the Health Center. A great majority of residents subsequently acknowledged the Health Center as their central or regular source of care.

The before-and-after studies described in the present report show, for example, marked increases in the reported use of such health services as asymptomatic checkups (from 17 per cent, prior to the establishment of the Health Center, to 59 per cent two years later), poliomyelitis immunizaiton in children (from 78 per cent to 92 per cent, reaching two children in three who previously had been without a polio vaccination), and a reduction in families that reported postponing needed medical care (from 23 per cent to 10 per cent).

Taken together, these and other reported findings demonstrate a major and significant change in behavior relating to medical care and utilization of numerous aspects of the health care system. One would anticipate that such a major behavioral change would be paralleled by and associated with significant change in attitudes, leaving aside for a moment the question of causality. The present study found that major attitudinal changes had occurred. Recognition of various signs and symptoms of illness as reasons for seeking medical care uniformly increased; this was particularly marked for symptoms of an earlier stage in the disease process, e.g., "sore throats" which increased from 30 to 50 per cent. The proportion of respondents who acknowledged the value of an asymptomatic checkup also increased from 47 to 62 per cent.

Attitudes toward sources of ambulatory care were also found to have improved markedly after the inception of the Health Center. The proportion of residents who reported that they were "very satisfied" with their (own) medical care increased from 56 to 81 per cent, and the proportion who rated health care services available at Columbia Point as "very good" or "good" increased from 24 to 91 per cent. Ninety-six per cent of survey respondents mentioned something they liked about the Health Center and only 37 per cent mentioned something they disliked.

Respondents were asked to rate physicians in general, on the basis of experience prior to the establishment of the Health Center, with those staffing the Health Center on a number of dimensions: competence, dedication, quality of care given, the personal manner in which care was given, and doctor-patient communication. Attitudes towards physicians at the Columbia Point Health Center were consistently more favorable than those expressed toward physicians prior ot the establishment of the Health Center. The proportion of respondents, for example, who complained of poor quality of care declined from 20 to 11 per cent, of the lack of personal interest by physicians from 31 to 12 per cent, and of the physicians' failure to explain what was the matter with the patient from 43 to 14 per cent.

Respondents were also asked systematically to compare the Health Center with two other alternative sources of care—the private practitioner and a hospital outpatient clinic or emergency service—on four major dimensions. A majority of residents preferred the Health Center over its closest rival by a ratio of at least 2 to 1 on each of the four dimensions. In response to a hypothetical situation in which medical care from any source would be free to the patient, the Health Center was favored by a ratio of 3 to 1.

Changes in a second set of variables might also be expected to accompany (or help account for) the changes in reported utilization of health care services— situational variables such as time, convenience, and money. The present study found that such factors did affect reported utilization of services. Almost uniformly, past problems in obtaining medical care were reported to have declined dramatically with the advent of the Health Center. For example, the proportion of residents who reported that they spent a minimum of two hours, door-to-door, in the typical effort to obtain medical care declined dramatically from 84 to 17 per cent. The percentage who complained about excessive waiting time in the doctor's office decreased from 53 to 20 per cent. Finally, financial indebtedness incurred for medical reasons declined from 11 to 3 per cent, a figure which is noteworthy when account is taken of the fact that a high proportion of this community was eligible for welfare or other third-party medical reimbursement.

Discussion

We have already shown that the advent and development of a Health Center which eliminates traditional barriers to comprehensive and community-relevant health services can significantly increase utilization of physicians and use of the health care system by a low income, urban population. We now find that advent of the Health Center also significantly changed attitudes, knowledge, and beliefs about health and health care, particularly in the critical areas of early diagnosis and treatment, and asymptomatic checkups, areas which in the past (probably for situational reasons), have received least attention from the poor. Since no systematic effort was made to modify beliefs and attitudes of the community through mass educational campaigns, we suggest that it is experience—the experience of the Health Center—which induced changes in attitudes as well as in actual behavior. In this respect, our inferences are paralleled by evidence from studies of racial integration, that it is not necessary to bring about changes in attitudes before achieving integration; both behavior and attitudes are likely to change in a positive direction as a *consequence* of social integration. The new health experience, however, has to meet the situational needs (time, cost, convenience, etc.) of the health consumers to be meaningful and to facilitate attitudinal and behavioral change. This may be the root issue of the failure of many "health educational" campaigns aimed at the poor in the past—efforts which tried to change the health attitudes and behaviors of the poor without changing the health care system. For many low income consumers, this must have seemed to be an attempt to lead them back into a grossly unsatisfactory system—and into a set of experiences which merely reinforced their previous negative attitudes. But if, in contrast, there is a change in the available health care system, then both attitudes and behavior may change.

If this is so, then something even more important than changes in utilization may have been occurring among the residents of Columbia Point after the advent of the Health Center with its situational advantages. One may at least hope that the changes in health-related attitudes and knowledge described in this study may persist beyond the consumer's length of residence at Columbia Point. A major effect of a Health Center, then, may be to increase the continuing and informed demands by the poor for significant improvement in the health care system available to them—improvement not only with respect to situational factors but also to meet their new expectations of early diagnosis and treatment, good preventive care, and high quality professional services delivered with concern and respect.

The significance of a new institution like a health center thus may extend beyond its immediate effects on (or advantages to) its target population; it may additionally create informed dissatisfaction with the present system and informed demands for change in the system to meet newly perceived needs for good primary and preventive care. Perhaps, for the health consumers as well, experience is the best teacher.

Reference

1.   Bellin, S.S., and Geiger, H.J.: Actual public acceptance of the neighborhood health center by the urban poor. *JAMA 214:*2147, 1970.

18

Basic Utilization Experience of OEO Comprehensive Health Services Projects

Mark A. Strauss and Gerald Sparer

This article is based on a study of eight comprehensive health services (CHS) projects receiving grants from the Office of Economic Opportunity (OEO). Five of the projects are representative examples of neighborhood health centers, in which the health care practitioners are employees of the centers. These centers cater almost entirely to persons with low incomes. The remaining three projects are associated with established group practices which provide services to OEO-assisted persons as well as to private patients. All the comprehensive health services projects provide a variety of health-related services to residents of specified geographical areas.

This paper describes utilization experiences of persons in impoverished communities who were registered with CHS projects. In search for early clues that the program provides adequate access to acceptable outpatient health services, utilization rates of the project registrants are shown together with rates obtained from a national survey and from several communities not assisted by the program.

In searching for these clues, it is assumed that utilization experience of individuals who depend for outpatient services on CHS projects is one of the important indicators of accessibility of the services. This assumption is based on beliefs that:

1. The studied projects function in a manner consistent with operational guidelines established by OEO, and, therefore, have similar outreach effectiveness, comparable health care plans and follow-up practices.
2. Populations of the studied projects and populations in communities not assisted by the CHS programs had similar morbidity patterns.

Furthermore, a comparison between utilization experiences of the studied projects is limited by the lack of knowledge of what were the utilization rates of the studied project populations prior to establishment of the projects. This

Reprinted from *Inquiry* 8, 4 (December 1971): 36–49. The original version of this paper contains a detailed description of the methodology used to compute the denominator of active registrants and to calculate registrant utilization rates. This chapter has been edited from the original.

limitation applies also to inferences drawn from utilization experiences of project populations and populations in communities which were not assisted by the CHS program. In addition, any utilization comparison between these communities and project populations is weakened by the inability to ascertain how extensive and selective was the penetration of communities served by the projects. The projects' patients may not be representative samples of the eligible residents in the served communities.

The discussion is presented in the following sequence: First, the critical and difficult issue of the denominator for utilization rates is broached. A concept of an "active registrant" is postulated. Then, utilization rates of the studied projects are shown and are collectively compared to rates obtained from past surveys. Differences in individual rates of the eight studied projects are examined. Lastly, evidence is shown that an initial surge of services provided to patients newly introduced into CHS projects subsides after six months of the patients' use of the projects.

In general, our findings were:

1. The concept of an "active registrant" is a useful denominator for utilization rates in making comparisons between health care delivery systems as well as in planning. The concept also serves as a meaningful bridge to a broader denominator, the "registrant."
2. The studied OEO-assisted projects are generally characterized by relatively high utilization rates for "users" and "active registrants"; the utilization rates of "registrants" are comparable to national averages for all persons. These findings imply adequate accessibility of medical services in OEO-assisted communities.
3. Patients newly registered with the projects initially utilize service at a higher rate than later during their enrollment. Services are made readily accessible to new registrants who, very likely, require prompt medical attention.

In order to compare utilization experiences for all of the studied projects, it was necessary to develop a technique for estimating the number of bona fide registrants from inflated registration files and then to calculate their utilization rates.[a]

Studied Projects and Their Utilization Experience

Important descriptives of the eight studied CHS projects and of their registrants are shown in Table 18-1. In three projects, X, Y, and Z, the OEO-assisted fami-

---

[a]For a detailed description of this methodology, see the original article's section on the problem of selecting the denominator, pp. 37–41.

lies receive medical services from group practices which existed 10 or more years prior to the establishment of ties with OEO. These groups continue to engage in private practice and presently provide services to all the patients on truly integrated bases. Their OEO patients range from less than 10 percent to as many as 40 percent of the total clientele. Two of these groups serve rural populations and one serves an urban community. The fiscal arrangement between OEO and these group practices ranges from fee-for-service reimbursement to capitation rate.

The selected neighborhood health centers are representative examples of this particular mode of health care delivery. The selected urban centers deliver different volumes of services, ranging from 20,000 to 67,000 encounters with

Table 18-1
Comprehensive Health Services Projects Selected for Study

	Rural				Urban			
		Neighborhood health centers						
		Previously existing group practices						
	A	X	Y	Z	B	C	D	E
M.D. encounters in clinic per year	18,000	17,000*	16,000*	25,000*	27,000	20,000	49,000	67,000
Age of projects at time of study	1-2	0-1	½-1½	1-2	3-4	0-1	2-3	½-1½
Approximate year of studied services	1969	1968	1968	1969	1969	1969	1969	1969
Age/sex categories of registrants								
Both sexes: 0-15	25**	41	43	64	55	62	49	49
16-44	26	29	43	32	31	28	35	41
45-64	31	18	12	4	5	6	13	4
65+	18	12	2	0	9	4	3	6
Males: All	40		47	45	42	42	45	39
16-44	7		16	11	12	7	18	11
Females: All	60		53	55	58	58	55	61
16-44	19		27	21	19	21	17	30

*Encounters with OEO-assisted patients
**Percent of all individuals

physicians per year. The one rural center selected is considered typical.

The ages of projects at the time of study varied from zero to four years. In the case of group practices, the age represents the period after instituting OEO's assistance program. It can be noted in table 18-1 that only centers B and D were in operation two years prior to the service periods examined in the study; the other projects were younger. In all cases, utilization experiences were obtained for the period which generally coincided with either the 1968 or 1969 calendar year.

Utilization of Services in Studied Projects

Table 18-2 portrays the utilization experience of the OEO-assisted populations. Two sets of rates are presented for projects unable to satisfy the definition of a "registrant": observed-active-registrant utilization rates (upper limits) and those rates adjusted to approximate the rates for "registrants" (lower limits). The

Table 18-2
Encounters at Clinic per Year per "Registrant," Observed Active Registrant and User of Clinical Services

		Rural				Urban			
		Neighborhood health centers							
			Previously existing group practices						
		A	X	Y	Z	B	C	D	E
With M.D.	Per "registrant"	4.4	5.7	4.0	3.3	4.6	4.4	4.1	4.2
	Per observed active registrant	6.3		5.7			6.3	5.9	
	Per user	6.6	7.9	6.7	4.4	6.2	7.5	6.3	6.6
With R.N. or P.H.N.	Per "registrant"				0.3	0.7	0.6	0.5	0.7
	Per observed active registrant						0.8	0.6	
	Per user				0.3	0.9	1.0	0.6	1.1
Percent of total		(10)*	(10)*	(12)**	6	13	12	9	14
Total	Per "registrant"	4.8	6.3	4.4	3.6	5.3	5.0	4.6	4.9
	Per observed active registrant	6.9		6.3			7.1	6.5	
	Per user	7.3	8.8	7.6	4.7	7.1	8.5	6.9	7.7

*Assumed
**Estimated

other projects were assumed to have defined and controllable registrant populations. "User" rates are shown for all of the eight projects.

The experience of OEO-assisted populations was obtained for a period of at least a year in all projects. Encounters between patients and physicians or patients and nurses were used to measure medical experience. An attempt was made in the study to count encounters which had a similar meaning.

In requesting data from the projects, an encounter was defined as a face-to-face meeting between a patient and a health care provider in which some significant medical service was given to the patient. The provider of care who was credited with an encounter should have acted independently and not just assisted another provider. For example, if a nurse assisted a physician during a physical examination by taking a history or drawing a blood sample, the nurse should not have been credited with a separate encounter. The nurse was simply participating in an encounter in which a physician was conducting an examination—in this case the physician should have been credited with an encounter. On the other hand, if a patient came in every week for some medication that a nurse administered on a standing order of the physician (but without the physician's actually seeing the patient each time), then these visits should have been credited to the nurse. Since this is not always an easy distinction to make by the projects, in encounters where more than one provider participated, the most senior professional present should have been shown in the records as the provider. The definition of encounter and the advocated recording procedure insures that encounters have uniform meaning in this study and were not counted more than once.

Utilization of Services by "Registrants"

A remarkable uniformity in M.D. "registrant" rates is revealed in table 18-2. Encounters with M.D.s per "registrant" per year range from 4.0 to 4.6 except for project Z, which has a value of 3.3, and project X, which has a value of 5.7. Similar uniformity is also observed in the total medical encounter rates of "registrants."

The difference in utilization of X and Z may be explained in part by the age differences of the served populations (see table 18-1), and partly by the different nature of the health care delivery systems and the methods of registration. Project X initially enrolled all those persons who were medically most deprived, while project Z carefully selected its enrollees by assigning priority to young and large families with presumably lesser incidence of morbidity. Project Z's relatively low M.D. rate is accentuated by the fact that it uses its nursing staff in direct patient service to a lesser extent than other projects for which nurse rates were available. Furthermore, project Z encourages telephone consultations; these were excluded from the encounter definition and, therefore, were not counted in this study.

The extent to which nurses contribute to the total utilization rates varies from 8 percent for project Z to 14 percent for project E. No relationships can be identified between individual percentages and the types of corresponding projects because, unfortunately, nurse rates were not available for projects A and X, while the rate for Y is an estimate based on the ratio of injections to other provided medical services.

The utilization rates of "registrants" of rural projects do not appear to differ significantly from the rates of urban projects. If the "more utilized" rural project X and the "less utilized" urban project Z were excluded from considerations, then the two other rural and four other urban projects would have averages that are much alike: 4.2 M.D. encounters per year per "registrant" for rural projects versus 4.3 for urban projects. Excluding populations of projects X and Z, the age/sex distributions of the remaining rural and urban projects (table 18-1) do not exhibit a pattern which can be useful in interpretation of the closeness of these two averages.

However, it is interesting to note among the rural projects that project X has a somewhat younger population than project A and yet the respective utilization rates do not reflect the difference. The opposite of what is expected is true—project A has a considerably lower "registrant" utilization rate than X. The explanation for this may be the same as that offered in a previous discussion—population of X has a greater incidence of morbidity.

The urban projects present an interesting contrast. Project Z with the lowest urban rate of 3.3 M.D. encounters per year per "registrant" has a slightly younger population than project B with the highest urban rate of 4.6. However, the difference between the age/sex distributions alone is insufficient to explain the rather large difference in utilization rates of these projects. Therefore, it is instructive to examine the frequency of M.D. encounters as a function of the percent of "registrants" for project Z, and to compare that frequency distribution with that of project B. Such a comparison is especially meaningful since both projects have well updated registrant rosters. To avoid assumptions needed in order to annualize experiences of new patients, distributions were based on exactly one year of services provided to individuals who, on the average, have been registered six months prior to the "experience period." When Z's and B's registrants with more than a six-month enrollment were separated from all the observed active registrants, their utilization rates were 3.0 and 4.5 M.D. encounters per year, respectively.

Figure 18-1 is a bar diagram which relates number of M.D. encounters per year per "registrant" to percent of "registrants" who were using services at the rates specified on the abscissa. The general shapes of the bar distributions for projects Z and B are nearly identical, except that Z has more low utilizers and B has more high utilizers. The bars for the "zero rate" show a difference of only 1 percent between the two projects. However, B has about 5 percent of "registrants" who had more than 15 encounters per year in contrast to Z's 1 percent.

Figure 18-1. Comparative Distributions of M.D. Encounters

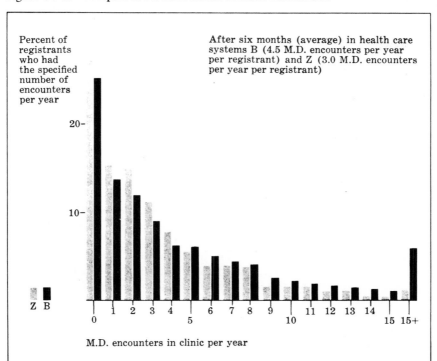

M.D. encounters in clinic per year

The difference of 1.5 M.D. encounters between these two projects is almost entirely due to utilization rates of *B*'s high utilizers. The fact that no-shows are a negligent factor in the low aevarge utilization rate of *Z* as related to the higher percentage of low utilizers in *Z*, does support the contention that *Z*'s "registrants" are generally healthier or that *B*'s "registrants" have a higher incidence of chronic illness.

Utilization of Services by Users

Utilization rates of "users" are also shown in table 18-2. The "user" rates exhibit the same relationships that were discerned in the "registrant" rates. Project *X* has again the highest value (7.9 M.D. encounters per year per user) and project *Z* has again the lowest rate (4.4 M.D. encounters per year per user). The "user" rates show a more striking uniformity than the "registrant" rates. Only the low value of *Z* stands apart from others; *X* is sufficiently close to the next highest value to be considered jointly with the other rates. Excluding project Z, M.D. encounters per year per user range from 6.2 to 7.9 for an average of 6.8.

Studied Projects Versus
Surveyed Populations

A number of surveys of selected communities with a large percentage of low-income people have been conducted by the National Opinion Research Center (NORC) of the University of Chicago. The selected urban and rural areas were surveyed prior to development of OEO-assisted health efforts. One of the questions addressed the number of contacts (visits and telephone calls) with physicians at home or in their offices, and visits to hospital clinics within the last 12 months. Utilization rates for nine urban and two rural communities were obtained from the surveys.[1]

It would require a thorough examination of the methodology used in the above surveys in order to meaningfully compare the medical experience derived from these surveys to the experience of project "registrants." Such a review of the methodology cannot be undertaken within the scope of this paper. Therefore, the utilization rates obtained from these surveys are merely presented as early clues to changes in accessibility patterns, possibly due to OEO's medical intervention.

The contact rate of the nine surveyed urban communities ranges from 2.8 to 4.7 with an average of 3.7. Most of these communities are located in the cities of the Eastern seaboard. Interestingly, the Southern cities contribute low values while the Northern cities contribute high values to the range of rates.

On the average, the contact rate of surveyed urban population is lower than the encounters with physicians and nurses per urban "registrant" (table 18-2). The average utilization of the urban CHS projects is 4.7 M.D., R.N., or P.H.N. encounters per "registrant." This average rate exceeds by one encounter the average utilization rate of the surveyed communities.

Although the surveyed urban areas are not the same as those of the studied projects, they are considered to be comparable. It is reasonable to assume that the utilization of medical services by residents in the five CHS project areas prior to the establishment of the projects was similar to that of the surveyed urban areas.

The difference in utilization between the two surveyed rural communities and the studied rural CHS projects is a considerable one; 3.2 and 2.6 contacts per year per resident versus an average of about 5.2 encounters with physicians or nurses per "registrant" for the three studied rural CHS projects. This difference is considered to be significant. However, because of diverse social and cultural settings of the compared surveyed rural communities and studied rural CHS projects, its magnitude is not readily generalizable.

Utilization rates derived from the U.S. health survey during the 1966-1967 period[2] are: 3.3 for non-S.M.S.A./farm, 4.1 for non-S.M.S.A./non-farm and 4.5 for S.M.S.A. populations. These rates are based on contacts with physicians, either in person or by telephone. The utilization experience of the studied urban OEO-assisted populations is close (except for project Z) to the national averages. Physician utilization rates of the studied rural CHS projects exceed the national average.

Initial Surge in Utilization of Project Services

As a part of the examination of accessibility, the following question was asked: "Are utilization rates of OEO-assisted populations affected by the length of exposure to comprehensive health care?"

To answer this, five of the eight populations studied in the previous section were divided into "newly introduced" and "after six months" observed active registrants. The experience of the individuals in the first group was recorded for a year (on the average) after their registration date. Because the experience of the individuals of this cohort was studied from the registration date, an annualization method was used to provide group utilization per year.

"After six months" cohorts consisted of observed active registrants who registered during a six-month period, selected in such a way that the middle of that period preceded the beginning of the examined "experience period" by six months. Experiences of these cohorts were recorded for exactly one year and, therefore, there was no need for annualization.

Comparisons of "registrant" and "active registrant" rates (table 18–3) between sets of these two cohorts show uniformly a drop in utilization rates after six months in the health care system. The same is true when "user" rates of those cohorts are examined.

Most probably, this finding indicates that the individuals who register tend to have an immediate need for physician services or that the new registrants receive initial "baseline" examinations in addition to the normal mix of needed services.

If either one or both of these assertions are true, the general availability of medical services is evidenced again. Specifically, the evidence points to priorities practiced by the studied projects—greater medical attention is focused on the new registrant.

Programmatic Implications of Findings

A national health maintenance strategy is emerging from current health planning activities. The concept of the health maintenance organization (HMO) appears

Table 18-3
Encounters at Clinic per Year per "Registrant" and per User of Clinical Services

		Newly introduced into the health care system							
		Rural					*Urban*		
		Neighborhood health centers							
		Previously existing group practices							
		A	X	Y	Z	B	C	D	E
With M.D.	Per "registrant"	5.1			3.8	6.9	4.5	4.7	
	Per user	7.3			4.9	7.3	7.6	6.7	
With R.N. or P.H.N.	Per "registrant"				0.3	1.0	0.4	0.4	
	Per user				0.3	1.0	1.0	0.6	
Total	Per "registrant"				4.1	7.9	4.9	5.1	
	Per user				5.2	8.3	8.6	7.3	
		After six months in the health care system							
With M.D.	Per "registrant"	3.5			3.0	4.5	4.5	3.6	
	Per user	5.6			4.1	6.1	7.4	5.8	
With R.N. or P.H.N.	Per "registrant"				0.2	0.6	0.3	0.6	
	Per user				0.3	1.0	0.9	0.9	
Total	Per "registrant"				3.2	5.1	4.8	4.2	
	Per user				4.4	7.0	8.3	6.8	

to be an attractive means of providing health services to a large segment of the U.S. population. The HMO combines health-insurance methods of payment with provider-group modes of practice. Although the viability of health maintenance organizations has been successfully tested by about two dozen existing institutions, an important question still remains to be answered: What will be the utilization pattern and, therefore, the cost of health care per capita when the HMO coverage is extended beyond the present five million consumers to include a large number of predominantly low-income persons?

Associated with this question is a subsidiary one: If the registered persons do not enter into contractual relationships as do enrollees in typical prepayment plans, what denominator should be used in order to derive a per-capita assessment of costs for low-income persons who themselves will not pay the received services?

Since the CHS projects are serving low-income communities, the findings of this study can be used to infer answers to the above questions.

HMOs which open their doors in medically indigent communities may expect new enrollees to utilize services at a higher rate than middle-income persons. This initial surge of services should eventually taper off to a utilization rate approximating the national experience. The pattern of initial surge and its later decline is consistent among all the studied projects although the actual utilization rates vary. How HMO providers can estimate the number of individuals or families as the basis for claiming reimbursement will be an important administrative issue. Little experience exists that provides clues regarding the behavior of registrants in "free" health projects. The absence of the contractual relationship between provider and consumer raises questions about the character and extent of services that registrants will expect from the provider. A continuous enrollment-verification mechanism, like quarterly or even monthly certification of registrants, will prove too cumbersome to administer. Frequent certification checks would be viewed as repugnant as the welfare screening procedures used in many jursidictions. Estimating techniques such as those used in this study will need to be extended and tested in order to address this difficult issue.

References

1. Partly published results of surveys conducted by the National Opinion Research Center of University of Chicago for selected projects funded by the Office of Economic Opportunity, and analyzed by System Sciences, Inc., Bethesda, Maryland.
2. National Health Survey Statistics, Series 10, Number 49, Table 1.

19

A Neighborhood Health Center: What the Patients Know and Think of its Operation

Bruce Hillman and Evan Charney

The Rochester Neighborhood Health Center is an OEO-supported program designed to provide comprehensive medical and dental care to an urban indigent population residing in a defined central city area in Rochester, New York. The services are administered jointly by the University of Rochester and Rochester Action for a Better Community, under the auspices of a community advisory board. To be eligible for registration at the Center, a family must reside within the geographic borders of the area (approximately 21,000 persons were so identified in the 1970 census), and also be eligible (or close to eligibility) for New York State Medicaid. Although eligibility criteria have steadily and progressively been narrowed in New York State, there were approximately 11,000 Medicaid recipients in the target area at the time of this study (summer and fall of 1970), and the Center had slightly over 9,000 registered patients. Like most central northern city areas in the United States, this population is poor (median annual income $5,000), lives in highly dilapidated housing (50 per cent so defined in 1964 census), and is composed mostly of black or Spanish families. Prior to the Health Center's opening in July 1968, health services were provided largely by distant hospital clinics or emergency rooms, or by Health Department-administered well-child stations. Only 23 per cent of the population used private practitioners for their medical care. Into this by-now familiar situation a center opened which promised comprehensive ambulatory and hospital services in an accessible, centrally located facility, open daily from 8:30 A.M. to 9:30 P.M., with physician on-call services 24 hours a day. In addition to having their own private physician (from a largely full-time salaried staff), patients would have a team nurse to provide preventive and home services, and a Family Health Worker drawn from the community and trained to act in a social service and health advocacy role. Both nurse and health assistant stress a moderately aggressive outreach role with follow-up of broken appointments, transportation, and direct health education.

Reprinted from *Medical Care* 10, 4 (July-Aug. 1972): 336–344.

Evaluation

Research on neighborhood health centers, one of the major innovations in
health care during the 1960s, has been meager. As part of an evaluation of the
effectiveness of this program, the present study was designed to assess how, in
fact, the Center was perceived by its registered clientele. Although patient
knowledge and satisfaction are not the sole determinants of a program's success,
failure to engage, satisfy, and communicate with patients would be a serious
condemnation of the Health Center concept, regardless of the quality of care
provided. It is as yet an unanswered question as to whether a poor family, often
with diverse and numbing social and economic problems, can appropriately
utilize sophisticated and highly organized modern group medical practice.[7]
Certainly most prepaid programs have shunned this costly and frustrating group
and, although evidence of success has been suggested by several programs,[1,2] it
is far from an established fact.

The questions this study sought to answer, therefore, are: 1. how well do
registered patients know and understand the roles of the people and services of
their Center, and 2. what do they like and dislike about the program? A portion
of the study sought further to identify differences between those highly satisfied
with their care, and those less enchanted.

Earlier studies of the impact of this Health Center had identified a 39 per
cent reduction in use of Hospital Emergency services for target area children,[4]
presumably due to availability of the Center as an alternative, and a less impressive but palpable shift in the pattern of hospitalization after two years; this last
includes reduced admissions for infections and respiratory disease, and increased
admissions for elective and corrective surgery.[5]

Methods

Families selected for study were drawn from among those registered with the
Center for more than six months. This was to insure adequate time for attitudes
to develop. A sample list of names was selected by random number assignment
from the Center's computer list. Home interviews were conducted until 20
families were interviewed in each of the Center's five team areas (a total of 100
families, or approximately 5 per cent of the Health Center role). To be included,
the respondent (in almost all cases the mother) must have indicated that the
family used the NHC for *at least part* of its care. The interviews were carried out
by three individuals, one black and one Spanish resident of the target area,
neither of whom were registered patients, and a freshman medical student
(B.H.). Each conducted a series of tape-recorded pilot interviews, both in order
to develop an appropriate open-ended interview schedule and to insure uniformity of technique with minimal bias. During the actual four-week period of

the study, tape-recorded interviews were reviewed periodically by one of the two authors (E.C.) to further monitor technique. The final interview schedule was evolved through the pilot interviews and a series of open-ended discussions with Health Center patients.

Families selected for the actual study were initially contacted by mail and informed that the University of Rochester was conducting a study of available health services. No mention was made of the Neighborhood Health Center initially by the interviewer. Patients were informed that their identity would not be transmitted to any health provider.

The final interview consisted of 56 questions, with ample opportunity for further elaboration by the patient. Areas covered included what sources of health care were regularly used by all family members, the names of their health providers, the patient's perception of the nature and hours of operation of the health facility, and opportunity for detailed comment on their satisfactions and dislikes. Health Center users were asked about the Center's Neighborhood Advisory Council, as well as who they thought did and should administer and direct the Center.

Results

The three interviewers visited 213 households. Of these, 76 families had moved and 19 were not home on several visits at different times of the day or evening. Comparison (based on demographic data obtained at their initial registration) revealed no difference between these 95 families and the 118 interviewed for the following variables: age and education of head of household, number in household, length of time at present address and in the county, and level of family income. None of the families who were contacted refused to be interviewed. One hundred and eighteen registered families needed to be interviewed before 100 respondents were found who identified the Neighborhood Health Center as responsible for part or all of their family's care.

Of the 118 families interviewed, 76 (65 per cent) named the Center as the *main or primary* health care resource for all family members; 24 (20 per cent) said that the Center was the primary source for *some* but not all family members, and 18 (15 per cent) said they did not use the Center at all for care, despite being registered there.

Access to the Center was considered very convenient by 93 per cent of those interviewed: 69 per cent walk there, 20 per cent use private cars, and only 11 per cent use transportation provided by the Center. Although a surprisingly high 86 per cent had the Center's telephone number memorized or could produce it, somewhat fewer (70 per cent) knew of the after-hour doctor availability, and only 47 per cent said they would use this call service if they felt they "needed to see a doctor during the night." Fully 63 per cent designated various hospital emergency departments as their source of after-hour care. Interestingly, a previous study indicated that Center families do not overuse hospital emergency facilities after 10 P.M. or on weekends.[4] Nonetheless, either the real or imagined barrier of a telephone answering service or the felt need to proceed directly to a hospital late at night have not been overcome in the minds of many patients. The fact that only 50 per cent of registered patients have private telephones could well be an important factor. Of the 100 Health Center users, 28 said they actually had obtained care outside of the Center for some family member since they had been registered.

Each health team—the unit responsible for a family's health and related social or economic problems—is composed of an internist, a pediatrician, an obstetrician-gynecologist, two nurses, and four or five family health assistants (who reside in the community). Patient knowledge of the names of those who specifically serve them varies considerably with the health provider's role. As will be shown, this is of no small importance since there is a high correlation between knowledge of an employee's name and satisfaction with the job he does. Seventy-three per cent of patients correctly named their internist or obstetrician, or both, and 71 per cent could name their children's pediatrician. This is in contrast to the 51 per cent who knew their nurse's name and 36 per cent who could name the family health assistant. Both nurse and family health assistant are not necessarily active with all families, and indeed it is this factor of activity with a family which correlated with knowledge of the health assistant's name. In interviews with the staff about selected families, 18 to 24 families visited by the health assistant at least monthly knew her name, whereas only three of 11 families with less than monthly contact could correctly identify her.

The patients were asked to define in their own words the roles of the nurse and health assistant. The nurses and health assistants were then asked to define their own roles. Tables 19-1 and 19-2 indicate how consumer and provider both view these roles. Patient's responses could generally be categorized under four or five major headings which were derived by the authors after reviewing what the patient had said. This condensation is helpful, but does not convey the intensity and feeling of many of the remarks. Essentially no negative feelings were expressed about these members of the health team. If they were only casually known to the family, the descriptions were usually rather neutral. Where the families had had a good deal of contact with either nurse or assistant (in about half of the cases), responses were warm and often exuberant. "She is God's gift to this earth," replied one elderly woman of her team nurse after some thought, a moving comment, if difficult to classify. From the interviews with the nurses, it is clear that the nurse views her job as closely matching the role projected for her by the Health Center, an expanded Public Health Nurse role to include direct preventive and some curative care to the patient; in essence, she is a family nurse practitioner. This also closely parallels the descriptions of her patients (table 19–1). She is seen as an autonomous health profes-

Table 19-1
Description of Job Role of Team Nurse by Patient and Nurse

Description	Number of patient comments	Rating of nurses' comments[8]
Provides well child, pregnancy and illness care in Center or home; offers health guidance	73	27
Helps cope with non-health problems: social, psychologic, economic; advocates for patient with community agencies	24	16
Makes appointments and reminds family; arranges transportation and checks when appointment broken	16	11
Miscellaneous	20	

sional and somewhat surprisingly none of the patients saw her as "the doctor's helper."

There is a greater discrepancy concerning the role of the family health assistant, as viewed by the Center, the patient, and the health assistants themselves. The intended concept of this job was to fulfill the community's special needs for health, economic, and social advocates. The health assistant was to help people cope with the often complicated bureaucratic systems of private and public agencies. In addition, they would serve as outreach personnel to register, orient, and help supply their patients with Health Center care. As shown in table 19-2, the indigenous health workers rate their job in general accordance with these principles. The patients, on the other hand, most often

Table 19-2
Description of Job Role of Family Health Assistant by Patient and FHA

Description	Number of patient comments	Number of HA comments
Makes appointments and reminds family, arranges transportation, babysitting, translates	45 (32%)	28 (26%)
Registers family for care; explains available services and how to use them	34 (24%)	16 (15%)
Helps cope with non-health problems: social, psychologic, economic; advocates for patients with community agencies	18 (13%)	42 (40%)
Helps cope with health problems: care of illness or carrying out medical care plans	15 (11%)	7 (6%)
Miscellaneous	28 (20%)	13 (13%)
TOTAL	140	106

name the more tangible aspects of their work when asked to list the services rendered to them. As was earlier mentioned, only 36 per cent of those interviewed knew their family health assistant by name; a sizable number of patients responded in ignorance of the existence of such a person altogether, despite acknowledged contact (often considerable) by the health assistant. It would appear, therefore, that the patients are not properly identifying the person with her role as a representative of the Neighborhood Health Center. As shall be shown later, sufficient contact between health assistant and patient appears to be a powerful determinant of satisfaction with the Center. A major limitation on their work, mentioned by several health assistants, would seem to be the present overload of patients designated to each health worker. Each was able to cite one or more projects—from helping to secure better housing to the formation of cooking and sewing get-togethers—which they have been unable to initiate for lack of time. This, indeed, is probably the dominant factor in the health assistants' failure to more fully assume their projected role. They unanimously feel this role to be desirable and realistic for both themselves and the community.

Patients' satisfaction with their physicians was uniformly high. Ninety-four per cent rated the quality of pediatrics excellent or good, and 92 per cent thought that their pediatrician displayed warmth and concern about their children's health. The combined figures for internists and obstetricians are similar, with 90 per cent rating the care excellent or good, and 80 per cent found him warm and concerned in his manner. Ninety-five per cent of respondents felt they could easily make an appointment with their own physician "most of the time." This is consistent with actual experience at the Center; analysis of patient visits for the last three months of 1970 indicated that 78 per cent of patients saw their own team physician for either illness or preventive visits during that period.

Satisfaction with the team nurse and family health assistant was, if anything, more positive, with only one patient expressing negative feelings about a family health assistant among those who had contact with these health professionals. Comments on the job performance of other Health Center Staff (receptionists, center nurses, and assistants) were also strongly positive.

Dental services were used by only 59 per cent of registered patients, in large measure because private dentists, unlike physicians in the county, will accept Medicaid patients. Of those using Health Center dental services, over 90 per cent found the quality good or excellent, the service easily accessible, and the dental staff concerned and attentive to their needs.

At the end of each interview, the patient was asked to enumerate those things which he most liked and disliked about the Neighborhood Health Center. Sixty-three per cent of those responding said they were generally satisfied but could name no special reasons why. Fifteen per cent said they particularly liked a specific individual and another 15 per cent listed the doctors' apparent concern for them as their major satisfaction. Sixty-five per cent of the comments voicing dissatisfaction concerned the age and appearance of the facilities (which are in a cramped basement of a housing project) or cited a lack of completeness in services as compared to the larger general hospitals in the area. It is expected that these problems will become less apparent with the completion of the new Health Center for which ground was broken in July 1971. The only other sizable suggestion (16 per cent) was to hire a greater number of Spanish workers and translators. This was named in 50 per cent of Spanish interviews. Thus only a very small number of respondents cited specific evils within the system itself. These ranged from difficulty in getting an appointment (three patients) to one person who complained about a doctor's lack of respect for his patients. In general, then, it appears that the population is largely satisfied with the operation of the Neighborhood Health Center and that this satisfaction is likely to increase with the improvement of the facilities.

A point of major controversy in the formation of Health Centers and projected patient satisfaction has been the question of community control. A finding of some significance was that virtually none of those interviewed fully understood who is responsible for direction and control of the Center. Only 8 per cent were able to suggest the names of any of the groups involved (OEO, the University of Rochester or the local antipoverty agency). Seventy-two per cent said they had no idea at all who directed Center operations, and the remainder named the County Health Department, "the doctors," or "the community." In fact, 44 per cent of respondents said that they didn't care who ran it, and 37 per cent said it should be run by "whoever was controlling it now." Nine per cent wished for the Center to be under community control. Only one of the interviewed families knew of the existence of the consumer-representative advisory council. Thus it appears that, in the minds of patients, community control is an issue secondary to the quality and empathy of care. Nonetheless, it is likely that active community interest in Health Center control will be slowly forthcoming and that this issue will assume greater importance in the future.

In order the gauge the degree of identification patients have with the Center, patients were asked to compare it with care they previously received; they also were asked where they would choose to go "if you could go anywhere, and all care were free." Tables 19-3 and 19-4 show their responses to these questions based on whether or not the patient knew the name of any of their team physicians. Prior to the Center's opening, 75 per cent had used hospital clinic or area clinic and emergency services, 13 per cent had used private physicians, and 12 per cent had used combinations of these services. Those previously using clinic services tended to be more positive about Health Center care (41 of 67 rated it better) than those previously using private care (5 of 12 rated it better).

Although fewer patients knew the name of their health assistant, those who did know were clearly the most satisfied with the Center's care; 78 per cent of these patients would choose Health Center care in the future over private or

Table 19-3
Comparative Perceived Quality of Care vs. Knowledge of Their Physician's Name

Compared to prior care	NHC physician's name known	NHC physician's name unknown
NHC Better	46 (64%)	7 (47%)
NHC Same	21 (29%)	3 (20%)
NHC Worse	5 (7%)	5 (33%)

Table 19-4
Comparison of Where Patient Would Go "If All Care Were Free" with Knowledge of Physician's Name

If all care free, would choose:	NHC physician's name known	NHC physician's name unknown
NHC	51 (65%)	5 (27%)
Private physician	21 (27%)	11 (61%)
Hospital clinic	7 (8%)	2 (12%)

clinic care, while only 45 per cent of those who didn't know their assistant's name would choose Center care.

When asked why they chose their hypothetical future site of care, the 56 per cent who named the Health Center cited both factors of easy accessibility and the personal warmth of the staff. Those who would choose a private physician (less than 50 per cent had actually used one) commented largely on the personal care they would anticipate receiving, and the 9 per cent who favored hospital clinics thought they would offer a broader range of services.

An attempt was made to study more closely the characteristics of highly satisfied and dissatisfied patients. Respondents who considered the Health Center superior to prior care and also would choose it over private or clinic care in the future—32 families in all—were placed in a "satisfied" group. The 19 families who considered it equal or inferior to prior care and who would not choose it in the future were considered "dissatisfied." These two subgroups were compared on the basis of various demorgaphic factors and their pattern of actual use of Center services over the previous year. In addition, their team nurse and health assistant were independently asked to comment about the family's social problems such as employment and housing difficulties, internal functioning, and integration into community activities. As previously noted, the family's own responses about the Center were not revealed to the health workers.

No differences between these two groups were noted in the following variables: number of persons in household, age and educational level of head of household, duration of residence at present address or in the county, and family income. Differences were evident in the frequency of visits to the Health Center, frequency of home contacts by team nurse and health assistant, and their estimates of the families' social and medical problems. Tables 19-5 and 19-6 summarize this data. It is evident that the satisfied family has used the Health Center services more extensively than the dissatisfied one, both for in-Center care and for outreach services. Somewhat surprisingly both groups break appointments equally often, and the satisfied group contains a higher number of families with multiple or complex social problems. Of course, it is likely that a satisfying relationship at the Center will result in increasing use and familiarity, and to this extent the results are expected. What is clear, however, is that the "multi-problem famliy" can be reached by a Health Center organization, can develop respectable frequency of contacts (though often continuing to break appointments) and can respond positively and enthusiastically to comprehensive care efforts. Whether or not such families could be equally well engaged

Table 19-5
Satisfied and Dissatisfied Families: Visits to Health Center

	Satisfied families n = 32	Dissatisfied families n = 19
Total NHC medical visits per family member in 1970	3.8	2.1
Per cent broken appointments	33%	36%
Per cent of children under five years in family with at least one well child visit in 1970	50-75%	0-25%

Table 19-6
Satisfied and Dissatisfied Families: Outreach Staff Contacts and Social Evaluation

		Satisfied families	Dissatisfied families
Family health assistant contact	At least monthly	16	5
	Minimal or no contact	10	12
Family health assistant estimate of problems	Many problems	8	3
	Average or less	13	11
Team nurse contact	At least monthly	10	2
	Minimal or no contact	19	17
Team nurse estimate of social problems	Many problems	7	1
	Average or less	12	9

with less extensive outreach efforts is not as clear. At least it seems evident that simple demographic factors do not predict with precision which families are likely to use and be satisfied with Neighborhood Health Center care.

Conclusions

In summary, these data support the idea that comprehensive Health Center care is accepted with enthusiasm by a large majority of urban indigent patients, many of whom have complicating social problems. Despite this fact, a significant minority have not been weaned from emeregncy room usage, and at least one quarter admit to going outside the system at some time for care. While this compares favorably with the 31 per cent who went outside a prepaid program at some time in a study reported a decade ago by subscribers to the Health Insurance Plan of Greater New York,[7] it does indicate that Neighborhood Health Centers may not meet all of their patients' primary care demands. Although the community control issue has not been a fiercely contested one at present in the Rochester Program, patients seemed more concerned with the availability, quality and attitudes of Center staff than they were with issues of Center control or direction. Unless health problems become central or overwhelming to a community, this may be a true reflection of patients' feelings, regardless of social class.

References

1. Bellin, S.S., and Geiger, H.J.: Actual public acceptance of the Neighborhood Health Center by the urban poor. *JAMA 214*:2147, 1970.
2. Columbo, T.J., Saward, E.W., and Greenlick, M.R.: The integration of an OEO health program into a prepaid comprehensive group practice plan. *Am. J. Public Health 59*:641, 1969.
3. Friedson: Patients' views of medical practice, New York, Russell Sage Foundation, 1961.
4. Hochheiser, L.J., Woodward, J., and Charney, E.: Effect of the Neighborhood Health Center on the use of Pediatric emergency departments in Rochester, New York. *N. Engl. J. Med. 285*:148, 1971.
5. Klein, M.: In press.
6. Roghmann, K.J., Haggerty, R.J., and Hochheiser, L.J.: Child health services: volume and flow patterns in a metropolitan community. Unpublished.
7. Roghmann, K.J., Haggarty, R.J., and Lorenz, R.: Anticipated and actual effects of Medicaid on the medical care patterns of children. In press.
8. The data on nurses were accumulated at a later date, when the nurses were asked to rate in importance the various facets of their role.

Part IX
Quality of Care

Introduction

Neighborhood health centers have had to contend from the outset with charges that they were delivering a substandard quality of health care. Mildred Morehead, Rose Donaldson, and Mary Seravelli, in Chapter 20, report on the most systematic attempt to date to evaluate the quality of care at OEO neighborhood health centers, and to compare it with the quality of care given by other health care providers. Critics of the quality of care at the centers have failed to level the same criticisms or apply the same standards of quality to other providers—hospital outpatient departments, private physicians, group practices—or they tacitly assume the quality of the care delivered in those settings to be superior.

The Morehead data provide much more accurate and systematic information than the casual observations and quick visits upon which critics of the quality of care have based their remarks. It is ironic that criticisms of the quality of care are voiced as vigorously as they have been with regard to a set of programs which gives care to persons who were previously not served at all or were served inadequately. Many of the centers have been established in areas where any new medical services was a substantial improvement.

Morehead and her associates conclude that neighborhood health centers measure up well against other providers and are in some ways superior to them. The ratings of the quality of care at the centers vary considerably. Their record could be better, but on the whole, it is a creditable one.

The Morehead study was financed by OEO and consisted of sampling and abstracting patient records and rating the care reported, mostly be noting the presence or absence and the timing of various procedures. The authors admit the methodological limitations of their study, but their methods are much more thorough and careful than other attempts to measure quality of care on such a large scale. To improve upon the methods of review employed would require a much more expensive undertaking. This one is itself quite costly.

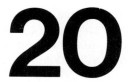

20 Comparisons between OEO Neighborhood Health Centers and Other Health Care Providers of Ratings of the Quality of Health Care

Mildred A. Morehead, Rose S. Donaldson, and Mary R. Seravalli

The OEO neighborhood health center programs were carefully designed to overcome many of the deficiencies that had existed in the health services that were previously available to the disadvantaged. Their goals included accessibility, a broad range of specialist and supportive services under one roof, participation of the community in decisions relating to the delivery model, treatment of the family as a unit and implied, of course, was the assumption that the services would be of high quality. Since the inception of the OEO health center program there has been a great deal of interest in evaluation of the quality of services provided; this interest has been manifested by a variety of activities of the OEO Office of Planning and Evaluation and has included communitywide surveys, development of cost and reporting systems and scheduled site evaluation visits. The Evaluation Unit of the Department of Community Health at the Albert Einstein College of Medicine has participated in this latter activity by conducting varying types of medical audits within the health centers and by encouraging internal review.

One of the methods employed to determine the quality of medical care has been to measure the extent to which infants, adult patients and pregnant and recently delivered women receive medical services in accord with generally accepted standards of care; these reviews have been designated as "baseline medical audits." This type of audit has been conducted in 35 OEO neighborhood health center programs. As the neighborhood health center programs are a relatively recent addition to the medical care scene, there is considerable interest in determining just how their performance compares with other forms of medical service organization. Indeed, very few studies are available for any form of medical practice to help answer the increasingly important questions: What is the effect of organization on the quality of medical care? What are the variations of the level of care among different providers? and the repetitive question, What standard should be used with which to compare findings?—the ideal, the average or performance of recognized providers of quality?

In this study, the decision was made to accept the level of care in medical school outpatient departments as the standard and to examine performance of

Reprinted from *American Journal of Public Health*, published by the American Public Health Association, 61,7 (July 1971): 1294-1306.

257

other providers in relation to the findings in these institutions. Sufficient data is not available to explore in depth the effect of the many aspects of organizational structure on professional performance, but by comparing the end product of baseline medical care, speculations can be made about the relationship between the goals and method of operation of the health providers and their performance in these areas.

Method of Review

An earlier paper[1] describes in greater detail the methods used for sample selection, abstracting of patient records and the scoring process applied to the findings. To summarize, registration files have been systematically searched for patients meeting the age criteria: 30–70 years for adult patients and 8–26 months of age for children. To remain in the sample, the patients must have paid at least three visits to the program, spanning at least a four-month period of time. This assures that they are using the facility for more than an isolated casual visit. This approach, adapted to hospitals, includes the additional criteria that adult patients be registered within the past three years (the maximum time span of operation of most of the OEO centers, which also precludes the possibility of a patient having received credit for a physical examination which was performed on a piecemeal basis over a span of five years or more). In addition, only patients presenting for ambulatory care have been reviewed (the majority of hospitalized patients would automatically receive many of the items receiving credit). The sample of obstetrical patients was obtained by requesting a consecutive list of patients who delivered going backward in time from a period eight weeks prior to the review date. (In hospitals, this was generally obtained from the delivery log.) To remain in the sample, the patients had to have made at least one prenatal visit to the facility.

Nurses, physicians, record librarians and a social worker have been engaged in the abstracting of medical records.[a] Data from each patient chart is abstracted into appropriate areas on a sheet specific for each patient. For each abstract, within the components of care, a numerator and denominator are computed and produce a score. The denominator is the expected care for that patient; the numerator, the extent to which that expectation is met. Some specific examples are: sickle cell screening is not expected for Caucasian patients, EKGs are not routinely expected for patients under age 50. These component figures for all patients reviewed are combined by adding the numerators and denominators to give a provider component score.

The numbers attached to the expected care for components within a

[a] Medical students Charles Ingardia, Jonathan Kotch, and Dennis Cryer also participated in this activity.

specialty were not equal to each other but instead reflected their relative importance (or weight) in the total baseline care.

In the presentation of this data the scores of the medical school affiliated hospital outpatient departments have been used as a standard against which to measure the performance ratings in the other programs reviewed. In the data presented, the percentages are the ratios of the average scores for the specific type of provider to the hospital outpatient average score multiplied by 100. For an overview, the average of the three outpatient over-all specialty scores is the base; interspecialty comparison is the focus. In examination of the component parts of each specialty, the hospital outpatient over-all specialty score is the base for both the over-all provider percentage and the component percentages: all comparisons are within the specialty.

The placement of the average of the medical school hospital outpatient department as a standard of 100 has comfortable implications concerning the provision of medical services that are, in fact, not justified by review of the actual data. In almost all programs reviewed, there is need for considerable improvement in performance to meet the minimal standards employed in measurement of the three specialty fields. Furthermore, the averaging of the findings within different groups of providers conceals wide ranges in performance of individual facilities or providers. It is also difficult to say how representative the non-OEO providers are of the group from which they were selected. Of the 50 OEO neighborhood health centers, 35 have been reviewed, and the findings should be quite reflective of the average performance in these centers. The other providers reviewed, however, are obviously only a small fraction of the total number of such resources in the country.

Other limitations of this method of measurement should be kept in mind. The ratings employed do not encompass judgments of clinical management or follow-up of potential pathology. The use and availability of resources required for adequate comprehensive care are not included; e.g., therapeutic care for children attending well-baby clinics or the use of community aides or other supportive personnel in the group practice plans. These scores do, however, reflect the adequacy of health assessments, a prerequisite for adequate medical care, and, in the case of pediatrics and obstetrics, the adherence to acceptable maintenance programs over a period of time.

The Health Providers Reviewed

Medical care in ten medical school affiliated hospital outpatient departments was reviewed. The bed-size of these institutions ranged from 260 to 1,500. All of them have traditionally provided care to the indigent and half serve as back-up facilities for neighborhood health centers in their areas. The findings in these institutions served as a standard against which to measure performance in the other programs. Five of these facilities were located on the eastern seaboard (in three different cities), one in the Midwest and the remainder in the Far West.

Care was reviewed in six Maternal and Infant Care Programs (M&I) and four Children and Youth Programs (C&Y) sponsored by the Children's Bureau. Three of the M&I programs were in different large cities and were part of the urban network for this service. Three functioned in rural areas. All but one of the C&Y programs were quite small, serving less than 2,000 children at the time of review. Records of infant care from health department well-baby clinics were reviewed in five different areas. One group of cases was from a major city, the other from county health departments, two of which were predominantly rural. With one exception, the sample selection in the health departments differed from that of other providers as the records sought were those of children who were obtaining their care at other institutions where they had paid at least three visits for illness. In these instances, the institutions providing care for ill children did not undertake to provide monitoring of growth and development or immunizations.

Records were reviewed in seven group practice programs. Two of these were established solely to serve the indigent; all but one of the others had an ongoing program of care for the disadvantaged in addition to their usual members who generally can be characterized as employed members of lower- to middle-income families. Three of the programs were also serving OEO populations, but the findings reported in this section reflect the performance ratings of care provided to their non-OEO populations. The method of financing varied: two were fee-for-service, two prepayment plans, two prefunded and one was supported by different types of financing methods.

The 22 nonhospital programs reviewed were dispersed throughout the country: nine were located on the eastern seaboard, four in the Midwest, one in the South and eight in the Far West. There were 14 urban and eight rural programs represented.

Of the 35 OEO centers reviewed, ten were located on the eastern seaboard, ten in the Midwest, nine in the South and six in the Far West. There were 25 urban and ten rural programs represented.

Eight of the programs reviewed were located in the state of Hawaii. The State legislature had authorized a study of the medical assistance program because of concern about cost as well as quality of care provided to Title XIX recipients. Greenleigh Associates conducted the over-all study[2] and requested the Evaluation Unit to perform the studies of the quality of medical care. A systematic approach was used to sample performance of the major providers of care to the indigent.

The other non-OEO health providers that were reviewed cannot be said to have been selected on other than an ad hoc basis. The facilities which permitted access responded to the personal request of either the senior author or the Director of Program Planning and Evaluation of OEO during the course of the OEO site evaluation visits or as a result of personal contact.

This report is based on a review of 3,040 patient records (table 20-1). The majority of these (1,700) were from the OEO health centers. Of the remaining records, 46 per cent were from the medical school affiliated hospital outpatient departments, 23 per cent from the group practice programs, 18 per cent from health departments and 13 per cent from the Children's Bureau Programs.

The Findings

When the average score of the three different specialties reviewed in the medical school affiliated hospital outpatient departments is considered the standard (100 points), both the OEO centers and the group practice plans had averages that were slightly higher (107 and 103 respectively) (table 20-2). The extent to which the scores varied from this arbitrary standard varied among the specialties. In general, the scores of obstetrical care reflected performance that was closer to the ideal standards than care in pediatrics or adult medicine. Pediatric care among these three providers received the lowest ratings. The OEO centers had the highest ratings for assessment of adult patients and the ratings of all three groups were similar for obstetrics. The specialized programs all received higher ratings in their fields than that of the other providers. The Children's Bureau Programs in particular (C&Y and M&I) were rated considerably above all other programs reviewed.

　When the ratings for adult medicine from the hospital outpatient departments are considered a standard of 100, the ratings for the OEO centers were 18 per cent higher and that of the group practice plans 7 per cent higher (tables

Table 20-1

Number of Patient Records Reviewed by Type of Provider and Specialty in Baseline Medical Audit

		Number of charts reviewed		
Type of provider	*Number of programs*	*Medicine*	*Obstetrics*	*Pediatrics*
Medical school Affiliated Hospital Outpatient Departments	10	183	222	214
OEO Neighborhood Health Centers	35	619	487	594
Group practices	7	124	68	113
Health Department Well-Baby Clinics	5	—	—	240
Children's Bureau Programs				
Maternal and infant care	6	—	73	—
Children and youth	4	—	—	103

Table 20-2

Baseline Medical Audit Scores of Selected Health Providers as Per Cents of the Over-all Average for Medical School Affiliated Hospital Outpatient Departments

Type of provider	Number of programs	Over-all average	Medicine	Obstetrics	Pediatrics
Medical School Affiliated Hospital Outpatient Departments	10	100	94	124	83
OEO Centers	35	107	112	121	90
Group practices	7	103	102	122	84
Health Department Well-Baby-Clinics	5	–	–	–	93
Children's Bureau Programs					
Maternal and Infant Care	6	–	–	138	–
Children and Youth	4	–	–	–	133

20-3 and 20-4). Examination of the scores by their component areas and the weights assigned to those areas gives an indication of relative strengths and weaknesses. The performance of routine laboratory studies (hemoglobin, urinalysis and serological test for syphilis) along with a routine chest x-ray was one of the principal reasons that the OEO centers received higher scores in medicine than the other providers. The OEO ratings for adequacy of histories and physical examinations were also higher than those observed in the outpatient departments, while the group practice ratings were slightly higher than OEO.

Table 20-3

Components of Average Baseline Adult Medicine Scores of Selected Health Providers as Per Cents of the Average for Medical School Affiliated Hospital Outpatient Departments

Components*	Weights	Medical school affiliated hospital outpatient departments	OEO centers	Group practices
History	20	114	120	122
Physical examination	20	98	100	107
Rectal and vaginal	10	64	91	98
Vital signs	5	118	144	116
Laboratory and x-ray	40	100	122	98
Time to assessment	5	93	125	118
Over-all average	100	100	118	107
Number of Programs		8	35	7

*See table 20-4 for details of each component.

Table 20-4

Components of Adult Medicine Baseline Audit

Records Reviewed: Patients between the ages of 30-70 paying at least three visits to the center over a four-month period of time.

Index items in each area:
  History:
    Family history
    Past illness
    Cardiac review
    Gastrointestinal review
    Genitourinary review
    Contraceptive advice (women under 45)
    Social history
    Chief complaint and present illness
  Physcial Examination:
    Fundoscopic
    Thyroid
    Heart
    Lungs
    Breasts
    Abdomen
    Reflexes

    Rectal examination
    Vaginal examination

    Vital signs:
      Blood pressure
      Pulse rate
      Height
      Weight
  Laboratory and X-Ray Examinations:
    Chest film
    Hemoglobin (HCT)
    Complete urinalysis
    Serological test for syphilis
    Sickle cell preparation (non-white)
    Papanicolaou smear
    EKG (over 50 years of age)
  Time between first visit and completed health assessment:
    Maximum credit if completed within three months after the first visit

The recording of blood pressures, pulse rates, weights and heights (an area receiving only 5 per cent of the allocated points) was higher than the over-all average for all providers, and noticeably high in the OEO centers. The OEO centers also had the highest ratings for the rapidity with which assessments were completed after initial contact was made with the centers.

The Children's Bureau Maternal and Infant Care Programs received ratings 11 per cent higher than the average of the medical school outpatient departments for care provided to the pregnant and recently delivered woman (tables 20-5 and 20-6). The ratings for OEO and the group practice plans were slightly

Table 20-5

Components of average baseline obstetrical scores of selected health providers as per cents of the average for medical school affiliated hospital outpatient departments

Components*	Weights	Medical school affiliated hospital outpatient departments	OEO centers	Group practices	Children's bureau maternal and infant care programs
Registration in first trimester	5	31	40	59	31
Prenatal work-up	50	108	107	106	119
Prenatal visits	20	106	108	115	119
Delivery records	5	129	82	78	133
Postpartum visits	10	83	83	89	103
Family planning	10	86	79	89	100
Over-all average	100	100	97	99	111
Number of programs		9	33	6	6

*See table 20-6 for details of each component.

below the hospital average. All of the programs received relatively low ratings for the proportion of pregnant women who registered in the first trimester of care, although the group practice plans, most of whom had a stable population of working families, had a higher proportion of women registering earlier. The completeness of the prenatal laboratory work-up and the adherence to prenatal visit schedules with concomitant recordings of weight, blood pressure and urine testing was most complete in the M&I programs, but performance in these areas was above the average of the over-all hospital performance in all programs. The M&I programs were equally effective in achieving the highest ratings for the number of women who returned for postpartum care as well as the offering of contraceptive advice to these women. The other programs fell below the over-all hospital average in these two areas.

The Children's Bureau Children and Youth programs received a total rating for pediatric care that was 60 per cent higher than the average of the hospital outpatient departments (tables 20-7 and 20-8). Their ratings were considerably higher in all areas than those of the other programs reviewed. The OEO centers, the well-baby clinics of the health departments and the group practices received ratings above that of the hospitals, but the differences were not as marked. One of the weakest areas for the hospital outpatient departments was the performance of immunizations, as many of the institutions did not consider this activity part of their function. The lowest area in the health department clinics was the performance of routine hemoglobins and urinalyses, apparently a screening tool that is not uniformly used by health departments; group practice plans were also low in this area.

Private Solo Practitioners

During the course of these reviews, the Evaluation Unit had occasion to conduct these baseline reviews in the offices of 20 solo practitioners. A total of
128 records were reviewed in medicine, 129 in pediatrics and 98 in obstetrics.
This small number of physicians can in no manner be considered representative
of what is really the largest source of ambulatory care in the country, namely
the solo practitioner's office where care is provided on a fee-for-service basis.

Table 20-6
Components of obstetrical baseline audit

*Records Reviewed: Women delivering 8 weeks prior to the date of review who
made at least one prenatal visit to the facility.*

Index items in each area:
   Registration in the first trimester of pregnancy
     Prenatal work-up:
       History:
         System review
         Past obstetrical history
         Family history
       Laboratory:
         Hemoglobin (HCT)
         Rh factor and blood typing
         Serological test for syphilis
         Chest film or negative skin test for tuberculosis
         Complete urinalysis
         Repeat third trimester hemoglobin
         Repeat third trimester serology
          (Indicated if the first one is done before the sixth month.)
         Papanicolaou smear
         Vaginal smear
         Sickle cell preparation (non-white)
         Nutrition discussion
         Dental care
       Measurements:
         Recordings of weight, blood pressure and urine for sugar and
          albumin on each prenatal visit.
     Visits:
       Frequency of prenatal visits in relation to the month of gestation.[*]
     Delivery Records:
       Place of delivery
       Type of delivery
       Weight of infant
       Condition of infant or Apgar score
     Postpartum Visits: (Related to the delivery date)
       Blood pressure
       Vaginal examination
     Family Planning:
       Contraceptive advice or indication of refusal

[*]Based on recommendations of the American College of Obstetrics and Gynecology.

Table 20-7

Components of Average Baseline Pediatric Scores of Selected Health Providers as Per Cent of the Average for Medical School Affiliated Hospital Outpatient Departments

Components*	Weights	Medical school affiliated hospital outpatient departments	OEO centers	Group practices	Health department well-baby clinic	Children's bureau children and youth programs
History and physical examination	30	140	133	119	125	173
Routine measurements	15	90	85	79	98	125
Hemoglobin and urinalysis	15	92	94	62	56	169
Immunizations	25	46	108	119	131	160
Screening for tuberculosis	5	119	96	87	117	156
Time to assessment	5	137	152	108	125	190
Frequency of visits	5	108	127	144	115	154
Over-all average	100	100	108	102	112	160
Number of Programs		9	35	7	5	4

*See table 20–8 for details of each component.

Table 20-8
Components of Pediatric Baseline Audit

Records Reviewed: Children between the ages of 8 and 26 months paying at least three visits to the facility over a four-month period of time.

Index items in each area:
  History:
    Birth History:
      Place of birth
      Type of delivery
      Birth weight
      Condition at birth
    Family history
    Feeding habits
    Development
    Past history
  Physical Examination:
    Ears
    Heart
    Lungs
    Abdomen
    Extremities
  Measurements: (Related to the number of visits)
    Height
    Weight
    Head Circumference
  Laboratory:
    .Hemoglobin (HCT)
    Urinalysis
    Sickle cell preparation (non-white)
  Immunizations: (Dependent on age)
    DPT. polio and boosters
    Measles
    Smallpox vaccination
  Screening for tuberculosis:
    Chest film or negative skin test
  Frequency of visits:
    Seven recommended for the first year of life
  Time between first visit and completed health assessment
    Maximum credit if completed before the fourth visit

The physicians reviewed can be characterized as general practitioners, practicing on a fee-for-service basis in rural areas. The patient reviewed records were those of the indigent population for whom payment was made from public funds. There were no constraints placed on the amount or kinds of services that could be provided.

The physicians' performance ratings in all fields were considerably lower than the medical school affiliated hospital outpatient department averages as well as those of the other providers reviewed. Findings for medicine were 29 per cent lower than the hospital outpatient department average, 24 per cent lower in obstetrics and 50 per cent lower in pediatrics. In medicine, the completion of laboratory tests, a chest film and the recording of an adequate history and physical examination were the areas that showed the greatest disparity in levels of performance when examined in relation to other providers. Pediatric care also suffered because of inadequate recording of histories and physical examinations and failure to perform routine measurements and laboratory studies. The private practitioners' completion of immunizations was similar to the ratings obtained in the hospital outpatient departments, and the assumption was said to be that children were obtaining this service at the local health department clinic. When the records of these children were looked for in the well-baby clinics, only 59 per cent were under care. The obstetrical ratings showed the greatest dificiencies in the failure to complete all of the components of a prenatal work-up and in the failure of as many women to return for postpartum care as occurred in the hospital clinics. A slightly higher proportion of women registered with the private practitioners during their first trimester than registered in the hospitals during this period.

A series of questions can be asked about the level of practice observed in these offices; questions that can have no definitive answers until more widespread access to private physicians' offices can be obtained. Are the deplorable record-keeping practices observed in these few offices typical of the average practitioner? How many physicians keep their records solely for billing purposes where entries consist only of charges and the drugs distributed? How does the practice of the physician dispensing and being paid for medications alter his practice? How is the quality of care affected by patient volumes which may go as high as 100 patients per day? Are these difficulties more inherent in rural practice than in urban areas?

As measured by these baseline audits, the health care provided by these private practitioners was woefully inadequate. The reasons for this are undoubtedly multiple and only speculation as to their order of importance can be made on the present data. It is apparent that the majority of the physicians did not see, or did not accept as their responsibility, the provision of this type of baseline care to the patients under their care. Whether this was from lack of direction provided by the funding agency, lack of conviction as to the importance of such type of care, lack of time to provide such services, lack of sufficient financial incentive or lack of supervision can only be speculative. What results, however, is a picture of medical care that viewed from minimal standards of care can only be regarded as unacceptable.

Discussion

The medical school affiliated institutions that were used as a standard in these studies have long been considered citadels of clinical excellence. This reputation, however, has not always extended to their ambulatory care services. There have been complaints about attitudes towards patients, long waiting periods, unattractive decor and fragmentation of service due to multiple specialty clinics. Examination of these important factors was outside the scope of this review. From the standpoint of health maintenance and assessment, these institutions have not traditionally considered their responsibility to be the provision of such care to a given population with concomitant outreach and follow-up. This has been less true for care provided to the pregnant and recently delivered woman. In this field their performance was slightly superior to the OEO centers and the group practice plans. Care to children and adult patients, however, was of a more sporadic nature, with attention directed toward the presenting problem and efforts were not always made to assess the patient as a whole. Adult patients who were under care of general medical clinics had excellent detailed work-ups. Others, whose initial complaint was readily identifiable as belonging to a specialty area, were sent immediately to such clinics and rarely achieved a complete examination. In general, infants, unless they had special problems which kept them under ongoing surveillance of special clinics, also received sporadic care directed towards the specific problems.

There was one striking exception to this pattern: one of the largest institutions reviewed has long had a practice of having all infants seen in the emergency room either referred immediately for a complete examination or having the examination performed in that area. Efforts (which were generally successful) were made to offer ongoing services to the family if they were without another source of care, and preventive health measures were built into their program for care. The ratings for pediatrics in this institution were superior to the others received. Generally, however, such services as immunizations and monitoring of growth and development were not part of hospital pediatric care and the assumption was made, with various degrees of validity, that the local health departments were providing such services.

As hospitals represent one of the major resources for medical care, it is important that the issues be addressed that will enable their services more readily to serve as a source of high quality care in this day of manpower shortages. There is need to identify patients who use such facilities as their sole source of care and to assure that their contacts are not a series of isolated specialty services. Collection of utilization data that will identify characteristics of patients under care is long overdue. The existence of multiple specialty clinics, many established and maintained in the name of teaching and research, needs to be reviewed in the light of total patient care needs. Several of the institutions in the sample are moving away from this concept, others are building in mechanisms that assure that total assessment occurs, even though specialty clinics continue to be maintained. The most important factor, however, would seem to be a commitment to the provision of total health care; there is little question that the institutions have the resources to implement such policies once the goals are accepted.

Among the health care providers whose performance was measured by these baseline standards, the care provided by the Children's Bureau Children and Youth and Maternal and Infant Care programs received the highest ratings. These highly organized programs, generally with full-time professional staff, are amply funded and have a broad range of paraprofessional resources. In addition, they are dealing with programs whose standards of care have had professional acceptance and patient understanding for some years. The extent to which patients understand and cooperate in obtaining health care is another area omitted from these reviews which is of extreme importance in completion of preventive health measures. The M&I programs did not succeed in reaching their populations earlier in pregnancy than the other providers serving the disadvantaged (the group practice plans did better in this regard), but quite obviously once a patient became part of the program, education about the need for ongoing care and implementation of follow-up procedures were successful in having patients adhere to the program's goals.

One important question may be raised about the smaller C&Y programs that were examined; namely, their economic viability as a national model. Although this is also a question raised about the OEO centers, the staff-patient ratios appear even higher in these programs. At the time of review, for example, one of the programs had 1,000 children enrolled (500 families). There were the equivalent of three and three-quarter full-time pediatricians, two public health nurses and a supervisor, two social workers and a supervisor, the equivalent of one and one-quarter psychiatrists and a part-time nutritionist. Other clinic staff such as aides and technicians were also available. The program's performance was outstanding, but the need to conserve resources makes it desirable that, having achieved excellence, such programs take into consideration how such quality can be maintained with more realistic patient loads and staff-patient ratios.

The health department clinics were performing at an adequate level the functions that were part of their program design. In all of the programs, the follow-up contacts of the public health nurses were evident and effective. Such contacts were generally related to the department's routines and because information was not readily available about serious pathology that was being cared for elsewhere, an over-all picture of fragmentation of services and limitation of functions resulted. These institutions need either a closer merger of their functions with those of the providers of therapeutic care or to assume responsibility for total care before their contributions to the health system can be most effective.

The group practice plans with their relatively stable population bases and with objectives of comprehensive care and economy of operation had performance ratings that were above those of the hospital outpatient departments but somewhat below those of OEO. There were a few indications that the emphasis on economy may have perhaps been overemphasized on occasion at the expense of quality. Ratings were considerably lower than OEO in some areas where unit costs play a factor; for example, laboratory and x-ray studies on adult patients and hemoglobins and urinalyses on infants. One program went so far as to state they did not provide measles immunizations because of the expense of this agent.

It is unfortunate that so little is known about the general level of medical practice in solo practitioners' offices. Without more detailed information about performance, it is not possible to balance the worth of the undeniable asset of a close physician-patient relationship (operative to a considerable extent when patients have "free choice") with the price that may have to be paid in terms of professional excellence. Certainly within the group reviewed in this study, the levels of care were unacceptable by any standards. Yet, as with other providers, ranges in performance were observed. One isolated general practitioner had superior performance ratings in all fields examined.

Perhaps one of the most important implications of these reviews results from the wide variation of performance that was observed within any one group of providers, variations that cannot be explained by the organizational pattern alone. To be sure, goals and policies are important; the hospital, a medical group or private practitioner needs to have the stated or implied goal of providing preventive health care. Yet even within this framework, the variation in large part seems to reflect individual commitment and performance; the isolated general practitioner referred to, the outpatient department where frequently the excellence of health assessments depends on the individual doctor, or the group plans where the work of a few physicians was observed to be outstanding. Administrative efficiency, organizational patterns and methods of financing undoubtedly have important effects on quality, yet without the conscientiousness, knowledge and sustained performance of the individual physician, one of the cornerstones of quality service will be lacking irrespective of the setting. However, the health needs of the country are too great to depend upon the integrity of the individual professional alone to provide services of high quality. Even if more was known about factors influencing and creating professional motivation and performance, the need for continued surveillance and the improvement of health service organizational structure would exist.

The OEO neighborhood health centers have attempted in a few years' time to encompass all of the positive aspects of the nation's existing health providers; clinical excellence, provision of preventive and comprehensive services, organization of medical and the equally important social services, efficiency and economy of operation, the maintenance of close continuity between a patient and his health provider and the fostering of attitudes and environment that will be conducive to patient acceptance. There are wide ranges in the extent to which these goals are reached by the centers. Program design, access to back-up resources, isolation in conservative rural areas and the ability to implement policies and practices with administrative efficiency all play a part in the level of achievement. The team concept, which has tended to blur specialty professional administrative lines, may be one factor in the unevenness of achievement of health procedures directed at a specific age group or type of condition (pediatrics and obstetrics).

This series of reviews undertook to measure only one parameter of performance: the adherence to standards of preventive health care. The ratings of the OEO centers in this area compared to the medical school outpatient departments, and indeed to the other providers reviewed, indicate that the neighborhood health centers are performing at a creditable level. This is not to say that there are not areas of concern about performance in these centers as well as among the others reviewed that require further analysis in relation to cost, quality and efficiency of operation.

Summary

Audits of the quality of care provided to adult patients, infants and pregnant and recently delivered women were conducted in a variety of programs. These reviews consisted of abstracting from patient records data which indicated the extent to which standards of care appropriate for the individual patient were met. Analysis of the data resulted in a score for each provider in each specialty. A total of 3,040 records were examined among medical school affiliated hospital outpatient departments (10), OEO neighborhood health center programs (35), Children's Bureau Maternal and Infant Care programs (6), Children and Youth programs (4), health department well-baby clinics (5), group practice programs (7), and 20 rural private practitioners.

The findings from the medical school hospital outpatient departments were used as a standard against which to measure performance of the other providers. The performance ratings of the Children's Bureau programs were outstanding; the other providers had ratings above that of the hospitals in the fields of medicine and pediatrics and slightly below in obstetrical care. Performance in the few solo practitioners' offices was judged to be below the hospital standard in all areas. In general, performance in obstetrical care was closer to the ideal for all providers, while pediatric care received the lowest ratings.

The conclusion reached from review of this data is that at the present time, with the exception of the few small, highly organized and richly staffed Children's Bureau programs, the neighborhood health center program performance is generally equal to and in some instances superior to that of other established providers of health care. When tools are available to measure the other important parameters of health care, one can be hopeful that these programs will have achieved no small measure of success in the demonstration of an effective model for the delivery of health services, particularly to the nation's disadvantaged.

References

1. Morehead, Mildred, A. Evaluating Quality of Medical Care in the Neighbor-hood Health Center Program of the Office of Economic Opportunity. M. Care 8,2:118–131 (Mar.–Apr.), 1970.
2. Greenleigh Associates, Inc. Audit of the Medical Assistance Program of the State of Hawaii. Audit Rep. No. 70-3, (Mar.), 1970 (Legislative Auditor, State Capitol, Honolulu, Hawaii).

Part X
Allied Health Workers and Health Teams

Introduction

The allied health workers and health teams are key innovations implemented through the neighborhood health centers.[1] The early proponents of the centers waxed particularly enthusiastic about these roles and new structures for the delivery of care. Neither the allied health workers nor the team approach are tied exclusively to neighborhood health centers, but the centers have been the facilities through which these concepts have been tested most vigorously. The two articles which follow report the experience of health workers and teams at one center where these approaches have been tried out with unusual vigor and follow-through. They express the reasons behind these attempts at reform, and discuss the successes and problems which each has encountered.[2]

The linked concepts of the family health workers and the teams have worked out rather differently than it was supposed and proposed that they would. The process of trying out and adjusting has not been an easy one. The Martin Luther King, Jr. Health Center has implemented the concepts more successfully than most. It has demonstrated a great deal about the potentialities and limitations of these concepts. The Center's experience can be immensely useful for improving the functioning of existing centers and guiding the development of new primary care services.

Harold Wise and his co-workers report on the early experience of the family health workers who comprise an integral part of the teams studied by Irwin Rubin and Richard Beckhard later on. "The Family Health Worker" discusses "the methods of the selection and training of the family health workers and is a preliminary report on their functioning as part of the family health team."[3] It includes an excellent description of the kinds of tasks included in the famliy health worker's job.

Rubin and Beckhard report on an action research process in which they not only systematically observed the functioning of health teams in neighborhood health centers, but also tried a variety of techniques to improve the effectiveness of these teams. Their research applies the analytical perspective of behavioral science and small group functioning. Their article focuses on a series of factors which determine the effectiveness of health teams: goals or mission, internal and external role expectations, decision-making, communication patterns, leadership, and norms. It frequently contrasts the working situation and job demands of the health center with those of hospitals, where, for example, goals and role expectations are clearer and more definite.

There is a fair amount of anecdotal evidence that patients of the health centers have not cottoned to the team approach. Patients who have never had a private physician are reported to have balked at the idea of being asked to relate to nurses and family health workers rather than exclusively with doctors. It is natural that they would seek standard middle-class medical care. The extent and duration of this reaction is still hard to measure. Wise et al. maintain that this had not been a problem at the Martin Luther King Center.

The factors which Rubin and Beckhard identify as important in determining the effectiveness of the teams are affected greatly by much larger forces—conflicts about the goals of the centers themselves, and the training and cultural backgrounds of team members, for example. Short-term intervention to improve the functioning of the team is not designed to resolve these conflicts and to overcome these forces. By focusing on issues of team functioning, this kind of analysis and training of this sort clarifies the larger issues. The research provides routes for continuing to grapple with these dilemmas, and may help to build pressure for resolving them. For instance, the inquiries into team effectiveness and efforts to help them can contribute to revisions of the curricula of professional schools so that over time, physicians, nurses and others will receive training in the new roles of team practice earlier on in their careers and be encouraged to have greater interest in, and accord greater respect to, these options for practice. At the local level, mechanisms for helping teams to work through issues of their own effectiveness may support movement toward fulfilling the center's promise as a vehicle for addressing the social and economic problems which so directly affect the health of its patients. In these ways, the issues of team functioning are tied to the question of what are the means by which the centers have, and can, serve as instruments of change in other health agencies and institutions.

Articles appearing in other sections of this reader include additional information on the allied health workers and teams. Hillman and Charney, in "A Neighborhood Health Center: What the Patients Know and Think of Its Operation," document patients' perceptions of the family health assistants who work at the Rochester Neighborhood Health Center. Torrens, in "Administrative Problems of Neighborhood Health Center," records problems which many centers have encountered in implementing the team approach and family-centered care. The experience of these centers indicates that many of them have contrived flexible, more ad hoc team approaches. Torrens notes widespread enthusiasm for, and endorsement of, the contributions of the family health workers.

References

1. For a comprehensive review of issues in team practice, see: Alberta W. Parker, "The Team Approach to Primary Health Care," Neighborhood Health Center Seminar Program, Monograph Series No. 3, University Extension, Univ. of California, Berkeley. January 1972.

2. A pair of articles about the Denver neighborhood health program offers additional information on health centers' experiences with allied health workers and health teams: James A. Kent and C. Harvey Smith, "Involving the Urban Poor in Health Services through Accommodation—The Employment of Neighborhood Representatives," *American Journal of Public Health 57,* 6 (June 1967): 997–1003; David L. Cowen and John A. Sbarbaro, "Family-centered Health Care—A Viable Reality?: The Denver Experience," *Medical Care 10,* 2 (March–April 1972): 164–172. Cowen and Sbarbaro recount how the Denver program departed from the formal model of team care and evolved over time a more flexible approach in which a fraction of the patients see a team and the rest are given comprehensive care, but not through a team practice mode. They identify and discuss factors which caused them to move away from the formal team model.

3. A more recent account of the experience of the family health workers at the Martin Luther King, Jr. Health Center is presented in E. Fulley Torrey, Deloris Smith, and Harold Wise, "The Family Health Worker Revisited: A Five-Year Follow-up." *American Journal of Public Health 63,* 1 (January 1973): 71–74. The editors learned of this article too late to include it in the present volume.

21

The Family Health Worker

Harold B. Wise, E. Fuller Torrey, Adrienne McDade, Gloria Perry, and Harriet Bograd

Although multipurpose workers with medical and social service skills have been proposed in the past,[1] few attempts have been made to train and integrate them into a functioning health care team. This report describes the family health worker who is trained in patient care and social-advocacy skills. In particular, the description concerns the philosophy behind their creation, the methods of selection, the training curriculum, and their early functioning as part of a family-care team

Background and Philosophy

In July, 1966, the Montefiore Hospital Neighborhood Medical Care Demonstration (NMCD)[2] was funded for 1.9 million dollars by the federal Office of Economic Opportunity. The program was developed in the Division of Social Medicine of Montefiore Hospital in the Bronx, and was designed to demonstrate a new approach to comprehensive medical care.

The neighborhood chosen for the project is a 55-square-block area — two health districts — located in a low-income neighborhood in the Southeast Bronx. Approximately 11,000 families (45,000 people) live there; this population is equally divided between Afro-Americans and Latin-Americans, with about 5 per cent white. The area is blighted with run-down factory buildings, empty tenements, and garbage-strewn streets. The gross "social statistics" confirm what the eye sees: there is a high unemployment rate, many families on welfare, crowded housing, high crime and drug use rates.

The vast majority of people in this neighborhood have received their medical care from the clinics and emergency rooms of nearby hospitals, from the five practitioners in the area, and from pharmacists and faith healers. Continuity, follow-up, and preventive medicine are almost unknown. There is a high infant mortality rate and a high incidence of tuberculosis.

Reprinted from *American Journal of Public Health,* published by the American Public Health Association, 58, 10 (October 1968): 1828-1838.

The complexity of modern medicine challenges the most sophisticated; for the poor it can be a nightmare. The typical outpatient department is an anachronism. The clinics are organized for the convenience of the professional staff — to accommodate the part-time physician, the intern, or resident interested in pursuing a disease specialty; they are not geared to provide ongoing medical care and have not been structured to offer a coordinated service. At the present time the poor must make their way through the bureaucratic maze of hospital, health, and welfare services, located in different buildings and in different parts of town. More disturbing has been the ever-increasing use of the emergency room as the prime, and sometimes only, focus for a variety of nonurgent, routine medical and social problems.

The Neighborhood Medical Care Demonstration was developed to answer some of these problems. It is organized around a main health center centrally located in the neighborhood[a] and smaller satellite centers (the first of which opened in June, 1967). The aim is twofold: to provide a facility which coordinates for the patient all outpatient services, preventive as well as therapeutic, in areas where the poor predominate; and to encourage "intensive participation" of neighborhood people in the operation of the health center. The family health worker was created as part of the effort to achieve these goals.

The medical manpower shortage is particularly grave in the neighborhoods where there is a high incidence of poverty. While there is more than one physician for every 600 persons in the borough of the Bronx as a whole, in the 55 blocks served by this project there were (before the arrival of the NMCD) only five physicians available to 45,000 people. To cope with the manpower shortage, the NMCD is utilizing group practice of physicians and team practice of physicians, nurses, and family health workers. In the context of team practice traditional roles have been examined and redefined.

The family physician is the team manager responsible for the medical care delivered by the team. The "family physician" is usually a team of internist and pediatrician or a general practitioner. The expanded role of the public health nurse is an innovation. She is responsible for the preventive care of the family: to carry out this mandate she receives additional training in well-baby, pre- and postnatal care as well as preventive care for the adult.[3] Her major responsibility is to coordinate the medical and social care of a family. She has the primary responsibility for the supervision of the family health workers on her team.

The family health worker, the third member of the team, has incorporated into her role some of the functions of the public health nurse, the lawyer, the social worker, the physician, and the health educator. This article deals with the methods of the selection and training of the family health workers and is a preliminary report on their functioning as part of the family health team.

---

[a] Opened in July, 1968

Selection

In making the selection of family health workers, preference was given to unemployed heads of households and to those trainees who, during the eight-week core training program,[4] showed maturity, warmth and interest in social advocacy, and who demonstrated ability to function as a team member. Many of the family health workers were already informal health advisers in their particular neighborhoods.

They were chosen on the basis of a group interview, an individual interview, and several written tests; two-thirds had high school diplomas. On the revised Beta examination (a "culture-free" IQ test), their average score was 102 (range 81 to 121, with a norm of 91). During the training program they were paid $55 and $60 a week; as graduates the family health workers began at $90 a week.

The first eight family health workers were selected in November, 1966, and six more were selected three months later. These first 14 had all completed their six-month training by the end of July, 1967. A third group of eight is presently in training.[b]

The family health workers are in their early thirties (the range has been from 21 to 47). They all live in the two health areas served by NMCD. To date all have been women. There is now one man in the third group. Most of them have several school-age children (range from one to six). All except one are married; they therefore reflect a more stable family pattern than the average in this neighborhood. Their past employment included jobs as cleaning woman, key punch operator, and nurse's aide.

Job Description

The family health worker's base is the health center, but much of her time is involved in making home visits in the community. She is the third member of the medical team, along with the physician and the public health nurse. She is assigned from 40 to 60 families. Her day-to-day supervision comes from the public health nurse on her team; continuing inservice training comes from a family health worker supervisor — a public health nurse whose prime assignment is training.

Daily activities of the family health worker include a variety of health education, patient care, and social advocacy activities. She instructs the new mother how to bathe and feed the baby, and is alert to household hazards such as fire traps and broken paint on walls. In her training strong emphasis is placed on patient education, case finding, the preventive aspects of medical care, and the

---

[b] As of September, 1968, there are 28 family health workers.

emotional factors influencing illness.

Her patient care activities include checking blood pressure and pulse (as on a known hypertensive patient recently discharged from the hospital); instructing relatives of bed-bound patients (bathing, skin care, changing dressings, irrigating catheters, giving enemas); carrying out the exercises prescribed by a physiatrist; checking whether a new diabetic patient understands how to check his urine and is following his diet. She is able to collect a midstream urine and is being taught how to collect venous blood samples. In addition, she administers a check list health inventory.

During the course of her home visits the family health worker deals with a variety of social and environmental problems. She assists a patient with heart disease to obtain a telephone through the Welfare Department, or to obtain more suitable, low-income housing for a large young family. Initiative and imagination in the family health workers are stressed as part of their patient advocacy role.

Every morning the family health worker meets with her public health nurse to go over daily assignments. Once a week she meets with the physician, public health nurse, lawyer, and other resource personnel at the health team conference; here they develop a health plan for each family seen in the past week.

Training

The family health worker is trained for eight hours a day for 24 weeks. The first eight weeks of the course consists of the core curriculum, which covers basic health skills, a survey of health careers, community resources, and remedial training in English and mathematics. Of the remaining 16 weeks, two-thirds of the time is allotted to health skills and one-third to community resources.

Health skills are taught by nurses, all with public health training or experience. The community resources part of the training is taught by a lawyer who is on the training staff. Seminars are given by a community organizer, a health educator, an anthropologist, internists, pediatricians, obstetricians, a psychiatrist, and a physical therapist. Many guest lecturers and members of the health center staff participate.

After graduation from the training course, the family health worker spends several hours a week continuing her inservice training and, if required, her work toward the high school equivalency.

Patient Care Activities

Most of the patient care activities are taught in the home situation, the health center, hospital outpatient department, and emergency room. Some time is spent learning technical procedures on the hospital wards. Lectures, discussions and demonstrations are used in a classroom setting. Throughout the program, the trainees are taught to improvise in the home situation. If the patient has no stove to sterilize an insulin syringe, a vegetable tin and Sterno are used as a substitute. If rubber sheets are not available, an oil cloth shower curtain is substituted.

Differences in cultural and religious practices are discussed, and the family health workers learn how the health team can accommodate to the patient.

> A family health worker noticed that, although the physician prescribed evaporated milk formula for a baby, the Latin-American mother was using whole milk prepared in the same proportions. (Whole milk is a status symbol among some Latin-American families.) After consultation with the doctor, the family health worker attempted to convinc e the family to use evaporated milk; failing that, she taught them to use whole milk in the correct proportions.

Emphasis is placed on preventive medicine, rehabilitation, and maternal and child health. The aim is to reach all household members. For example, if the family health worker is visiting the home for general health supervision of a diabetic amputee, she may find the following:

> He is not taking his insulin properly.
> He is not using his prosthesis or exercising his stump as advised.
> He is not following the prescribed diet because of insufficient funds.
> There is a pregnant mother not under medical supervision.
> There is a child with cerebral palsy neither attending school nor under medical supervision.
> There is inadequate space in the apartment for the number in the family.

To complete the routine health inventory forms, the family health worker evaluates the family both medically and socially, and writes a report which is presented at the team conference. Under the supervision of the public health nurse, she provides bedside patient care and general health supervision, or offers referral to the appropriate social agency to carry out part of the family health plan.

Community Resources

During the training of the family health worker, four basic principles are stressed in all patient encounters: problem formulation, planning a course of action, investigation, and utilization of available resources.

Problem Formulation. The family health worker is trained to help people face their problems. The approach is the same whether it is a health, social, or legal problem: A 14-year-old girl with diabetes is unreliable in taking her insulin; a father of four is being laid off from work; a young mother is being sued by a credit company.

In each case the family health worker must first help the patient face the reality of the problem and gather courage to seek assistance.

Planning a Course of Action. The family health worker is trained to listen carefully, and to think through what the patient wants to do before looking for solutions to the problem: A woman complains that her husband is a drug addict. Before making any suggestions, the family health worker must know more about the situation: Does the wife want to take any action? Does she want only to get him out of the house? Would she force him into an institution against his will? Does her family need money? Is she afraid the landlord will put her out? How does her husband feel about this? Does he want help? May the family health worker speak to him? The family health worker learns not to make decisions for people, but rather to help them make their own decisions.

Finding Available Resources. A multitude of agencies claim to deal with the same special problems. There are, for instance, at least ten different agencies to which a person in the Bronx might be referred if there are rats in his apartment.[c] Some of these agencies are ineffective; others deal only with one aspect of the problem. A woman whose husband is an alcoholic must choose between many different agencies which may, among other things, help her sue him for support, offer voluntary treatment, or assist her in getting a divorce or a job to support her family.

The family health workers are trained to be familiar with many agencies and to evaluate which is appropriate for a particular family with a particular problem. They visit at least 16 agencies during their training, including a Welfare Center, the Family Court, the Legal Aid Society, the Criminal Court, the Probation Department, a school, a mental hospital, a social work agency, and

[c]The landlord; Department of Buildings; Rent and Rehabilitation Administration; Claremont Area Services; League of Autonomous Bronx Organizations for Renewal (LABOR); Project Rescue; Department of Health; Legal Aid Society; Bronx Community Self-Improvement Association; Morrisania Community Progress Center; Welfare Department.

the Social Security Administration. After each trip the group uses discussion, role play, and written assignments to learn how to get more information about this and other agencies and resources. The group may use role play, for example, to learn what to say to a switchboard operator to get directly to a supervisor; the process of role play helps to develop the necessary confidence to obtain information over the telephone and to deal with a bureaucracy.

Making Use of Available Resources. Although private agencies claim to offer many services, and government agencies are required by law to dispense certain benefits, yet people are often bullied or ignored when they ask for something to which they are entitled. The family health worker is trained to help people negotiate with agencies to get the help they need.

If a welfare recipient needs a crib for a new baby, the law requires that she be granted money for the crib within 30 days. What if three months have passed and the request has been ignored? The family health worker learns many alternative approaches to such a problem: whether the person concerned should call the caseworker or the administrator, whether to request a fair hearing or to contact a welfare action group. The family health worker learns to encourage people to take such actions on their own, however, she also knows that, in order to teach a timid or unskilled person to help himself, she may first have to provide concrete support.

The family health worker trainee needs new skills to help people utilize available resources. Many new trainees have to learn simple office procedures such as writing a business letter, making carbon copies, and recording telephone messages. The family health worker trainee needs to gain self-confidence in order not to be intimidated by professionals and agency officials. The field trips to other agencies provide a valuable opportunity for family health workers to meet with directors and key staff members of agencies, to explain what the family health worker's role is, to ask questions about the agency, and to explore ways in which they can cooperate. By the end of the 16 field trips most of the family health workers are ready to call or visit a new agency on their own.

Anecdotal Material

Some idea of the functions of the family health worker may be obtained from the following material taken from the health center's records.

A 34-year-old Spanish speaking man, father of two, appeared at the health center complaining that his 24-year-old wife had been ill for five days with swollen joints and was unable to move. The family health worker visited the home and reported to the internist on her team that the patient appeared acutely ill, had swollen tender joints, a fever, and rapid pulse. The physician saw the patient and had her hospitalized. She had rheumatic fever with carditis.

> The family health worker visited the patient at the hospital, interpreting and assisting in persuading the patient to remain in the hospital for six weeks. She arranged homemaking services for the two children. She has written the Housing Authority to get the patient into an elevator building. She visits the patient three times a week − checks vital signs and emphasizes the need for bed rest and the monthly injections of long-acting penicillin.

An elderly woman with terminal carcinoma of the breast was able to go home from the hospital. A family health worker visited her daily to change the dressings and supervise her diet.

A six-year-old retarded child was not attending school and was under no medical supervision; the mother was Spanish speaking. The family health worker, acting as interpreter, arranged for the child to get medical treatment and assisted the mother to get the child into special classes.

A family of 11 lived in a dilapidated apartment with only six beds. The three-year-old had been eating large quantities of broken plaster. The family health worker persuaded the fearful mother to have the child hospitalized for examination and explained the dangers of lead poisoning. She also helped her to get a special grant for new beds from the Welfare Department, showed her how to shop economically, and helped her to contact a local group which would arrange to have repairs made in her apartment.

Problems

Creating a new group of health workers has not been without its problems. Perhaps the major one was the difficulty that the first group of trainees had in envisioning a job that for them had no model. This difficulty was compounded by varying perceptions of the job by members of the teaching staff. During early discussion, it became apparent that each professional on the staff (e.g., lawyer, nurse, health educator, community organizer, anthropologist) looked upon the newly emerging family health workers as their own subprofessional staff. The result, of course, was increased job anxiety for the family health workers.

Those staff members who at first wanted to create subprofessional specialists gradually became convinced that the creation of a competent group of generalists was more important. Each family at the neighborhood health center can now confide in one family health worker, rather than a home health aide, a social work aide, a legal aide, and a health education aide. The family health worker gets to know family members intimately and provide coordination, continuity of care, follow-up, and preventive education.

More anxiety arose when it became clear to professionals on the staff, especially the nurses, that these new health workers were crossing rather sacred guild lines. Although most of the staff believed that family health workers should be equal members of the team, they had to make conscious efforts to allow them a voice in decision-making. At first the family health workers remained silent at health team conferences, unsure themselves of the value of their opinions, and unsure whether professionals would listen to them. They have since become much more vocal at team conferences and make significant contributions to the family health plans.

Originally, the proposed base of the family health worker was her own apartment; she was to be given a desk and chair, some nurse-aide equipment, a contribution to her apartment rental, and a shingle for her door.[d] Because of the small number of family health workers, and because of some resistance on their part to look after close friends or neighbors, the plan for "geographic" placement of family health workers has been postponed for the time being.

Some felt the family health worker would face the same community antipathy experienced by the welfare caseworker. Early experience has been quite the contrary. The remarkably friendly reception the family health worker has received is in part due to her entree as a health (rather than social) worker, her status as a member of the community, and her "advocacy" role for the patient — against the establishment including, if necessary, the NMCD. There has been little expression of the uneasiness felt by some community residents that family health workers (i.e., nonprofessionals) would be used in lieu of physicians. The team concept is beginning to be understood, as the family health worker's role as a member of that team and her access to the doctor and public health nurse.

Another problem area concerned the training curriculum. The temptation to fix the curriculum, and thereby produce a clearer definition of the expected role, had to be balanced against the need for flexibility as the role evolved in practice. The curriculum is reviewed on a regular basis to provide feedback from the functioning family health workers to those responsible for the training.

Future Plans

The Neighborhood Medical Care Demonstration plans to train 60 more family health workers over the next three years. There will be a simultaneous program of evaluation of the family health workers, comparing social and health data on the families for which they are providing care and on a control group not receiving such care.

---

[d] Suggested by Dr. Ray Elling, Department of Sociology, University of Pittsburgh.

Efforts will continue to arrange affiliation of the family health worker training program with an academic institution or to obtain accreditation toward a
college degree. The NMCD is involved in discussions with five local colleges and
universities on this issue. Licensure for family health workers is another goal, and
will be pursued through established channels. (In September, 1968, seven family
health workers entered a two and a half-year associates arts degree program at
the City University of New York, working as family health workers half the time,
with half-time for college training, allowing them at the end of the two and a half
years to take the registered nurse examinations.)

Early impressions by the professional staff of NMCD is that the family health
worker is successful in carrying out her job mandate; a few have shown the ability
to take on considerably more responsibility. As a group they have consistently
surprised the doctors and nurses with their grasp of complex medical and social
problems.

The creation of the family health worker may point the way to a new kind
of profession, nursing performed in the social context. It presumes a health
worker can enter the system on the entry level and with training — on-the-job
and in the traditional classroom setting — would work as a health team member
specifically in the ambulatory and home care situations. Her role would be that
of the generalist, coordinating and providing nursing and social service functions
for whole families.

Summary

An initial report is made of a program to train and employ family health workers
in a neighborhood health center program located in an impoverished area of the
Bronx. The program demonstrates how a neighborhood resident, trained for six
months and supervised by public health nurses, can perform many of the
functions traditionally assigned to public health nurses and social workers. The
effect should be to simplify the complexity of health and social services now
available to poor patients who have become dissected into clinic cards and social
work records.

References

1. Blum, H.L. The Multipurpose Worker — A Family Specialist. A.J.P.H.
    55:267-376 (Mar.). 1965.
2. Wise, H.B. Neighborhood Medical Care Demonstration — Proposal to the
    Office of Economic Opportunity. (Apr.). 1966.
3. Expanded Role of Public Health Nurse. NMCD (mimeo.).
4. Zahn, Stella, Core Curriculum. (Nov.), 1966 (mimeo.).

22

Factors Influencing the Effectiveness of Health Teams

Irwin M. Rubin and Richard Beckhard

Group practice in health care delivery takes many forms. The term "group practice" usually refers to a group of professionals who combine their resources in delivering treatment care to a patient population. Some of these groups are actively involved in preventive medicine efforts. Because of heavy work loads, more and more activities are being delegated to nurses, physicians assistants and, in some cases, community-based family health workers. One common condition in all of these settings is that a group is doing the "practicing."

The effectiveness of any group in any setting is related to *both* its capabilities to do the work and its ability to manage itself as an interdependent group of people. The central focus of this paper will be upon the internal dynamics involved when a collection of individuals attempts to function as a group. The objective is to provide a framework that will facilitate consideration of several important issues involved in the more effective utilization of groups in delivering health care.

We will begin by drawing upon the general body of knowledge about groups and their dynamics developed within the behavioral sciences. Several key variables known to be of prime importance in any group situation will be discussed. Next, we will discuss the particular relevance of these variables to group medical practice.

Third, we will draw upon our own experience in helping several health teams improve their effectiveness. The setting for this effort was a community health center, located in a low income urban area, concerned with providing comprehensive, family centered health care using health teams[1] as the main "delivery system."[2]

We will then discuss some issues that apply to a variety of health care delivery settings, where groups are collaborating on the delivery. Finally, we will indicate some issues for the education and training of health workers who will be functioning in groups.

Reprinted from *Milbank Memorial Fund Quarterly* 50, 3 Part I (July 1972): 317-335. The action-research intervention discussed in this paper was carried out at the Dr. Martin Luther King, Jr. Health Center in the Bronx, New York. The effort was supported through grants from Montefiore Hospital and the Carnegie Corporation.

The Dynamics of Groups

This section will present and briefly define seven selected characteristics or variables known to be of importance in any group situation.[3] Each characteristic can be viewed as a scale or yardstick against which one can ask the question: is this particular group (made up of certain kinds of people, trying to do a given task in this situation) located where it needs to be on each of these scales to function most effectively?

Goals or Mission

A team or group has a purpose. There exists a reason (or reasons) for the formation of the group in the first place. Any group, therefore, will be confronted with issues such as:

1. how clearly defined are the goals? Who sets the goals?
2. how much agreement is there among members concerning the goals? How much commitment?
3. how clearly measurable is goal achievement?
4. how do group goals relate to broader organizational goals? To personal goals?

Since a group's very existence is to achieve some goal or mission, these issues are of central importance.

Role Expectations: Internal

In working to achieve their goals, group members will play a variety of roles. Among the members of a group a set of multiple expectations exists concerning role behavior. Each person, in effect, has a set of expectations of how each of the other members[4] should behave as the group works to achieve its goals. In any group, therefore, questions exist about: (1) the extent to which such expectations are clearly defined and communicated (role ambiguity); (2) the extent to which such expectations are compatible or in conflict (role conflict); (3) the extent to which any individual is capable of meeting these multiple expectations (role overload).

These role expectations are messages "sent" between the members of a group. Generally, the more uncertain and complex the task, the more salient are issues of role expectations.

Role Expectations: External

Any individual is a member of several groups. Each group of which he is a member has expectations that can influence his behavior. The director of pediatrics in a hospital, for example, is "simultaneously" the manager of his group, a subordinate, a member in a group of peers (directors of the functional areas), a member of a hospital staff, a father, husband and so forth

Each of these "reference" groups, as they are called, holds expectations of a person's behavior. Together they can be ambiguous, in conflict or create overload. These multiple reference group loyalties can create significant problems for an individual in terms of his behavior as a member of a particular group. Although the source of the conflicts involved in the question of reference group loyalties is external to a particular group, it can have significant internal effects.

Decision-making

A group is a problem-solving, decision-making mechanism. This is not to imply that an entire group must always make all decisions as a group. The issue is one of relevance and appropriateness; who has the relevant information and who will have to implement the decision. A group can choose from a range of decision-making mechanisms including decision by default (lack of group response), unilateral decision (authority rule), majority vote, consensus or unanimity. Each form is appropriate under certain conditions. Each will have different consequences both in terms of the amount of information available for use in making the decision, and the subsequent commitment of members to implement the decision.

Similarly, when a group faces a conflict it can choose to ignore it, smooth over it, allow one person to force a decision, create a compromise or confront all the realities of the conflict (facts and feelings) and attempt to develop an innovative solution. The choices it makes in both of these areas will significantly influence group functioning.

Communication Patterns

If, indeed, a group is a problem-solving decision-making mechanism, then the effective flow of information is central to its functioning. Anything that acts to inhibit the flow of information will detract from the group effectiveness. A range of factors affects information flow. At a very simple level are the architectural and geographic issues. Meeting space can be designed to facilitate or hinder the flow of communication. Geographically separated facilities may be a barrier to rapid information exchange. Numerous subtler factors must also be considered. Participation — frequency, order and content — may follow formal lines of authority or status. High-status members may speak first, most and most convincingly on all issues. The best sources of information needed to solve a problem will, however, vary with the problem. Patterns of communication based exclusively on formal lines of status will not meet many of the group's information needs. People's feelings of freedom to participate, to challenge, to express opinions also significantly affect information flow.

Leadership

Very much related to the processes of decision-making and communication is the area of leadership. To function effectively, a group needs many acts of leadership; not necessarily one "leader" but many leaders. People often misinterpret such a statement as saying "good groups are leaderless." This is not the intent. Depending on the situation and the problem to be solved, different people can and should assume leadership. The formal leader of a group may be in the best position to reflect the "organization's" position on a particular problem. Someone else may be a resource in helping the formal leader and another member clarify a point of disagreement. All are examples of necessary acts of leadership. It is highly unlikely that in any group one person will be capable of meeting all of a group's leadership needs.

Norms

Norms are unwritten (often untested explicitly) rules governing the behavior of people in groups. They define what behavior is "good or bad," "acceptable or unacceptable" if one is to be a functioning member of this group. As such, they become very powerful determinants of group behavior and take on the quality of laws — "it's the way we do things around here!" Their existence is most clear when they are violated; quiet uneasiness, shifting in one's seat, joking reminders, are observable. Repeated violation of norms often leads to expulsion, psychological or physical.

Norms take on particular potency because they influence all of the other areas previously discussed. Groups develop norms gorverning leadership, influence, communication patterns, decision-making, conflict resolution and the like. Inherently, norms are not good or bad. The issue is one of appropriateness — does a particular norm help or hinder a group's ability to work?

These seven factors, then, are characteristics of any group situation. Where a particular group needs to be on each of these "yardsticks" is a function of the situation. We turn now to look at these factors within the setting of health terms.

The Dynamics of a Health Team

Our intention in this section is to look at these factors affecting group functioning and to relate them to a group[5] setting (community based, total health care).

The center in which we have worked[6] is the particular situation from which we will draw examples and observations. However, the issues raised are broadly relevant.

Goals or Mission

A health team striving to provide "comprehensive family centered health care" faces uncertainties substantially different from those one might find in a hospital setting. The goals[7] in a hospital are relatively clear: remove the gall stone, deliver the baby. Success is measurable and clear. Seldom are social factors of prime importance. The thrust is curative and the emphasis is medical.

The community oriented health teams we have studied experience considerable uncertainty over their mission. "Comprehensive" means the team can not ignore social problems and emphasize the "relative security and certainty" of medical problems. Considerable anxiety is generated because the team does not really know when and if it is succeeding. The questions of priorities and time allocations become complicated; how does one decide between competing activities in the absence of clearly defined goals? A team member wonders whether to spend one-half a day trying to arrange for a school transfer for a child or see the other patients scheduled for visits.

No one member of the team has been trained to be knowledgeable in all the areas required. Yet, the complexity of the task demands that doctors become involved in social problems; nurses become the supervisors of paraprofessional family health workers who are an integral part of the team; and these community based family health workers become knowledgeable in diagnosing and treating psychiatric problems. This is not to say everyone should become an expert at solving all problems. The requirements are for considerable information collection, sharing and group planning so that the team has all the available information to deploy its total resources to the task.

The anxieties and frustrations created by the complexity of the task are inevitable — an inherent part of providing "comprehensive" care.[8] A major team dilemma is one of managing short- versus long-run considerations — to give itself short-run security and direction while not losing sight of its long-run, vague and global goal.

Role Expectations: Internal and External

The nature of the task — comprehensive family centered health care — demands a highly diverse set of skills, knowledge and backgrounds. In creating a team, many "cultures" are of necessity being mixed and asked to work together.

As a result of educational background and training, the doctors are accustomed to being primary (if not sole) authority and most expert in medical issues. The specialist role for which they have been so well trained and that is so appropriate in a hospital setting comes under pressure. As a team member, in addition to his specialist skills, the doctor is asked to become more of a generalist. He needs to teach other health workers some of his medical knowledge. He also needs to learn from them more about the social problems facing the community and the character, mores and values of the particular patient population.

Doctors tend to maintain strong psychologic ties with their professional speciality groups. The stronger these ties for a physician the more difficult it will be for him to develop needed team loyalty. His sense of professionalism stems from these external reference groups. The careful hospital-type workup he has been so well trained to do may not be feasible or appropriate in the face of the hectic schedule generated by large numbers of patients. The conflict may become one around "professional standards." Comprehensive group practice may require a redefinition of these standards and perhaps even the redefinition of a professional.

Both the nurses and family health workers tend to bring a history of submissiveness. The nurses have been trained to be submissive to doctors. In this setting nurses find themselves as coordinators of the work of a team including doctors — a complete role reversal.

Family health workers in this case are local community residents, who, after six months of clinical training, suddenly find themselves defined as "colleagues" with middle-class physicians. They bring a deep concern for social problems coupled with the best understanding of what will or will not work with patients (their friends and relatives). The team needs their knowledge of the cultural norms of the community and their commitment to social issues. Their background and passive posture is often a barrier to the realization of these expectations.

Whereas the nurses and doctors have a professional reference group, the family health workers as yet have none. The resulting feelings of "homelessness" are heightened by their liaison role at the interface between the team and the community.[a] Their membership and acceptance in the community is crucial to the team's ability to be of service. They alone can serve to bridge the cultural gaps that exist.[9]

This set of conditions differs markedly from the hospital setting where strong reference group loyalties and clearly defined role expectations are common. Behaviors learned during one's individual preparation are appropriately applicable in the vast majority of situations. Although professionals and paraprofessionals work in the same organization, seldom, if ever, are they asked to work in highly interdependent on-going stable groups.

---

[a]Such people have been called marginal men. A foreman in a factory is another example — caught between the management culture and the worker culture.

A part of being a member of a highly interdependent team is the need to develop new loyalties and learn some new skills not anticipated or covered during individual training. In fact, it is unlikely that, in the face of the mission of providing "comprehensive family-centered health care," clearly defined, complete job descriptions will ever be feasible.[10] This reality puts great stress on a team's ability to learn and adapt by itself. In response to a particular problem, the question cannot be "Whose job is it?" but may instead have to be "Who on the team is capable?" or "Who needs to learn how to handle the situation?"

Decision-Making

The inherent uncertainties in its mission and the diverse mix of skills represented on a health team suggest that decisions can seldom be appropriately made in a routine, programmable or unilateral manner. This is in sharp contrast to the majority of cases in the hospital setting in which is found the relative clarity and certainty of the goals and clearly defined roles and lines of authority.

One difficulty in any on-going team is the need to differentiate a variety of decision-making situations. In an attempt to be "democratic and participative" a team might try to make all decisions by consensus as a team. This represents a failure to distinguish, for example, (a) who has the information necessary to make a decision, (b) who needs to be consulted before certain decisions get made and (c) who needs to be informed of a decision after it has been made. Under certain circumstances the team may need to strive for unanimity or consensus; in other cases majority vote may be appropriate.

Perhaps the greatest barrier to effective decision-making in highly interdependent health teams stems again from the "cultural" backgrounds of team members. Doctors are used to making decisions by themselves or in collaboration with peers of equal status – other doctors or highly educated professionals. At the other extreme, the community residents who work on the team are used to being passive dependent recipients of others' decisions. Yet many times, on a health team, the doctor and the community workers are and must behave as peers, neither one possessing all the information needed to solve a particular problem or make a particular decision. Furthermore, many times the doctor is the one who needs information held by another health worker. When a conflict develops, the required discussion that will lead to consensus is difficult to achieve; forcing, compromise or decision by default may result. Commitment to decisions is low with the result being that many decisions have to be remade several times – "I thought we decided that last week!" or "Didn't we decide that you would do such and such?"

The team approach to delivery of health care puts great stress on the need for numerous and various inputs to many decisions. When the decision-making process is inappropriate less information is shared, commitment is lowered and anxiety and frustration are increased.

Communication Patterns and Leadership

Issues of communication patterns and leadership can be handled together for, as was true in the case of decision-making as well, the central theme is one of "influence." The leadership or influence structure — to which we have all become so accustomed via family, educational and organizational experiences and that is appropriate for, say, a hospital operating room — will be incapable of responding to the diversity of issues with which a health team must deal. In this setting each member is a resource. He must have open channels to all the other members. Because of the complexities in this type of group, a number of communication norms are required: openness (leveling) and a person-to-person relationship with enough mutual trust to enable each person to "tell it like it is."

Team practice can not work if roles talk to roles; a much more personal mutual dependency is required. Influence, communication frequency and leadership should be determined by the nature of the problem to be solved and not by hierarchical position, educational background or social status.

With respect to leadership, in particular, the teams we have studied relied on the model they knew best — in this case "follow the doctor." Continued reliance on that model will result in an overemphasis on medical instead of social issues, a lack of shared commitment to decisions (which doctors sometimes interpret as "lack of professional attitude") and less than complete sharing of information, all of which directly affect the task performance.

Norms

Much of what has been described is reflected in a group's norms. The teams studied have exhibited several powerful norms:
1. "In making a decision silence means consent";
2. "Doctors are more important than other team members"; "we don't disagree with them"; "we wait for them to lead";
3. Conflict is dangerous, both task conflicts and interpersonal disagreements; "it's best to leave sleeping dogs lie";
4. Positive feelings, praise, support are not to be shared; — "we're all 'professionals' here to do a job."
5. The precision and exactness demanded by our task negate the opportunity to be flexible with respect to our own internal group processes (this may be a carry-over from the hospital operating room environment where the last thing needed is an innovative idea as to how to do things better.

The effects of these norms, and others like them, is to guarantee that a team gets caught in a negative spiral.[11] The norms are those of rigidity, but the complexity of the environment and the task to be done demand flexibility. The frustrating, anxiety-provoking quality of the task places great demands for some place to recharge one's emotional battery. The team is potentially such a place.

In addition to these specific norms of flexibility, support and openness of communication, a set of higher order norms is essential. Task uncertainty and environmental changes require that a team develop a capacity to become self-renewing — become a learning organism. Learning requires a climate that legitimizes controlled experimentation, risk taking, failure and evaluation of outcomes. In the absence of norms that support and reinforce these kinds of behaviors, a team will end up fighting two enemies — its tasks and itself.

In other words, a unique connection exists between what a team does (its task) and how it goes about doing it (its internal group processes). At a simple level, the health care analogy would be: if a team is to treat a family as an integrated unit (its task), the team itself must, in many ways, operate as a highly integrated "family unit" (its internal group processes). Without this ability to maintain itself a health team will, like many other "pieces of equipment" eventually burn itself out. In the interim, work continues to get done, but more and more energy is demanded to "move the machine forward."

To summarize, the "internal process" issues that have been discussed will occur in any group. They can not be wished away or ignored for long without some cost. Nor are they the result — as is frequently assumed — of basic personality problems. More often team members have difficulty functioning together because of ambiguous goal orientations, unclear role expectations, dysfunctional decision-making procedures and other such process issues.

If a health team is first to survive and second to grow, it must develop an attitude and a capability for building and renewing itself as a team. It can do this first by becoming aware of how its internal group processes influence its ability to function and second by learning how to manage these processes or maintenance needs in a more productive manner.

We turn now to a brief case illustration of an effort aimed at helping health teams move closer to this ideal of becoming self-renewing or learning organisms.

A Case Study of a Health Team Improvement Effort

Our efforts at helping teams improve their functioning[12] relied heavily upon a simple but powerful model: the action research approach.[13] The basic flow of activities can be depicted in the following manner:

$$\text{Data Collection} \longrightarrow \text{Summarization and Feedback} \longrightarrow \text{Action Planning} \longrightarrow \text{Evaluation}$$

In this setting, the initial activity with a health team involved interviewing each member individually using both open-ended questions and check list ratings. Questions asked related directly to the seven process factors discussed earlier such as team goals, levels of participation, decision-making styles and so forth. These data were then summarized and fed back anonymously to the entire team.

Team members' reactions to the data presented during this feedback session were varied. For some, the result was one of surprise — "I didn't realize people felt that way about this team!" Others were surprised to find many of their own concerns widely shared. Before the feedback session, many people believed they were the only ones experiencing certain difficulties. The most frequent reaction could be characterized as follows: "These problems have been around — under the surface — for a long time. Now they have been collected, summarized and are out on the table for all of us to see."

The teams, in other words, were provided with an image or picture of their present state based on information (feelings as well as facts) collected from the most valid sources available, the team members themselves. As a result of the interview feedback process, teams owned the information (verbatim quotes were used to exemplify a particular issue) and shared the image of their present state — "it's out on the table for all of us to see." These two elements of shared owner-ship helped to create a heightened desire and commitment on the part of team members to solve their problems.

To cope with the large number of complex problems reflected in the infor-mation and to move most effectively into action planning, the health teams had to:

1. Assign priorities to the multiple issues reflected in their data;
2. Decide upon the most appropriate format to use (total group, homogeneous versus heterogeneous subgroups and so forth) to generate solution alterna-tives;
3. Develop a clear and shared set of change objectives or goals; an image of what a more ideal or improved state would be;
4. Allocate individual and subgroup responsibilities to implement chosen actions;
5. Specify mechanisms and procedures for checking progress (follow-up).

The problem-solving skills, attitudes and norms needed to accomplish the above "process work" were similar to behaviors needed to successfully accom-plish "task work." This unique connection between task and process can be clarified with the following example.

A salient problem in each health team concerned their regularly scheduled 90-minute weekly team conference meetings. These meetings represented the one time each week when the entire team met together. The intent was to discuss patient family cases, learn from each other's experiences, work on common problems and the like. The pervasive feeling with regard to these meetings was one of frustration and dissatisfaction. They were dull, a waste of time and a time for some people to "lecture" about their pet topics.

The way the team managed itself (its process) during these meetings in fact made the situation more difficult. The negative spiral to which we referred earlier was operating to drain energy and commitment required to solve patient problems.

The specific action plans developed and subsequent team improvement interventions were, in each case, a product of the particular issues reflected in the data collected initially from a team. Regardless of the problem, the same action research model, with minor variations, was applied. For example, action plans aimed at improving the team conference meeting included: (a) the formation of agenda planning committees; (b) systems of rotating chairmen to help all team members enhance their skills at running a meeting; (c) designation of observers, on a rotating basis, to help the team evaluate, at the end of each meeting, the impact of its own group dynamics.[14]

Many consultant interventions were aimed at helping a team to solve problems it presently felt; longer run considerations also guided consultant behavior. Whenever feasible, a team was helped to see the connection between what they were doing (their task) and how they were going about it (their internal group process). This expanded awareness helped to develop an attitude (norm) toward change, which legitimized managed experimentation and learning. In other words, if a team is to become self-renewing, it must be willing to experiment in a controlled way — to try new ways of working, evaluate and learn from the consequences of these efforts, and use this new learning in planning and implementing future efforts. On the assumption that the action research approach we used represented a general problem-solving model, we continuously worked to help the teams to adapt this model so that they could apply it when confronted with future problems.

The short time frame within which we worked dictated limited and modest objectives. Short-run changes have been observed and documented in terms of:

1. Greater work productivity, particularly with respect to team conference meetings;
2. Increased clarity of role expectations plus mechanisms for negotiating changes in role behavior as they are needed;
3. Greater flexibility in decision-making;
4. More widely shared influence and participation among all team members.

Implications for Health Team Operations

Based on an understanding of groups in general and our experiences with health teams working in an urban community, several significant lessons are beginning to emerge with implications for the delivery of health care using groups or teams.

1. Some conscious program that helps team members look at their particular goals, tasks, relationships, decision-making, norms, backgrounds and values is essential for team effectivness. It is naive to bring together a highly diverse group of people and to expect that, by calling them a team, they will in fact behave as a team.

2. Behavioral science knowledge and techniques, developed in a variety of nonmedical settings are relevant and appear to be transferable to organizations involved in the delivery of health care. The action research approach is one such example. It reflects a methodology and set of values that can help a team become a self-renewing organism. In some ways, it demands of a team that it treat itself as a patient, periodically diagnosing its own state of health, prescribing medication, and subjecting itself to the check-ups to insure that the prescription is working. Although this process may require the assistance of a "third party" initially, the "patient team" can learn to do many of the things itself.

3. Ideally, every team member can be a participant in the group's task and an observer of the group's process. At a minimum, such capability for helping teams look at their own working should be built into the training of team leaders.

4. The organizations in which health teams are imbedded will need to develop an internal capability to help groups manage their own process. Outside resources are appropriate to initate such activities, but internal specialists are needed to provide needed continuity, follow-up and reinforcement.

5. Programs need to be developed that focus specifically on the problems of helping people cope with cultural discrepancies whether these be between a team and its client population or between team members; e.g., the professionally based physician and the community based family health worker.

6. Certain team members will need particular leadership skills. If nurses are expected to act as team coordinators, they will need special training. All team members will need to develop membership skills; e.g., listening, collaborating.

7. Although some of this needed training may be accomplished during individual preparation,[15] some training needs to be done with the team as a unit. In addition, more of this training needs to be goal related — e.g., treating a family as an integrated unit — as compared to technique related — e.g., taking histories, doing EKG's. (This does not imply that such skills are unimportant, only that they should be learned in relation to specific goals.)

8. The socialization of new team members needs to be examined. Programs need to be developed that in fact orient a new family health worker, for example, to her role as a team member as well as a specialist with particular skills.

9. There is great value in initiating team development activities, of the kind described, at the point of a team's formation. Teams, like individuals, develop their own cultures or personalities. In "older teams" a considerable amount of unfreezing may have to take place before new changes can be tried. Early team

development efforts would have several distinct advantages: (a) the period of initial socialization has a significant effect on the team's future development — early experiences set a very strong tone that influence future events; (b) a group can more easily create the kind of culture, norms and procedures it deems useful if it is starting fresh rather than having to "undo" a long history of past experiences; (c) perhaps most important would be the early recognition that the team really has two equally important tasks — to deliver health care and to continuously work to develop and maintain itself as a well-functioning team to improve its services.

The focus of this paper has been upon the working of existing health teams in a community setting where entire families are "the patient." We have explored some ways in which one might help such a team learn more about its own "internal dynamics" and use these learnings to improve the way it functions in delivering health care.

We will, in all likelihood, see an increasing number of models for delivering health care in which groups of some form play an integral part. The effectiveness of these groups in accomplishing their tasks will be, in part, a function of how well they manage themselves with respect to the "process variables" discussed in this paper.

References

1. The average team in this center consisted of a full-time internist, a full-time pediatrician, two full-time nurses and four to six full-time family health workers drawn from the community. Available on a part-time basis were a dentist and a psychiatrist, in addition to the back-up support of x-rays, laboratories and the like. A team was responsible for 1,500 families in a particular geographic area.

2. We pay little attention in this paper to the important question of the organization of which the health team is a part. For an intensive discussion of the organizational issues involved in the delivery of health care see Beckhard, R., Organizational Issues in Team Delivery of Health Care, *Milbank Memorial Fund Quarterly 50,* 3 Part I (July 1972): 287-316.

3. For an excellent and readable description of group process see Schein, E.H., *Process Consultation,* Reading, Massachusetts, Addison-Wesley Publishing Co., Inc., 1969; for a more general introduction to the field of organizational psychology see Schein, E.H., *Organizational Psychology,* Englewood Cliffs, New Jersey, Prentice-Hall, Inc., 1965.

4. For a study of role sets see Kahn, R.N., *et al., Organizational Stress: Studies in Role Conflict and Ambiguity,* New York, John Wiley & Sons, Inc., 1964.

5. Group practice here means situations in which people are together over long periods of time working on a common task. More temporary groups such as the group formed to do a particular operation in a hospital are not included in the discussion. Even in many temporary groups, such as short-

duration task forces or committees, many of the process factors discussed can be observed to be in operation.

6. For a more detailed preliminary report of activities in this setting see Fry, R.E. and Lech, B.A., An Organizational Development Approach to Improving the Effectiveness of Neighborhood Health Care Teams: A Pilot Program, unpublished masters thesis, Massachusetts Institute of Technology, June, 1971.

7. If one takes a total hospital as a group many similar issues appear. Revens, for example, argues that the central task in a hospital is the management of anxiety. This is analogous to the position we take vis-a-vis a health team. The only difference is that the problems are more visible in the smaller social system of an ongoing group. See Revens, R.W., *Standards for Morale: Cause and Effect in Hospitals,* London, Oxford University Press, 1964.

8. A useful tool for diagnosing the forces impinging upon a team is called force field analysis. For more detail see Fry and Lech, *op. cit.;* and an article by Lewin, K., in Bennis, W., Benne, K. and Chin, R., *The Planning of Change,* second edition, New York, Holt, Rinehart & Winston, Inc., 1969.

9. The notion of a team approach to the delivery of health care may, for example, force a redefinition of the norm of privacy between doctor and patient. The norm may need to be adapted to encompass team and patient.

10. Many organizations are realizing the needs for such fluid role relations. A job is now viewed as a "man in action in a particular situation at a particular moment." Such "job descriptions" must be constantly renegotiated and updated to account for both changes in the man and the situation.

11. It is in this regard that our thinking is similar to Revens'. The ineffective management of inherent anxiety results in more anxiety creating a negative feedback loop and a self-reinforcing downward spiral. See Fry and Lech, *op. cit.*

12. Initial efforts at intervening into two health teams are reported in detail in Fry and Lech, *op. cit.* We have to date completed initial interventions with six health teams. Similar activities are planned for other teams in the future as well as follow-up activities to reinforce initial efforts. Four of our students — Ron Fry, Bern Lech, Marc Gerstein and Mark Plovnick — have worked closely with us in these efforts.

13. For a description of this model and its applicability in a wide variety of situations see Beckhard, R., *Organization Development: Strategies and Models,* Reading, Massachusetts, Addison-Wesley Publishing Co., Inc., 1969.

14. In several cases, these observers were part of the next agenda-planning committee. The data collected by the observers, in other words, were quickly used as an input into the next action planning phase.

15. It is clear that existing educational and training institutions — medical schools, nursing schools, teaching hospitals — will need to bear part of this responsibility. In addition to the content areas of psychology, social psychology, sociology and the like, increasing emphasis must be placed on such areas as group dynamics, organizational behavior, social intervention and the theory and process of planned change.

Part XI
Neighborhood Health Centers As
Instruments of Change —
Relationships With, and Impacts
On, Other Health Institutions

Introduction

Among the objectives which various actors had in mind for the neighborhood health centers at the time of their inception were that the centers would effect changes in other parts of the health care system. It was hoped, for instance, that the opening of a neighborhood health center would alleviate overcrowding of hospital outpatient clinics and emergency rooms in the vicinity. Some saw the health centers as levers to accomplish broader changes — strengthening community medicine offerings in medical school curricula, securing greater emphasis by medical schools of their community service functions, creating more open and more responsive associations of health professionals. There is an increasing accumulation of anecdotal evidence on the issue of the broader impacts of the centers. Some partisans of the health center movement claim as an indication of the success of the centers in this regard the fact that "we have captured the rhetoric." They mean that key aspects of the health centers which were highly innovative a few years ago are now accepted procedure and are endorsed by parties who opposed, or were ignorant of, these features and approaches when the health centers were getting started.

To some extent, discussion about whether or not the centers have functioned effectively as catalysts of change in the larger health system hinges upon philosophical and political differences of opinion about what is significant change and how one measures it. Very often persons who have been actually involved in bringing about change are disappointed not to have achieved more than they have. They tend not to have notched, or not to recognize, benchmarks which allow perception of change. Mentally, their benchmarks shift so that they profess to see no significant movement.

The increasingly significant volume of evidence on the health centers as instruments of change includes the fact of tremendous growth in the number of departments of community medicine in medical schools and new residency programs in family medicine, a field popularized by the health centers. Another example of impact — department chiefs know what consumer participation is and play by the new rules of the game in dealing with communities even if they do not like the new rules.

There does exist hard evidence about the ways in which some individual neighborhood health centers have effected hospitals. Two of the articles reprinted below document the effects which services delivered by a neighborhood health center have had in reducing or otherwise altering their patients' use of various hospital services. In "Impact of Ambulatory-Health-Care Services on the Demand for Hospital Beds," Seymour Bellin, H. Jack Geiger, and Count Gibson report that the opening of the Columbia Point Health Center resulted in a dramatic decline in admission of residents of the Columbia Point housing project to Boston City Hospital and in the number of bed days spent at the hospital during the first two years of the Center's operation. Louis Hochheiser, Kenneth Woodward and Evan Charney, in "Effect of the Neighborhood Health Center on the Use of Pediatric Emergency Departments in Rochester, New York," conclude that the services of the Rochester center resulted in a 38 percent reduction in child visits by the service population to emergency departments from 1967 to 1970.[1,2]

Anthony Kovner et al., in "Relating a Neighborhood Health Center to a General Hospital: A Case History," examine "the question of whether a formally structured relationship with a general hospital is necessary for the neighborhood health center to achieve its goals and to function as a viable organization." In addressing this question they document the effects of the Gouverneur Health Services Program, a neighborhood health center built on a restructured hospital which had ceased to provide inpatient services, on the Beth Israel Hospital of New York City. They also discuss the impact of the hospital on the neighborhood health center.

References

1. A later article by Gordon T. Moore, Roberta Bernstein, and Rosemary A. Bonanno, "Effect of a Neighborhood Health Center on Hospital Emergency Room Use," *Medical Care, 10,* 3 (May-June 1972): 240-247, concludes that the operation of the Bunker Hill Health Center in Boston has not changed the level of use of emergency services at Massachusetts General Hospital by residents of the area served by the center. They did find that health center registrants who used the emergency room of the hospital were more likely to have been referred there by a physician, to have a regular source of primary medical care, and to be using the emergency room as back-up for their regular care than were those patients who were not registered at the health center.
2. Another paper by persons associated with the Rochester Neighborhood Health Center compares hospital admissions patterns between children who are users of the center, nonusers who lived in the center's target area and a comparison group. See: Michael Klein, Klaus Roghmann, Kenneth Woodward, and Evan Charney, "The Impact of the Rochester Neighborhood Health Center on Hospitalization of Children, 1968 to 1970," *Pediatrics 51,* 5 (May 1973) 833-839.

23

Impact of Ambulatory-Health-Care Services on the Demand for Hospital Beds

A Study of the Tufts Neighborhood Health Center at Columbia Point in Boston

Seymour S. Bellin, H. Jack Geiger and Count D. Gibson

The focus of this paper is to measure the effect of the Columbia Point Neighborhood Health Center on the demand for hospital beds.

The Study Design

Sources of Data

Data on hospitalization were obtained for a sample of residents at Columbia Point from two sources: medical records at Boston City Hospital; and medical billing records at the Boston City Welfare Department. The Hospital furnishes us with hospital inpatient utilization for *all* residents so far as they are hospitalized at that facility. The base-line health survey reveals, on the basis of respondents' reports, that over three of five of all admissions were to City Hospital. A relatively complete history of hospitalization during this period can be constructed for the families who were continuously on welfare — about 30 percent of the study families. Unfortunately, welfare medical records, unlike hospital records, do not contain information on diagnoses.

The Study Population

The population for this inquiry into hospitalization was limited to the residents who took part in the original study panel of 357 families, randomly chosen to provide a base-line picture of health-care beliefs, attitudes and practices prevailing just before the Health Center opened its doors.[a] To hold constant time at risk, families that were not in residence in this community for the full 30 months of

Reprinted from *New England Journal of Medicine* 280, 15 (April 10, 1969): 808-812. Introductory material about the Columbia Point Health Center and its community setting contained in the original version of this paper has been deleted because comparable information appears at the beginning of Chapter 16.

[a] An original census of all residents of Columbia Point and the baseline Health Survey was designed by Daniel Yankelovich, Inc., in co-operation with the staff of the Tufts Department of Preventive Medicine. The firm also assisted in the design of the repeat Health Survey and carried out all the data collection and processing.

the study period — from 12 months before to 18 months after the advent of the Health Center — were excluded. To eliminate the bias introduced by the passage of Medicare legislation early during the study, which undoubtedly affected both the rate and the site of hospitalization, all persons 65 years of age and over were also excluded. Thus, the final study sample consisted of 209 families containing 980 members. Sixty-one of these households — a total of 296 persons, excluding the elderly — were continuously on welfare during the study period.

The Findings

In the 12 months before the Health Center opened its doors the demand for hospital beds by the Columbia Point Community approximated that of the general population of the United States whether calculated in terms of hospital admissions, total hospital days or average length of a hospital stay (table 23-1).

The 10.7 reported hospital admissions per 100 persons in table 23-1, derived from a survey of a random sample of households at Columbia Point just before the Health Center opened in 1965, compares with the rate of 9.3 reported in the National Health Survey.[1] On the basis of hospital records, the admissions rate of 11.7 per 100 persons estimated for Columbia Point compares with a comparable figure of 12.9 for the general population.[2]

Boston City Hospital Admissions

Boston City Hospital accounted for nearly two of three hospital admissions in the year before the Neighborhood Health Center was established. Excluding the

Table 23-1

Annual Number of Hospital Admissions and Total Hospital Days per Hundred Persons for Columbia Point (Boston) and the United States

Source of Data	Annual No. of Admissions/100 Persons	Annual Hospital Days/100 Persons
Hospital records:		
USA, 1960[2]	12.9	98.3
Columbia Point*	11.7	81.4
Health survey:		
USA, 1960-62[1]	9.3	—
Columbia Point†	10.7	—

*Rates estimated on basis of admissions to Boston City Hospital adjusted for ratio of Boston City admissions to all hospital admissions derived from 1965 Health Survey.

†Based on self-reported hospitalizations in random sample survey of 357 households before establishment of Health Center in 1965.

elderly, the number of admissions to Boston City Hospital inpatient facilities and the total number of bed days spent there, on the basis of hospital medical records, markedly declined after the Center was opened (table 23-2). The sharpest reduction took place in the Health Center's second year of operation. Admissions to the hospital for all diagnoses declined by 41 percent during the Center's first year. In the second year, there was a further reduction of 75 percent from the figure for the first year. Thus, by the end of the second full year of operation, admissions to Boston City Hospital had been reduced by 84 percent of those occurring in the 12 months before the advent of the Center. These findings hold for type of medical problem: for obstetric, general medical and surgical admission. Whereas surgical admissions also declined in both years, they did so at a constant rate.

Although the pattern for total hospital bed days is similar for all admissions, there are differences according to type of medical problem. During the Center's initial year, the decline in total bed days spent in the hospital by Columbia Point residents is largely accounted for by surgical cases. Total hospital bed days for general medical and obstetric admissions declined only slightly: except for normal deliveries, which showed no change, the drop in the number of general medical admissions and admissions for complications associated with pregnancy was offset by an increase in average length of stay. During the second year, however, our projected figures reveal a sharp decline in total hospital bed days for general medical and obstetric, as well as surgical, admissions.

The dramatic decline in admissions to Boston City Hospital, of course, may merely reflect a change in *site of* hospitalization rather than a true drop in the total demand for hospital beds. Since ambulatory health services are major gatekeepers in the pathways to hospitals and the great majority of Columbia Point residents rely on the Neighborhood Health Center as their central source of care, the possibility must be considered that the Tufts-sponsored Center,

Table 23-2
Annual Admissions to and Total Days Spent in Boston City Hospital According to Type of Medical Condition for Columbia Point Families Continuously in Residence for Persons under 65 Years of Age*

| | All Diagnoses | | | | Medical Cases | | | | Surgical Cases | | | |
| | admissions | | hospital days | | admissions | | hospital days | | admissions | | hospital days | |
Year	no.	% of base yr	no.	% of base yr	no.	% of base yr	no.	% of base yr	no.	% of base yr	no.	% of base yr
1965 (base)	69	100.0	461	100.0	15	100.0	138	100.0	33	100.0	245	100.0
1966	41	59.4	322	68.8	11	73.3	132	95.7	16	48.4	120	49.0
1967*	11	15.9	66	14.3	0	0	0	0	8	24.2	55	22.4

Table 23-2
(Concluded)

	Obstetric cases					
	Total		Normal deliveries		Complications	
	admissions	hospital days	admissions	hospital days	admissions	hospital days
Year	no. / % of base yr	no. / % of base yr	no. / % of base yr	no. / % of base yr	no. / % of base yr	no. / % of base yr
1965 (base)	21 100.0	78 100.0	14 100.0	56 100.0	7 100.0	22 100.0
1966	14 66.7	70 89.7	11 78.6	52 92.9	3 −†	18 81.8
1967*	3 14.3	11 14.1	3 −†	11 19.6	0 0	0 0

*Statistics for yr based on utilization figures for 1st 6 mo; projections derived from average relation of 1st 6 mo to 2d 6 mo for preceeding yr.
†Percentages not calculated for denominators <10.

with its affiliated hospital, may have affected the pattern of inpatient hospital referrals. An examination of hospital referrals for families on welfare on the basis of welfare records reveals only negligible differences in the distribution of admissions among Boston hospitals before and after the Center opened. Although such third-party payment mechanisms as Medicaid have made voluntary hospitals more receptive to fiscally risky patients, this legislation was not effectively implemented until well after the close of the study period.

A change in site of hospitalization is not a likely explanation for the observed decline in hospital admissions; only data on admissions to all general hospitals can definitively lay to rest any nagging doubts on this point. Welfare medical billings afford precisely such data.

Welfare Medical Records

Both the patients eligible for welfare medical benefits and the hospitals to which they are admitted, including Boston City Hospital, have every incentive to file claims arising out of a hospital admission. Consequently, welfare medical billing records furnishes for families *continuously* on welfare throughout the thirty-month study period, about three in 10 of the study sample, a fairly complete history of admissions to all hospitals.

The findings concerning the demand for hospital beds by these families are similar to those previously reported for all patients on the basis of admissions to Boston City Hospital alone. There was a drop in number of hospital admissions and in total number of bed days spent in the hospital in the first year of the Center's operation that was accelerated in the second year (table 23–3). By contrast with the year before the Neighborhood Health Center opened, the total number of hospital admissions in the second year had dropped by 69 percent,

Table 23-3

Annual Admissions to and Total Days Spent at All Hospitals, for 61 Households Continuously on Welfare, for 296 Persons Under Age of 65[*]

Year	No. of Admissions		Hospital Days	
	no.	% of base yr	no.	% of base yr
1965 (base)	26	100.0	200	100.0
1966	20	76.9	110	55.0
1967[†]	8	30.8	40	20.0

[*]Total families with at least 1 hospitalization during study period 26.

[†]Statistics for yr based on utilization figures for 1st 6 mo; projections derived from average relation of 1st 6 mo to 2d 6 mo for preceding yr.

and the total number of hospital bed days by 80 percent. The corresponding figures for Boston City Hospital admissions alone reveal a decline of 84 percent in number of admissions and 86 percent in total bed days. Thus, the statistics on the welfare families confirm the essential findings of the Boston City Hospital data.

Before the reduction in hospitalization can be credited to the Center, one other alternative exaplanation needs to be given consideration: the possibility that a general decline in the frequency of illness and injury serious enough to warrant hospitalization coincided with the establishment of the Health Center. There is no evidence, however, to support such a hypothesis. Boston City Health Department statistics on mortality and reportable communicable diseases show no city-wide changes between 1965 and 1966.[3] Preliminary data on health conditions reported for a sample of families in a survey repeated two years after the Center opened reveals a *rise* rather than a decrease in prevalence, undoubtedly reflecting in large measure increasing health sophistication resulting from more frequent contact with health-care services on the part of low-income residents.

Finally, the decline in maternity admissions merits a special comment. The possibility that the birth rate declined during this period either generally or at Columbia Point is being explored. Although a family-planning service was made available in this community, its effects, obviously, could hardly be felt until the second year. A more likely explanation for the drop in births during the first year is the nature of the panel-study design: as an aging cohort, it is subject to diminishing fertility.

Discussion

The Neighborhood Health Center has demonstrated the potential effectiveness of comprehensive ambulatory health-care services in reducing the demand for hospital beds in a low-income community. The decline in the rate of hospital admissions, already evident in the first year of the Center's operation, was accelerated in its second year. This achievement is especially impressive in that it has taken place in a community that, hitherto, had been medically disadvantaged. Since this community had previously had a large pool of unrecognized and medically unattended health problems, the high volume of use of the Center's services might have been expected to inflate hospital admissions greatly. It is this identification of neglected medical conditions that undoubtedly explains the more modest reduction in admissions to hospitals from the community during the first year. Unquestionably, then, not only is the Neighbhorhood Health Center successful in achieving public acceptance and high utilization of its services, but these are effective in preventing conditions from becoming serious enough to require hospitalization. This is our most important conclusion.

Still further gains in the reduction of hospital admissions can be anticipated although, obviously, not on the dramatic scale as appears to have already been achieved. It should be appreciated that the decline in hospital admissions was accomplished primarily by the effective treatment of illness and injury rather than by their prevention. Although the Center staff has endeavored to incorporate a few basic preventive public-health measures into its routine health-care practices — immunizations and asymptomatic general physical examinations — and the community Health Association has initiated, with the co-operation of the Health Center and other community groups, a few campaigns aimed at eliminating health hazards from the community, these efforts have until recently been sporadic and fragmented. The backlog of unmet medical problems and the trials of institution building have placed preventive and community medicine second in the Center's scheme of priorities. Within the past few months, however, both the Center and the community Health Association have reached a point in their development and in their relations with each other that has enabled both to direct more systematic attention to these issues, and already a number of imaginative programs and proposals have been developed. A further reduction in hospital admission can be expected as these programs are implemented.

Beyond this, the reduction of hospital admissions depends on the extent to which new developments in the expanding frontier of medical and behavior sciences equip health-care practitioners with more effective treatment procedures. The Neighborhood Health Center has been more successful in treating and preventing hospital admissions for some conditions than others. For example, neurologic and psychologic disorders, for which a longer hospital stay is typical, made up only 8 percent of all nonmaternity admissions before but 22 percent after the Center opened its doors. Consistent with this finding is a decline in short-term stays in hospitals from 53 percent to 40 percent after the Center was established.

This study adds to the growing body of evidence that points to the value of ambulatory health-care services in preventing and effectively treating illnesses that otherwise might require hospital care. Not all ambulatory systems are equally effective in preventing hospitalization. For example, a recent study of federal employees revealed that those who receive health coverage through group practice have markedly lower levels of utilization of hospital beds than those covered by indemnity or Blue Cross-Blue Shield plans.[4] At the same time, there is considerable variability among the various group practices in the rate of utilization of inhospital facilities by their respective clienteles. Employees utilizing the group practice with the lowest level of utilization of hospital bed days were 59 percent below the comparable figure for those covered by Blue Cross-Blue Shield. Undoubtedly, neighborhood health centers, varying as they do in conception, internal organization and relations to their host community, are also likely to show variation in effectiveness in control and prevention of illness and injury. There is a need for systematic comparative study of these variations in delivering health care to establish and account for their relative efficacy.

It is evident that the neighborhood health center is one major system for delivering ambulatory health care that brings about a more rational use of the intensive-care facilities of a hospital. The spread of third-party payment plans such as Medicare and Medicaid has already increased nationwide pressure on costly hospital beds. Although there is room for more effective cost-reducing managerial strategies — the more intensive use of automation, further special tion and division of labor and creation of multihospital consortiums to achieve purchasing and other economies — intensive bed care can be expected to grow progressively more expensive with each advance in the medical and behavioral sciences. The dramatic reduction achieved by this Neighborhood Health Center and other group-health practices offers a much more fundamental solution in the long run to the problem of scarcity of hospital beds and high cost of hospital care.

In this connection, neighborhood health centers and other ambulatory health-care services can help greatly to reduce the number of days spent in the hospital by assuming responsibility for the supervision of the posthospital convalescent care of patients no longer requiring intensive hospital care. It is not unlikely that hospital staffs would be more disposed to discharge patients earlier if adequate ambulatory-care facilities existed with which they had good working relations.

Making more rational use of hospital beds requires comprehensive planning resulting in the development in each community of a full range of co-ordinated health-care facilities — from the neighborhood-based ambulatory-care facility that will prevent serious conditions requiring hospital care, the intensive-treatment hospital and the convalescent dormitory adjacent to the hospital, which, along with the ambulatory health service, can take responsibility for patients during their convalescence.

References

1. Ballo, L.E., and Gleeson. G.A. Persons Hospitalized by number of hospital episodes and days in year. United States — July 1960-June 1962. *Vital Health Statist. 10:*1-42, 1965.
2. United States Department of Health, Education and Welfare. Public Health Service. Health Economics Branch. Division of Community Health Services. Health Economics Series No. 1. *Medical Care Financing and Utilization: Source book of data through 1961.* Washington, D.C.: Government Printing Office, 1962. P. 160. (Publication No. 947.)
3. Department of Health and Hospitals, City of Boston. Personal communication.
4. Perrott, G.S. Federal Employees Health Benefits Program. III. Utilization of hospital services. *Am. J. Pub. Health 56:*57-64. 1966.

24 Effect of the Neighborhood Health Center on the Use of Pediatric Emergency Departments in Rochester, New York

Louis I. Hochheiser, Kenneth Woodward, and Evan Charney

In July, 1968, a Neighborhood Health Center sponsored by the Office of Economic Opportunity was established under the auspices of Action for a Better Community to provide comprehensive family-centered care to residents of a defined poverty area in Rochester, New York. The Center's administration is guided by the University of Rochester School of Medicine. One of several studies in progress to assess the effectiveness of the program measured the impact of the Center on visits to the pediatric emergency departments in hospitals in the Rochester area.

An important aspect of the current medical-care crisis is the reported alarming increase in emergency-room usage. Emergency care not only is expensive but also, by being episodic rather than comprehensive, lacks the prerequisites of quality care. One of the primary goals of neighborhood health centers is to provide continuity of care that will reduce the use of emergency departments.

The hypothesis that the Health Center would decrease child visits to all hospital emergency rooms was tested by comparison of the visits by Center-area children to the emergency departments before and after establishment of the Health Center. These changes were compared with emergency-department visits by other child populations residing outside the Center's catchment area.

Material and Methods

The Rochester Neighborhood Health Center was established in a geographically well defined poverty area that includes 22,000 residents, of whom about 12,000 are on Medicaid and therefore eligible for ongoing care at the Center. The Center replaced a smaller Settlement-House-sponsored clinic that had operated on a daily basis in the same building. In February, 1969, 7000 patients (about 2000 families) were registered with the Health Center. By February, 1970, the number of registered patients had increased to 9000. Pediatric coverage is pro-

Reprinted from *New England Journal of Medicine* 285, 3 (July 15, 1971): 148–152.

We are indebted to Klaus Roghmann, Ph.D., for advice on the design and statistics of the study, to Jane Annechiarico for computer programming and to the administration and record-room personnel of the four hospitals involved for co-operation.

vided by appointment at the Center from 8:30 A.M. to 9:30 P.M. daily and
from 8:30 A.M. to 12:30 P.M. on Saturdays. At all other times registered
patients may use a telephone exchange service to reach one of the Health Center
pediatricians available to advise or see patients. Eight census tracts comprise the
Center's catchment area. These tracts are assigned to five teams of doctors,
nurses and health assistants.

The study included four of the six Rochester hospitals, the remaining two
hospitals providing emergency care to only a few children. Strong Memorial,
Genesee and Rochester General hospitals have pediatric emergency departments
and both inpatient and outpatient pediatric services; St. Mary's Hospital cares for
a large pediatric emergency-department population, but has no pediatric inpatient service.

Three periods of identical length were considered: February 24 to March
30, 1967 (15 months before the Health Center was established), February 24
to March 30, 1969 (nine months after the Center was in operation), and
February 24 to March 30, 1970 (nearly two years after the Center opened).
Because appropriate records were not kept at St. Mary's Hospital in 1967, that
time sample was omitted. Records were not available for February and March,
1967, from Genesee Hospital, and that hospital's sample for that year was taken
from November 1 to December 5 (this period was chosen because the number of

Table 24-1

Sample Sizes and Total Numbers of Pediatric Emergency-Department
Visits during the Periods Studied

Sample	No. of Visits in Sample	Total No. of Pediatric Visits to Emergency Department
Strong Memorial*:		
1967	320	1,600
1969	279	1,395
1970	283	1,413
Genesee†:		
1967	273	819
1969	357	1,071
1970	314	943
Rochester General†:		
1967	320	968
1969	334	1,012
1970	359	1,077
St. Mary's:		
1969	277	835
1970	259	782

*20% sampling fraction.
†33% sampling fraction.

pediatric visits and the weather were similar, and there were no known epidemics during either period).

The sample design included visits by every third child (under 15 years of age) during the five-week period under study at Genesee, Rochester General and St. Mary's emergency departments and visits by every fifth child to Strong Memorial emergency department. The sample sizes ranged from 273 to 359 visits (table 24-1). For the final analysis, the Strong Memorial Hospital figures were multiplied by weight factor of 1.66 to attain an overall sampling fraction of 33 percent (33/20 = 1.66).

The variables studied were census tract, age, sex, race, time of day, day of week, payment status and patient's complaint (table 24-2 presents grouping of complaints). "Complaint" was chosen rather than the physician's diagnosis in an attempt to determine the patient's reason for seeking medical care. The reliability of the complaint grouping was checked by recording of a 10 percent sample by another physician; disagreement was observed in less than 1 percent of the cases. Another variable, "registration status at the Health Center," could be included only for the 1969 and 1970 periods. The number of visits to the emergency departments for each of the three years was used as the dependent variable.

Results

Visits

There was a 38.3 percent reduction in pediatric emergency-department visits from Center-area children to three hospitals from 1967 to 1970 (table 24-3). A 27.9 percent reduction was noted from 1967 to 1969, and an additional 14.5

Table 24-2
Yearly Percentages of Sampled Pediatric Emergency-Department Visits from Center Area, According to Complaint

Complaint	1967	1969	1970
Infection	63.0	47.0	43.8
Injury	22.7	33.6	27.8
Foreign body	2.3	4.2	2.1
Ingestion	2.7	0.0	0.8
Malaise without other symptom	0.8	0.0	0.0
Allergies	2.7	4.5	6.6
Emotional	0.0	0.0	1.6
Unclassified*	5.8	10.7	17.2

*Includes no disease found, nonspecific rashes, abdominal pain, undetermined etiology, etc.

Table 24-3

Percentage Changes in Pediatric Emergency-Department Visits from Different Areas

Sample	Percentage Change				
	Center area	3d ward	Rest of city	Surburban areas	Totals
Hosp 1, 2 & 3					
1967-69	-27.9	- 5.9	+11.2	+13.1	+2.7
1969-70	-14.5	-15.1	- 9.3	+14.2	-3.5
Hosp 1, 2, 3, 4*					
1969-70	-19.2	-15.0	-10.1	+14.9	-4.0
Total for					
Hosp 1, 2, & 3					
1967-70	-38.3	-20.1	- 0.8	+29.1	-0.9

*Includes St. Mary's Hospital.

percent drop occurred between 1969 and 1970. Between 1967 and 1970 the number of visits by city children outside the catchment area remained stable; visits by the suburban children increased 29 percent, and the Third Ward, somewhat similar in size and socioeconomic status to the Center's area, showed a 20 percent drop in pediatric emergency-department visits.

Clearly, this change in Emergency Room use, with a large drop by Center-area patients and a rise in suburban use is not a change occurrence. The overall chi-square value for the four patient areas over the three-year period is 38.3, df= 6, p less than 0.01. More precisely, the drop in patient use from the Center area is significant both for 1967-1969 and 1969-1970 (p less than 0.0005 for both). the increase in suburban use is similarly significant for both years (p less than 0.01). The change in visit rates from the two other areas of the city were not statistically significant.

Two hospitals, Strong Memorial and Genesee, received over 85 percent of the Center-area emergency-department visits. Both hospitals showed a marked reduction in visits by the children from the Center area between 1967 and 1970. These changes, in addition to the percentage changes in emergency-room visits at three hospitals for the same period samples, are shown in table 24-4. St. Mary's emergency department did not see enough Center-area patients to note a significant change.

Center Area Visits

Table 24-5 reveals that the reduction in visits was fairly equally distributed among the eight census tracts from 1967 to 1970. There were two noticeable exceptions

Table 24-4

Percentage Changes* in Pediatric Emergency-Department Visits from Center Area to Individual Hospitals and Percentage Changes in Total Pediatric Emergency-Department Visits

Hospital	1967-69	1969-70	1967-70
Strong Memorial	-49.0 (-13†)	+10.7 (+ 1)	-44.5 (-15)
Genesee	+ 6.1 (+25)	-30.0 (-12)	-25.7 (+13)
Rochester General	-20.0 (+ 4)	-26.3 (+ 5)	-44.0 (+10)
Totals	-27.9	-14.5	-38.3 (+ 1)

*Figures in parentheses indicate change in total pediatric emergency room visits.
†Reduction in Center-area visits accounts for 78% of this drop.

with one census tract (8) having close to an 80 percent reduction in visits whereas another (44) showed essentially no change.

Day of Visit

There was a uniform daily number of emergency department visits, including Saturday and Sunday, regardless of the area of sample involved. Center-area children did not visit emergency rooms more frequently on Saturdays and Sundays when the Health Center was closed.

Health Center Registration Status

This variable is pertinent only for 1969 and 1970, after the Center began operation. Results showed that one fifth of the visits to the emergency departments from the Center area were made by children registered with the Center. Half the Center-area child visits were made by children who were unregistered at the time of their emergency-room visit but were eligible for care at the Health Center.

The remainder of the variables studied revealed no meaningful patterns of use.

Discussion

This study strongly suggests that the Neighborhood Health Center is responsible for the 38 percent decrease in emergency-department visits by Center-area children between 1967 and 1970. During the same period pediatric emergency visits from all other areas increased 7 percent. The effect of the Center in

Table 24-5
Number of Pediatric Emergency-Department Visits from Health Center
Census Tracts during Periods Studied

| Census Tract | Visits | | | Popula-tion (1964) | Change in Emergency Department Visits (%) 1967-70 |
	1967	1969	1970		
8	140	65	39	3,100	-79.0
11	13	22	6	670	-38.4
12	22	22	12	1,250	-45.5
13	116	61	75	4,300	-35.3
14	115	60	75	3,595	-34.8
15	70	82	57	3,590	-18.6
43	33	32	24	1,930	-27.2
44	94	93	93	3,680	- 1.1
Totals	603	437	375	22.115	-38.3*

*1967-69 change = -27.5%, 1969-70 change = -14.0%.

decreasing emergency-room visits is even more apparent when one considers that a clinic was in operation in the same setting before the Health Center's opening. However, this clinic did not provide comprehensive services and lacked an outreach program.

Two alternate hypotheses might also explain the data. The first is that there were fewer children residing in the Health Center area in 1970 than in 1967, and the second that there is less illness in that area now (or some combination of these). The latter hypothesis does not ring true from a common-sense point of view, and would mean an isolated drop in illness in this area while other areas of the community were unchanged. Furthermore, the Health Center sees 50 to 100 children daily for management of illness. Without accurate census figures it is difficult to be sure about the first hypothesis. Urban renewal has been progressing in both Third Ward and Health Center areas, but our distinct impression is that at present this has resulted in movement within these ghetto areas rather than outside. Preliminary 1970 census data indicate a reduction of approximately 3 percent in the child population in the Health Center Area from 1967 to 1970. Essentially no low-cost housing has been built in suburban areas during this time.

Six of the census tracts showed an overall reduction in visits from 1967 to 1970 between 23 percent and 45 percent. The large reduction in visits from census tract 8 may be related to the fact that this area lacks good public transportation to hospital facilities (and thus the Health Center is accessible), and that its large Spanish-speaking population had a strong advocate in a Spanish-speaking health assistant at the center. This woman was a member of the team serving this area and received night calls at her home to help patients obtain care. There are several possible explanations for the stable visit rate for census tract 44. This tract is situated farthest from the Health Center, and public transportation to Genesee and Strong Memorial hospitals is easily available whereas there is no public transportation to the Health Center. Census tract 44 is also the second most populous of the Center's tracts, and effective outreach to this area has only recently been established.

In 1970, 40 percent of all pediatric visits from the Center area to the emergency departments were made by patients not registered but eligible for care at the Health Center. Since these visits were made by a relatively small group of children (one fourth of the total number of eligible patients), regular Health Center care for them would probably reduce the number of emergency visits even further.

The greatest decline in visits to Strong Memorial Hospital was expected. The Center's physicians are all on the staff of this hospital, and most inpatient admissions and newborn deliveries of Center-area patients occurred there. In addition, residents of the census tracts showing large reduction in the number of pediatric emergency visits had primarily been users of Strong Memorial Hospital before establishment of the Health Center.

Genesee Hospital opened an enlarged and more attractive emergency department in March, 1968. This probably accounts for the 25 percent increase in pediatric visits to that emergency department, 6 percent of these being by Center-area children, between 1967 and 1969. In the following year the new facilities no longer attracted so many patients, and the overall number of pediatric emergency visits to Genesee declined. Center-area patients formerly using Genesee Emergency Department who began visiting the Health Center more frequently accounted for at least half the reduction in visits noted at Genesee.

Because the Health Center is closed after 9:30 P.M. on weekdays and after 12:30 P.M. on Saturdays, increased emergency-department visits at night and on weekends by children who regularly used the Center might be expected. The fact that there was no such increase is indirect evidence that the answering service method of reaching Center physicians on call is effective or that the security of knowing assistance is available precluded a visit to an emergency department.

Since the Health Center provides only limited injury treatment, a lesser reduction in the number of emergency-department visits for injury would be expected. Indeed, whereas the number of pediatric emergency visits for infection from the Center area declined 56 percent from 1967 to 1970, injury visits dropped only 34 percent. In addition, Center-registered children paid fewer emergency visits for infection than nonregistered Center-area children. That the other poverty area (Third Ward) did not show a corresponding shift supports the hypothesis that the Health Center is responsible for the decline in the number of visits for infections.

On the basis of total population figures,[a] and despite the noted reduction in the number of visits, when compared with the rest of the city and the suburban populations, children from both the Center area and the Third Ward "overuse" hospital emergency-department facilities. If the rest of the city were used as a base line, suburban children would be declared "underusers." However, this study identifies a strong trend developing in the opposite direction, with a 29.1 percent increase in emergency-room use by the suburban population. In part this reflects a growing suburban population, but in part suggests a change in the availability of private care in the suburbs.

Implications

Evaluation of Neighborhood Health Centers has been slow in coming. The important role of Health Centers in providing medical care for indigents makes the data presented here important in national assessment of the effectiveness of these centers. Two effects of the Rochester Neighborhood Health Center have been to reduce barriers to comprehensive medical care and to reverse the general trend of rising emergency-department use. The Health Center's proximity to the population that it serves seems to be an important but not an over-riding inducement to use. Simply providing quality care is not enough; it must be associated with aggressive outreach into the community and continuing consideration of cultural factors. The effectiveness of the Center's program is in large measure directly related to the health teams' effectiveness in communicating with the patients.

We still need to determine why children eligible for Center care continue to use emergency departments. This may be a function of the time required to change entrenched patterns of health care or there may be a substantial number of patients who will always prefer other sources of care such as emergency departments. This study suggests that although successful, Neighborhood Health Centers may not be able to provide all the health care that is deserved or required by residents of poverty areas.

[a]United States Commerce Department, Census Bureau: Special Census of Monroe County, New York, April 1, 1964.

25 Relating a Neighborhood Health Center to a General Hospital: A Case History

Anthony R. Kovner, Gerald Katz, Stanley B. Kahane, and Cecil G. Sheps

Organized personal health services for ambulatory patients are now being provided in a variety of settings, including hospital outpatient departments, private group practice facilities, and community or neighborhood health centers. The notion that comprehensive personal health services should be accessible, available, dignified, and provided by a team of health personnel on a continuous basis is slowly becoming generally accepted.[1]

Recently, mounting interest in organized neighborhood personal health services has developed. These services may be made available in a free-standing, completely independent neighborhood health center or in one which has a formal structured relationship with a general hospital. If newly organized, the independent health center is not constrained by historical factors in being responsive to community needs. In any event, decision-making in the independent center does not have to be governed by in-hospital considerations, and innovations in organization can be accomplished without taking into consideration possible effects on the general hospital's policies. Fewer hierarchical levels and specialized departments can result in decisions being made and implemented more quickly. Whereas the general hospital's goals of patient care, education and research will sometimes conflict with each other, the independent neighborhood health center's mandate to provide patient care for a designated population is clear and relatively unambiguous. Moreover, responsibility for inpatient care and specialized ambulatory services does not have to be assumed directly by the neighborhood health center, whose staff is therefore freed to devote all its energies to the provision of primary services to ambulatory patients.

This paper will examine the question of whether a formally structured relationship with a general hospital is necessary for the neighborhood health center to achieve its goals and continue to function as a viable organization. The ex-

Reprinted from *Medical Care* 7, 2 (March-April 1969): 118–123.

The original publication of this article stimulated a critical comment and responses to that comment: Samuel Standard, M.D., "Comment on the Neighborhood Health Center and the General Hospital," *Medical Care, 8,* 3 (May-June 1970): 252–253; "Comments on Surgical Services in The Beth Israel Medical Center - Gouverneur Affiliation," *Medical Care, 8,* 6 (Nov.-Dec. 1970): 523–525.

periences of the Gouverneur Health Services Program and the Beth Israel Hospital of New York City and their effects upon each other will be used to illustrate the relevant issues and considerations.

A Short History of Gouverneur-Beth Israel Affiliation

Today, the Beth Israel Medical Center is comprised of the Gouverneur Health Services Program, the Bernstein Institute for psychiatry and addictive diseases, and Beth Israel Hospital. Beth Israel Hospital, located ten minutes north of Gouverneur (about two miles) is a large (550 beds) voluntary general hospital with a full range of services, a teaching and research program, and active outpatient and emergency services departments. The General Director of the Medical Center is responsible for the overall direction of all three units, each of which has its own administrator. For the purpose of this paper, the history of the Gouverneur-Beth Israel relationship can be divided into three stages of development.

Stage I: 1961–1965

By 1961, the 70-year-old municipal Gouverneur Hospital, located in lower Manhattan, had lost both its hospital and its teaching accreditations. The Hospital Review and Planning Council of Southern New York and the Department of Hospitals of the City of New York recommended that the hospital be closed and that community residents use facilities farther away.

The community served by Gouverneur is unique in the strength and number of its well-organized, voluntary, social agencies with a long history of responding to the health and welfare needs of the Lower East Side. Community leaders influenced the municipal government and the planning agency. As a result, the City of New York contracted with Beth Israel Hospital to provide personal health and emergency services to ambulatory patients in the old facility. In contrast to other city voluntary hospital affiliations, the entire staff at Gouverneur, with the exception of the engineering crew, is subject to Medical Center-wide policies and is not employed by the city. At the time of affiliation, all civil service staff at the old Gouverneur Hospital was transferred to other city hospitals.

With funding provided by the City of New York, the Gouverneur Ambulatory Care Unit functioned as a "neighborhood health center" for some years before this concept was further developed and adopted nationally by the Office of Economic Opportunity.[a] Primary adult and pediatric medical care was emphasized. The services were organized so that patients were encouraged to maintain a continuing relationship with a personal physician rather than to receive fragmented services in numerous subspecialty clinics. An individual appointment system was instituted. The building was attractively painted and refurnished. Local community people were employed wherever possible, and a dialogue was established between staff and community leaders and organizations.[2]

During this period, program responsibility was largely delegated to the Gouverneur administration. The Director of the Gouverneur Ambulatory Care Unit was recognized as responsible for the entire pattern of service, and had to work out diverse arrangements with the directors of clinical departments at the hospital. Under the provisions of the contract with the City of New York, all Gouverneur physicians had to be specialists who were board-eligible, and they were appointed by and to the medical staff of the hospital. At first, no special attention was given to the admission of patients from the Gouverneur program to the general hospital. For example, patients referred to Beth Israel were, in some of the services, generally not admitted unless they were "interesting" teaching cases. When a patient was admitted, diagnostic work-up, which had been completed at the neighborhood health center was not uncommonly duplicated at the general hospital. The nature of the affiliation did permit Gouverneur to develop an innovative, flexible, responsive program. Members of the Gouverneur professional staff identified themselves as part of an organization committed to dignified personal service and responsibility to community needs, not governed by the traditional considerations of medical education and research.

Stage 2: 1965–1967

The Office of Economic Opportunity provided additional funding in early 1965 which permitted the amplification of dental, psychiatric and obstetrical services, and the extension of services into the evening hours. "Outreach" was organized by adding staff for community organization and health education. Affiliation with the Judson Health Center enabled services to be amplified in the western part of the Gouverneur district. The Judson Health Center had been a free-standing, ambulatory facility under voluntary auspices, and had provided preventive services only. Through affiliation, treatment services were added to the Judson program. In recognition of an expanded scope of services, the Gouver-

---

[a]The philosophy underlying the Office of Economic Opportunity's "neighborhood health center" concept drew heavily on the Gouverneur experience. Dr. Cecil G. Sheps, General Director, Beth Israel Medical Center, Dr. Howard Brown, Medical Director, and Mr. Harold Light, Associate Director, Gouverneur Health Services Program, served with others as consultants to the Office of Economic Opportunity.

neur Ambulatory Care Unit became at this time the Gouverneur Health Services Program. With the addition of the Bernstein Institute and Gouverneur, Beth Israel Hospital became Beth Israel Medical Center.

The response to the program which was organized at Gouverneur can be illustrated by the great growth in volume of services provided. The number of clinic visits more than trebled in the first four years, reaching 232,314 clinic visits made by 38,622 individuals in 1967.[b] Of there, 17,512 visits were made by 5,514 patients to the satellite Judson Health Center. The program budget for 1967 was approximately $3.5 million dollars. There was an employed medical and dental staff of 115, of whom 15 were fulltime and 23, halftime. This total staff was equivalent to 43 fulltime physicians or dentists. On-site medical services provided included internal medicine, pediatrics, psychiatry, obstetrics, gynecology, family planning, surgery, ophthalmology, orthopedics, dermatology, allergy, otolaryngology, urology, neurology, dentistry, podiatry and optometry.

During this period, also, the Medical Center became affiliated with the newly-established Mount Sinai School of Medicine of the City University of New York.

Stage 3: 1967–

Intensive integration of Gouverneur's program with that of the other Medical Center units is now taking place. The extent and pace of integration has been greater in certain departments because of specific interest and sufficient organizational resources. Integration is by no means complete, and the process has made manifest diverse interests and patterns of responsibility. In the following sections, the nature and consequences of integration are examined.

The Impact of the General Hospital on the Neighborhood Health Center

Gouverneur provides "front-line" or primary services, which include ongoing general family care and high-volume specialty services such as dental, obstetrical-gynecological and psychiatric. Highly specialized ambulatory services and in-patient care are provided at Beth Israel Hospital and at Bernstein Institute. Gouverneur's experience indicates that a formally structured relationship with a general hospital is necessary for neighborhood health center patients to receive high priority when referred for care. Without this relationship, communication will generally be indirect, uneven or limited, and the benefits of the relationships

---

[b]Because of the nature of development, longer history and mixed funding, Gouverneur is considerably larger than other OEO health centers, serving four times the suggested OEO target population of 30,000 persons.

which have developed between staff and patients are not used to facilitate mutual understanding of patient and staff at the hospital. Communication problems in the hospital may even have an adverse effect upon the relationships with patients developed at the neighborhood health center. A reliable referral and information system between Gouverneur and Beth Israel is now being developed to facilitate continuous patient care. Beth Israel Hospital makes arrangements with other institutions for the few specialized services it does not provide at present. Recently, for example, Beth Israel Hospital assumed direct responsibility for provision of rehabilitative medical services to all Gouverneur patients. Since this does not presently include the construction and fitting of prostheses, arrangements for these services were made with the Institute of Rehabilitation Medicine of New York City.

The personal physician and his team of allied health professionals and auxiliaries at Gouverneur provide continuity and coordinate all aspects of medical care for the patient.[c] In order to assure continuous and coordinated care, surgical procedures for Gouverneur patients are now performed and follow-up is provided under the personal supervision of Gouverneur surgeons. A block of operating room time has been set aside at Beth Israel Hospital for sugery on Gouverneur patients. The necessity for a structured interagency relationship applies as well to social service, nursing and other services. When a Gouverneur patient undergoing surgery at Beth Israel Hospital is worried about his child's performance at school, the problem is referred and followed up by social service staff and the personal physician at Gouverneur.

The neighborhood health center cannot easily attract and retain high-quality staff without providing opportunities for adequate professional career development. The neighborhood health center program by itself is not large enough to create an organizationally-separate educational component which would be viable. At Gouverneur, all physicians have staff privileges at Beth Israel Hospital and participate to varying extents in rounds, conferences, committee work and other departmental assignments. Members of the medical staff are being appointed currently to the faculty of the Mount Sinai School of Medicine on the same basis as other Medical Center physicians.

A patterned relationship with a general hospital gives the neighborhood health center access as well to the skilled services of hospital administrative and technical staff. A consultative relationship between staff experts from a central office and the line officers of operating administrative units is routine in organizations of large scale. The Beth Israel controller has been of great assistance to Gouverneur in recruitment of accounting staff, setting up of procedures, budget

[c]Sheps and Madison have specified three aspects of continuity of care: (a) among sources providing health care: (b) within and between clinical episodes of medical care, and (c) long-term (Evaluation of Neighborhood Health Center, Prepared for the Office of Economic Opportunity, pp. 36–50, 1967).

preparation, and in financial relationships with funding agencies. Similarly, Beth Israel's personnel director has provided Gouverneur with expert counsel concerning union negotiations, wage and salary administration, setting up of procedures, and personnel policy formulation.

Impact of the Neighborhood Health Center on the Hospital

Less easily discernible, perhaps, are the consequences of affiliation for the general hospital. General hospitals have had a traditional concern for the hospitalized patient which has not been paralleled for the same patient before he enters or after he leaves the hospital. The development of a relationship with a neighborhood health center is likely to alter this pattern of responsibility. Gouverneur organized a home-care program and arranged to provide medical services in a proprietary nursing home, a pattern of program responsibility which Beth Israel subsequently assumed as well. Like many large general hospitals, Beth Israel did not welcome patients for delivery on its ward service who had not received prenatal care at the hospital. The relationship with Gouverneur helped produce the understanding that these women are now considered to be high-risk, high-priority patients, who are delivered without question at Beth Israel, and followed up either at the hospital or at Gouverneur.

A review of the philosophy underlying graduate medical education has also resulted from the combined program. Hospital training programs no longer focus solely on the clinical "interest" of a patient's disease, but are concerned with the health and dignity of the patient independent of his financial status. If a bed is available, a Gouverneur patient is now admitted to Beth Israel Hospital directly upon the recommendation of the Gouverneur physician. He does not have to "clear" with the admitting resident, as before, regarding the desirability of the case for teaching and/or research purposes.

Affiliation with a neighborhood health center results in an increased demand on the hospital's communication and reporting system. It soon becomes apparent that comparable medical records with uniform input mechanisms must be developed for accurate, immediate and relevant feedback information on all referrals. Under the direction of a specially qualified medical records administrator, the Beth Israel Medical Center is now instituting a unit record system for all patients in all units. This will result in a single record available at the point of service. To facilitate the flow of patients, staff, services and information, jitney service between Gouverneur and Beth Israel, has been established, and a Medical Center-wide transportation service is to go into operation soon.

The general hospital may have to adjust its delivery of services to meet the expectations of neighborhood health center patients. Clearly the demonstration of patient and professional satisfaction with the Gouverneur pattern of service organization has influenced the development of plans and implementation of a comprehensive approach to dignified personal health care at Beth Israel Hospital. Beth Israel Hospital is now extending its ambulatory services program into the evening, is providing the ambulatory patient with the opportunity to enjoy the services of a personal physician, and has established an appointment system for the patient's convenience.

Conclusion

Based upon the six-year Gouverneur-Beth Israel experience, it is clear that the neighborhood health center and the general hospital can both benefit importantly through affiliation. Since patterns of responsibility differ, each should have major responsibility for its own program. Decision-making which concerns the integrated system must not be governed solely by considerations of inpatient care and disease-oriented research on the one hand, or by the political struggles of community interest groups on the other. A general hospital's program usually is made up of services provided by individual departments. The neighborhood health center starts with a commitment to provide services to a given population in terms of an integrated program. Therefore, while there must of course, be clinical departments at the neighborhood health center, the directors of the same clinical departments at the hospital must work with the director of the neighborhood health center in terms of developing an integrated neighborhood health center program as such. The Gouverneur-Beth Israel experience indicates that negotiation on mutual problems can lead to satisfactory solutions, and that this essential process takes considerable and continuous effort.

A formal structured relationship with a general hospital can result in increased patient access to a broad range of services, and improved continuity of care at the neighborhood health center level. High-quality care can be facilitated by the establishment of consistently reliable referral and feedback systems to and from a general hospital. Physicians and other staff can enjoy added opportunities for professional growth and career development within a larger health services system, and scarce health manpower and equipment can be used more efficiently. Through close affiliation, the neighborhood health center and the general hospital can have significant impact upon each other and the goals of each can be satisfied. Without such affiliation, the neighborhood health center's achievements will stand isolated from the general medical care system, and patients and staff will be denied access on a regular, reliable and continuous basis to important services and activities which can be provided only by general hospitals of large scale.

References

1. James, G.: Medical advances in the next 10 years. The implications for the organization and economics of medicine. The expanding role of ambulatory services in hospitals and health departments, *Bull. N.Y. Acad. Med. 41*: 23, 1965.
2. Light, H.L., and Brown, H.J.: The Gouverneur health services program, an historical view. *Milbank Mem. Fund Quart. 45*: 375, 1967.

Bibliography

The list of materials below supplements the chapters included in the reader. It is a selective bibliography which includes only items which are readily available in libraries. It is organized into sections according to the subject matter covered.

Evolution of Neighborhood Health Centers of the 1960s

General

Bamberger, Lisbeth. "Health Care and Poverty: What are the Dimensions of the Problem From the Community's Point of View?" *Bulletin of the New York Academy of Medicine* 42 (December 1966): 1140-1149.

Berry, Theodore M. "Recent Federal Legislation: Its Meaning for Public Health." *American Journal of Public Health and the Nation's Health* 56 (April 1966): 582-589.

Brooks, Wendy Goepel. "Health Care and Poor People." In Cahn, Edgar S., and Passett, Barry A. *Citizen Participation.* New York: New Jersey Community Action Training Institute, 1969, pp. 197-215.

Brown, Howard J. "Delivery of Personal Health Services and Medical Services for the Poor — Concessions or Prerogatives?" *Milbank Memorial Fund Quarterly* 66 (January 1968): 203-223.

Bryant, Thomas E. "Goals and Potential of the Neighborhood Health Center." *Medical Care* 8 (1970): 93-94.

English, Joseph T. "Is the OEO Concept — The Neighborhood Health Center — the Answer?" In Norman, John C. (ed.), *Medicine in the Ghetto.* New York: Appleton-Century-Crofts, 1969, pp. 261-266.

_____. "Office of Economic Opportunity Health Programs." *Inquiry* 5 (March 1968): 43-48.

English, Joseph T., and Scherl, Donald J. "Community Mental Health and Comprehensive Health Services Programs for the Poor." *American Journal of Psychiatry* 125 (June 1969): 12.

Ferguson, Allen, Jr. "National Health Proposals, The Neighborhood Health Center, and the Poor." Neighborhood Health Center Seminar Program Monograph Series No. 2, University Extension, Univ. of California, Berkeley, October 1971.

_____. "The Role of Neighborhood Health Centers in Economic Development." Neighborhood Health Center Seminar Program Monograph Series No. 4, University Extension, Univ. of California, Berkeley, January 1972.

Gibson, Count D. "The Neighborhood Health Center: The Primary Unit of Health Care." *American Journal of Public Health* 58 (1968): 1188-1191.

_____. "Will the Urban University Medical Center Join the Community?" *Journal of Medical Education* 45 (March 1970): 144-148.

Goldberg, George A.; Trowbridge, Frederick L.; and Buxbaum, Robert C. "Issues in the Development of Neighborhood Health Centers." *Inquiry* 6 (March 1969): 37-47.

Grant, J. "Health Centers in Urban and Rural Areas." In Seipp, C. *Health Care for the Community: Selected Papers of John B. Grant.* Baltimore: The Johns Hopkins Press, 1963, pp. 21-24.

Harper, Dean. "Providing Health Care to the Poor: Neighborhood Health Center." *New York State Journal of Medicine* 69 (July 15, 1969): 2048-2054.

Herman, Mary W. "The Poor: Their Medical Needs and the Health Services Available to Them." *Annals of the American Academy of Social and Political Science* 399 (January 1972): 12-21.

_____. "Health Services for the Poor and Neighborhood Health Centers." *Hospital Administration* 17 (Spring 1972): 50-64.

Hiatt, Howard H. "Medical Care for Northbridge: A Model for Teaching Hospital-Community Interaction." *New England Journal of Medicine* 284 (March 18, 1971): 593-602.

Humphrey, H. H. "Statement on Neighborhood Health Centers." Excerpts from "The Future of Health Services for the Poor," *Public Health Reports* 83 (1968): 1-10.

Kasanof, David. "The Medical Crisis in Our Cities: Antipoverty Medicine — Atlanta to Watts." *Medical Economics* 45 (July 8, 1968): 122-143.

Langston, J. H. *et al. Study to Evaluate the OEO Neighborhood Health Center Program at Selected Centers,* Vols. 1-3, Geomet, Inc., Rockville, Md. 1971.

Lashof, Joyce C. "Medical Care in the Urban Center." *Annals of Internal Medicine* 68 (January 1968): 242-245.

Madison, Donald L. "Organized Health Care and the Poor." *Medical Care* 26 (August 1969): 783-807.

_____. "The Structure of American Health Care Services." *Public Administration Review* 31 (September/October 1971): 518-527.

New, Peter Kong-ming, and Hessler, Richard M. "Neighborhood Health Centers: Traditional Medical Care at an Outpost." *Inquiry* 9 (December 1972): 45-58.

Paxton, Harry T. "Does Antipoverty Medicine Threaten Private Practice?" *Medical Economics* 47 (October 12, 1970): 142-160.

Randal, Judith. "The Bright Promise of Neighborhood Health Centers." *The Reporter,* March 1968, pp. 15-18.

Renthal, A. Gerald. "Comprehensive Health Centers in Large U.S. Cities." *American Journal of Public Health* 61 (February 1971): 324-336.

Safford, Frank K. "Health Centers for Preventive Medicine, Recreation, and Education." *Design Trends,* February 1968, pp. 66-71.

Schaefer, M. "Commentary on the Social Scientist's Views of the Neighborhood Health Center as a New Social Institution." *Medical Care* 8 (1970): 116-117.

Schwartz, Jerome L. "Early Histories of Selected Neighborhood Health Centers." *Inquiry* 7 (December 1970): 3-16.

Silver, George A. "What Has Been Learned From the Neighborhood Health Centers?" (Excerpts from "What has Been Learned About the Delivery of Health

Care Services to the Ghetto?"), in Norman, J. C. (ed.), *Medicine in the Ghetto.* New York: Appleton-Century-Crofts, 1969, pp. 65-72.

Simpson, George A. "What Is a Neighborhood Health Center?" *Urban Health* 1 (October 1972): 8-10+.

Sloane, Harvey. "Can We Cut the Red Tape? Or Must We Strangle?" *American Journal of Public Health* 61 (May 1971): 887-890.

Sparer, Gerald, and Johnson, Joyce. "Evaluation of OEO Neighborhood Health Centers." *American Journal of Public Health* 61 (May 1971): 931-942.

Stoeckle, John D. "The Future of Health Care." In Kosa, John; Antonovsky, Aaron; and Zola, Irving Kenneth (eds.), *Poverty and Health: A Sociological Analysis.* Cambridge, Massachusetts: Harvard University Press, 1969, pp. 292-318.

Walter, Charles. "Anti-Poverty Medicine: Another Big Sleeper." *Medical Economics* 43 (November 14, 1966): 74-82.

Weinerman, E. Richard. "The Response of the University Medical Center to Social Demands." *Journal of Medical Education* 45 (Part 2), (November 1970): 69-78.

Wood, Courtney B. "The Neighborhood Health Center — The Concept and the National Scene." *Journal of the National Medical Association* 63 (January 1971): 52-57.

Development and Experience of Individual Projects

"Alviso Clinic Exemplifies Grass Roots Community Organization." *California's Health* 25 (December 1967): 7-8.

Ames, Wendell R. "Redirection of Health Department Services in Rochester, New York." *American Journal of Public Health and the Nation's Health* 56 (April 1966): 599-602.

Bakst, H. J. "The Roxbury Comprehensive Community Health Center." *Public Welfare,* July 1969, pp. 227-231.

Beloff, Jerome S.; Snoke, Parnie S.; and Weinerman, E. Richard. "Yale Studies in Family Health Care: II. Organization of a Comprehensive Family Health Care Program." *Journal of the American Medical Association* 204 (April 29, 1968): 355-360.

Beloff, Jerome S., and Wienerman, E. Richard. "Yale Studies in Family Health Care: I. Planning and Pilot Test of a New Program." *Journal of the American Medical Association* 199 (February 6, 1967): 133-139.

Brown, Roy E. "Delivery of Pediatric Health Services in a Rural Health Center." *Pediatrics* 44 (September 1969): 333-337.

Butter, Irene; Moore, Gordon T.; Robertson, Robert L.; and Hall, Elizabeth. "Effects of Manpower Utilization on Cost and Productivity of a Neighborhood Health Center." *Milbank Memorial Fund Quarterly* 50 (October 1972): 421-452.

Chabot, Andre. "Improved Infant Mortality Rates in a Population Served by a Comprehensive Neighborhood Health Program." *Pediatrics* 47 (June 1971): 989-994.

Coleman, Arthur H. "The Hunters Point-Bayview Community Health Service." *California Medicine* 110 (March 1969): 253-255.

Collins, B. "Denver Builds Citywide Health Network." *Modern Hospital* 110 (May 1968): 102-106.

Cowen, David L. "Denver's Neighborhood Health Program." *Public Health Reports* 84 (December 1969): 1027-1031.

Creditor, Morton C. "The Neighborhood Health Center. Where Does the Hospital Fit?" *American Journal of Public Health* 61 (April 1971): 807-813.

de Diaz, Sharon Daniel. "Beyond Rhetoric — The NENA Health Center After One Year." *American Journal of Public Health* 62 (January 1972): 64-68.

Delaney, Paul. "Problems Plague Rural Care Units." *New York Times* 119:54c, 1 December 1969. Reprinted in *Medical Care Review* 27 (January 1970): 21-23.

Ferguson, Lloyd A. "The Medical Needs of the Ghetto and Inner City in Chicago." *Proceedings of the Institute of Medicine of Chicago* 28 (January 1970): 10-17.

Flynn, Ken. "Pressures for Change. A Response: Neighborhood Health Care Clinics." *Hospitals* 45 (February 1, 1971): 81-84.

Geiger, H. Jack. "The Endlessly Revolving Door." *American Journal of Nursing* 69 (1969): 2436-2445.

_____. "Health Center in Mississippi." *Hospital Practice* 4 (1969): 68-81.

_____. "The Neighborhood Health Center — Education of the Faculty in Preventive Medicine." *Archives of Environmental Health* 14 (1967): 912-916.

_____. "Of the Poor, By the Poor, or for the Poor: The Mental Health Implications of Social Control of Poverty Programs." *Psychiatric Research Report* 21, American Psychiatric Association, April 1967, pp. 55-65.

Giorgi, E. A. "What We've Learned from the Watts Health Center." *Medical Times* 98 (December 1970): 139-157.

Hall, R. "A Stir of Hope in Mound Bayou." *Life,* March 28, 1969.

Ingraham, Norman R., and Lear, Walter J. "A Big City Strives for Relevance in Its Community Health Services." *American Journal of Public Health* 60 (May 1970): 804-810.

James, A. "Tufts-Delta Administers Environmental Treatment." *Journal of Environmental Health* 31 (1969): 437-446.

Jessiman, Andrew G., and Crampton, Kathleen R. "A Directory of Boston Neighborhood Health Centers." *New England Journal of Medicine* 286 (March 9, 1972): 524-526.

Kovner, Anthony R., and Seacat, Milvoy S. "Continuity of Care Maintained in Family Centered Outpatient Unit." *Hospitals* 43 (July 1, 1969): 89-94.

Langer, Elinor. "Medicine for the Poor: A New Deal in Denver." *Science* 153 (July 29, 1966): 508-511.

Lashof, Joyce C. "Chicago Project Provides Health Care and Career Opportunities." *Hospitals* 43 (July 1, 1969): 105-108.

Lepper, Mark H.; Lashof, Joyce C.; Pisani, Albert; and Shannon, Iris. "An Approach to Reconciling the Poor and the System." *Inquiry* 5 (March 1968): 37-42.

Light, H. L., and Brown, H. J. "The Gouverneur Health Services Program: An Historical View." *Milbank Memorial Fund Quarterly* 65 (1967): 375-390.

Lloyd, William B., and Wise, Harold B. "The Montefiore Experience." *Bulletin of the New York Academy of Medicine,* Second Series 44 (November 1968): 1353-1362.

Maloney, William F. "The Tufts Comprehensive Community Health Action Program." *Journal of the American Medical Association* 202 (October 30, 1967): 411-414.

McLaughlin, Mary C. "Present Status and Problems of New York City's Comprehensive Neighborhood Family Care Health Centers." *Bulletin of the New York Academy of Medicine* 44 (November 1968): 1390-1395.

Powell, R. N. "What Has Happened in the Watts-Willowbrook Program." In Norman, J. C. (ed.), *Medicine in the Ghetto.* New York: Appleton-Century-Crofts, 1969, pp. 73-85.

Sanders, Marion K. "The Doctors Meet the People." *Harper's Magazine*, January 1968, pp. 56-62.

Sloane, Harvey. "Neighborhood Health Center, Louisville." *Journal of the Kentucky Medical Association* 66 (August 1968): 712-713.

Snyder, James D., and Enright, Michael J. "Free Neighborhood Health Centers Promise Big Impact for Hospitals." *Hospital Management* 103 (March 1967): 38-44.

Wise, Harold B. "Montefiore Hospital Neighborhood Medical Care Demonstration." *Milbank Memorial Fund Quarterly* 66 Part I (July 1968): 297-307.

Young, M. M. "Chattanooga's Experience With Reorganization for Delivery of Health Services." *American Journal of Public Health* 60 (September 1970): 1739-1748.

Patients' Use and Response

Christie, Robert W. "Public Acceptance of the Neighborhood Health Center." *Journal of the American Medical Association* 215 (March 8, 1971): 1669.

Greenlick, Merwyn R.; Freeborn, Donald K.; Colombo, Theodore J.; Prussin, Jeffrey A.; and Saward, Ernest A. "Comparing the Use of Medical Care Services by a Medically Indigent and a General Membership Population in a Comprehensive Prepaid Group Practice Program." *Medical Care* 10 (May-June 1972): 187-200.

Harrison, Ira E. "Patients' Evaluation of Neighborhood Health Centers." *Journal of the National Medical Association* 64 (July 1972): 348-352.

Klein, Michael; Roghmann, Klaus; Woodward, Kenneth; and Charney, Evan. "The Impact of the Rochester Neighborhood Health Center on Hospitalization of Children, 1968 to 1970," *Pediatrics* 51 (May 1973) 833-839.

Moore, Gordon T.; Bernstein, Roberta; and Bonanno, Rosemary A. "Effect of a Neighborhood Health Center on Hospital Emergency Room Use." *Medical Care* 10 (May-June 1972): 240-247.

Moore, Gordon T., and Bonanno, Rosemary. "Follow-up Care After Hospitalization: Health Center vs. Hospital." *Journal of the American Medical Association* 222 (October 16, 1972): 299-301.

Richardson, W. C. "Measuring the Urban Poor's Use of Physicians' Services in Response to Illness Episodes." *Medical Care* 8 (1970): 132-142.

Robertson, Leon S.; Kosa, John; Alpert, Joel J.; and Heagarty, Margaret C. "Anticipated Acceptance of Neighborhood Health Clinics by the Urban Poor." *Journal of the American Medical Association* 205 (September 16, 1968): 815-818.

Salber, Eva J.; Feldman, Jacob J.; Johnson, Helen; and McKenna, Elizabeth. "Health Practices and Attitudes of Consumers at a Neighborhood Health Center." *Inquiry* 9 (March 1972): 55-61.

Salber, Eva J.; Feldman, Jacob J.; Offenbacher, Hanna; and Williams, Shirley. "Characteristics of Patients Registered for Service at a Neighborhood Health Center." *American Journal of Public Health* 60 (December 1970): 2273-2283.

Salber, Eva J.; Feldman, Jacob J.; Rosenberg, Lynn A.; and Williams, Shirley. "Utilization of Services at a Neighborhood Health Center." *Pediatrics* 47 (February 1971): 415-423.

Schumaker, C. J., Jr. "Attitudes Toward Change of Health Center Sponsorship." *Inquiry* 9 (March 1972): 62-65.

_____ . "Change of Health Center Sponsorship: I. Impact on Patterns of Obtaining Medical Care." *American Journal of Public Health* 61 (August 1971): 1536-1544.

_____ . "How Change in Sponsorship Affected Use of Neighborhood Health Center." *Hospital Topics* 48 (May 1970): 69-72+.

Sparer, Gerald, and Anderson, Arne. "Utilization and Cost Experience of Low-Income Families in Four Prepaid Group Practice Plans 1970-1971." *New England Journal of Medicine,* 282 (July 12, 1973) 67-72.

Quality of Care

Brooke, Ronald. "An Audit of the Quality of Care in Social Medicine." *Milbank Memorial Fund Quarterly* 6 (July 1968): 351-376.

Dreyfus, Edward G.; Minson, Ronald; Sbarbaro, John A.; and Cowen, David L. "Internal Chart Audits in a Neighborhood Health Program: A Problem-Oriented Approach." *Medical Care* 9 (September/October 1971): 449-454.

Morehead, Mildred A. "Evaluating Quality of Medical Care in the Neighborhood Health Center Program of the Office of Economic Opportunity." *Medical Care* 8 (1970): 118-131.

Sheppard, James, Jr.; Haedke, Edna K.; Cornely, Paul B.; and Steen, James D. "Research and Evaluation in an OEO Neighborhood Health Center: Community Group Health Foundation, Inc." In U.S., Department of Health,

Education and Welfare, National Center for Health Services Research and Development, *University Medical Care Programs: Evaluation.* Washington, D.C.: U. S. Government Printing Office, 1971, pp. 17-26.

Health Workers and Allied Health Teams

Andrus, Len Hughes. "The Private Physician — Overcoming the Health Manpower Shortage." *Bulletin of the American College of Physicians,* August 1969, pp. 381-384.

Bates, James E.; Lieberman, Harry H.; and Powell, Rodney N. "Provisions for Health Care in the Ghetto: The Family Health Team." *American Journal of Public Health* 60 (July 1970): 1222-1224.

Brunetto, Eleanor, and Bink, Peter. "The Primary Care Nurse — The Generalist in a Structured Health Care Team." *American Journal of Public Health* 62 (June 1972): 785-794.

Beloff, Jerome S. and Willet, Marion. "Yale Studies in Family Health Care: III. The Health Care Team." *Journal of the American Medical Association* 205 (September 2, 1968): 663-669.

Caton, Myrtle U. "Problems of Neighborhood Health Center Employees in Watts." *American Journal of Public Health* 61 (April 1971): 814-819.

Cherkasky, Martin. "Medical Manpower Needs in Deprived Areas." *Journal of Medical Education.* 44 (February 1969): 126-131.

Cowen, David L., and Sbarbaro, John A. "Family-centered Health Care — A Viable Reality?: The Denver Experience." *Medical Care* 10 (March-April 1972): 164-172.

Crook, William G. "Personnel for Health Centers." *New England Journal of Medicine* 281 (December 11, 1969): 1372-1373.

Dedeaux, Paul J. "Training of Dental Assistants in a Comprehensive Family-Oriented Neighborhood Health Center." *New York State Dental Journal* 37 (December 1971): 614-618.

Kent, James A., and Smith, C. Harvey. "Involving the Urban Poor in Health Services Through Accommodation — The Employment of Neighborhood Representatives." *American Journal of Public Health* 57 (June 1967): 997-1003.

Lashof, Joyce C. "The Health Care Team in the Mile Square Area, Chicago." *Bulletin of the New York Academy of Medicine* 44 (November 1968): 1363-1369.

Lloyd, William. "Training and Use of Members of the Community That Is Served by the Center." *Bulletin of the New York Academy of Medicine* 45 (December 1969): 1357-1359.

Moore, Frank I., and Stewart, James C., Jr. "Important Variables Influencing Successful Use of Aides." *Health Services Reports* 87 (June/July 1972): 555-561.

Morehead, Mildred A. "Changing Roles of Personnel in Neighborhood Health Centers." *Postgraduate Medicine* 49 (April 1971): 193-197.

Parker, Alberta W. "The Team Approach to Primary Health Care." Neighborhood Health Center Seminar Program Monograph Series No. 3. University
Extension, Univ. of California, Berkeley, January 1972.

Simpson, George A. "The Family Health Worker at the Community Field
Level." *Annals of the New York Academy of Sciences* 166 (December 31,
1969): 916-926.

Torrey, E. Fuller; Smith, Deloris; and Wise, Harold. "The Family Health Worker
Revisited: A Five-Year Follow-up." *American Journal of Public Health,* 63
(January 1973) 71-74.

Wise, Harold. "The Primary Health Care Team." *Archives of Internal Medicine*
130 (September 1972): 438-444.

Wise, Harold, with Doyle, Nancy. "For Ghetto Families, Personal Medical Care
Is Something New." *National Tuberculosis and Respiratory Disease Association Bulletin* 55 (February 1969): 5-7.

Wolfe, Samuel, and Mann, Judith. "Interaction of Professionals and Neighborhood Trainees." *Comprehensive Health Services Career Development: Technical Assistance Bulletin* 1 (January 1970): 1+4.

Zahn, Stella. "Neighborhood Medical Care Demonstration Training Program."
Milbank Memorial Fund Quarterly 66 (Part I) (July 1968): 309-328.

Consumer Participation and Community Control

Anderson, Donna M., and Kerr, Markay. "Citizen Influence in Health Service
Programs." *American Journal of Public Health.* 61 (August 1971): 1518-
1523.

Brieland, Donald. "Community Advisory Boards and Maximum Feasible Participation." *American Journal of Public Health* 61 (February 1971): 292-296.

Bryant, Thomas E. "Discussion of the Role of the Health Professional in
Achieving Effective Consumer Participation." *Bulletin of the New York
Academy of Medicine* 46 (December 1970): 1054-1056.

Campbell, John. "Working Relationships Between Providers and Consumers in a
Neighborhood Health Center." *American Journal of Public Health* 61
(January 1971): 97-103.

Chenault, W. W., and Brown, D. K. *Consumer Participation in Neighborhood
Comprehensive Care Centers.* Vols. 1 and 2. National Technical Information
Services, Springfield, Va. 1971.

Cherkasky, Martin. "Medical Care: Doctors and Community Control." *Trans-
actions and Studies of the College of Physicians of Philadelphia* 38 (April
1971): 212-220.

Davis, James W. "Decentralization, Citizen Participation, and Ghetto Health
Care." *American Behavioral Scientist* 15 (September/October 1971): 94-107.

Davis, Milton S., and Tranquada, Robert E. "A Sociological Evaluation of the
Watts Neighborhood Health Center." *Medical Care* 7 (March-April 1969):
105-117.

Dumois, Ana. "Organizing a Community Around Health." *Social Policy* 1
(January/February 1971): 10-14.

Falk, Leslie A. "Community Participation in the Neighborhood Health Center."

Journal of the National Medical Association 61 (November 1969): 493-497.

Frankel, Mortimer. "In the Watts Health Center, the Customer Is Nearly Always Right." *National Tuberculosis and Respiratory Disease Association Bulletin* 55 (February 1969): 14-16.

Galiher, Claudia B.; Needleman, Jack; and Rolfe, Anne J. "Consumer Participation." *HSMHA Health Reports* 86 (February 1971): 99-106.

Hatch, John W. "Discussion of the 'How' of Community Participation in Delivering Health Care." *Bulletin of the New York Academy of Medicine* 46 (December 1970): 1084-1090.

Health Policy Advisory Center. "Eastside Story – Groups Seek Major Role." *Health/Pac Bulletin* 2 (July 1968).

Lash, Trude. "Community Attitudes: Medical and Community Partnership." *New York State Journal of Medicine* 68 (September 1, 1968): 2294-2297.

Moore, Mary L. "The Role of Hostility and Militancy in Indigenous Community Health Advisory Groups." *American Journal of Public Health* 61 (May 1971): 922-930.

New, Peter Kong-Ming; Hessler, Richard M.; and Cater, Phyllis Bagwell. "Consumer Control and Public Accountability." *Anthropological Quarterly* 46 (July 1973): 196-213.

Parker, Alberta W. "The Consumer as Policy-Maker – Issues of Training." *American Journal of Public Health* 60 (November 1970): 2139-2153.

Partridge, Kay B., and White, Paul E. "Community and Professional Participation in Decision Making at a Health Center." *HSMHA Health Reports* 87 (April 1972): 336-342.

Salber, Eva J. "Community Participation in Neighborhood Health Centers." *New England Journal of Medicine* 283 (September 3, 1970): 515-518.

Sheppard, James, Jr., and Kaedka, Edna K. "Impact of the Consumer on Inner City Health Centers." *Journal of the National Medical Association* 64 (July 1972): 370-371.

Sparer, Gerald; Dines, George B.; and Smith, Daniel. "Consumer Participation in OEO Assisted Neighborhood Health Centers." *American Journal of Public Health* 60 (June 1970): 1091-1102.

Stokes, Ann; Banta, David; And Putnam, Samuel. "The Columbia Point Health Association: Evolution of a Community Health Board." *American Journal of Public Health* 62 (September 1972): 1229-1234.

Waldron, Walter. "Discussion of the Role of the Health Profession in Achieving Effective Consumer Participation." *Bulletin of the New York Academy of Medicine* 46 (December 1970): 1071-1076.

Wolfe, Samuel. "Consumerism and Health Care." *Public Administration Review* 31 (September/October 1971): 528-536.

Medical and Nonmedical professions at Neighborhood Health Centers

Bograd. Harriet, "The Role of the Lawyer in the Neighborhood Medical Care Demonstration." *Milbank Memorial Fund Quarterly* 66 (July 1968): 341-350.

Budd, Matthew A. "The Challenge of the Neighborhood Health Center." *Harvard Medical Alumni Bulletin* 46 (March/April 1972): 18-19.

Cowin, Ruth. "Some New Dimensions of Social Work Practice in a Health Setting." *American Journal of Public Health* 60 (May 1970): 860-869.

Gaspard, Nancy J. "Director of Nursing in a Comprehensive Health Center." *Nursing Outlook* 19 (September 1971): 590-591.

Light, Harold L. "Social Work in Neighborhood Health Centers." *Bulletin of the New York Academy of Medicine* 44 (November 1968): 1378-1380.

"The Pediatric Nurse Practitioner in a Neighborhood Center." *American Journal of Nursing* 71 (March 1971): 513-515.

Shannon, Iris S. "More Nursing Per Square Mile." *Nursing Outlook* 18 (April 1970): 42-44.

Tilson, Hugh H. "Characteristics of Physicians in OEO Neighborhood Health Centers." *Inquiry* 10 (June 1973): 27-38.

_____ . "Stability of Physician Employment in Neighborhood Health Centers." *Medical Care* 11 (September/October 1973): 384-400.

Urvant, Penny. "Health Advocates." *Public Health Reports* 84 (September 1969): 761-766.

Pharmacists

American Pharmaceutical Association and Office of Economic Opportunity. "Pharmaceutical Services for the Neighborhood Health Center." 106 pages. Washington, D.C.: The Association, n.d.

Blatman, Morris E. "A Vendor System for Pharmaceutical Services." *Journal of the American Pharmaceutical Association* NS8 (1968): 536-538.

Cooper, C. "OEO's Tough Competition Shuts Stores, NARD National Association of Retail Druggists Finds." *Drug Topics,* September 29, 1969.

English, Joseph T. "Health Programs for the Poor — Pharmaceutical Services." *Journal of the American Pharmaceutical Association* NS8 (1968): 532-535.

Fagin, Carl. "Pharmacists' Role Expands in the Neighborhood Health Center." *Hospitals* 42, October 16, 1968.

Henley, A. J., and Blissitt, Charles W. "Involvement of the St. Louis College of Pharmacy in a Neighborhood Health Center." *American Journal of Pharmaceutical Education* 33 (August 1969): 343-347.

Howells, Albert. "Pharmacy Inside and Outside Health Centres." *Royal Society of Health Journal* 90 (January/February 1970): 14-15+.

Parris, Noel F., Jr. "OEO Program in Dorchester, Massachusetts." *Journal of the American Pharmaceutical Association* NS8 (October 1968): 546-548+.

Paul, Stephen H. "The Neighborhood Health Center: Pharmacy's First Frontier." *American Journal of Pharmaceutical Education* 33 (August 1969): 352-360.

Penna, Richard P. "OEO — A Challenge for Pharmacies." *Journal of the American Pharmaceutical Association* NS8 (1968): 531.

_____ . "Pharmacy Services in the Health Center." *Hospitals* 44 (July 16, 1970): 70-72.

Dentists

Bishop, Eric, and Christensen, Hal M. "Dentists and the War on Poverty: A Discussion on Neighborhood Health Centers." *Journal of the American Dental Association* 75 (July 1967): 45-54.

Dummett, Clifton O. "The South Central Multipurpose Health Services Center for Watts: Dentistry's Contributions." *Journal of the National Medical Association* 59 (May 1967): 206-208.

Gerrie, N. F., and Ferraro, R. H. "Organizing a Program for Dental Care in a Neighborhood Health Center." *Public Health Reports* 83 (August 1968): 633-638.

Henry, Joseph. "Role of Dental Schools in Neighborhood Health Centers." *Journal of Dental Education* 36 (April 1972): 61-62.

Jong, Anthony, and Field, Howard. "The Role of a Community Health Center in Dental Education." *Journal of Dental Education* 36 (March 1972): 36-39.

Jong, Anthony, and Leverett, Dennis H. "The Operation of a Community Dental Clinic in a Health Center: An Evaluation." *Journal of Public Health Dentistry* 31 (Winter 1971): 27-31.

"Neighborhood Health Centers." *Journal of the American Dental Association* 75 (July 1967): 25.

Sarda, Olda; Stallard, Richard E.; and Goldberg, Hyman J. "Dental Utilization of a Neighborhood Health Center." *Journal of Public Health Dentistry* 32 (Summer 1972): 175-179.

Mental Health Services at Neighborhood Health Centers

Mallory, George L. "The Role of the Psychiatrist in a Comprehensive Neighborhood Health Center." *Journal of the National Medical Association* 64 (September 1972): 438-439+.

Lowenkopf, Eugene L., and Zweling, Israel. "Psychiatric Services in a Neighborhood Health Center." *American Journal of Psychiatry* 127 (January 1971): 916-920.

Philippus, M. J. "Successful and Unsucessful Approaches to Mental Health Services for an Urban Hispano American Population." *American Journal of Public Health* 61 (April 1971): 820-830.

Sata, Lindberg S. "A Mental Health Center's Partnerships with the Community." *Hospital and Community Psychiatry* 23 (August 1972): 242-245.

Scherl, Donald J. "Mental Health Implications of the Economic Opportunity Act." In *Proceedings of Psychology Program Directors and Consultants in State, Federal, and Territorial Mental Health Programs,* August 1966.

Scherl, Donald J., and English, Joseph T. "Community Mental Health and Comprehensive Health Service Programs for the Poor." *American Journal of Psychiatry* 125 (June 1969): 1666-1674.

Free Clinics

Bloomfield, Constance, and Levy, Howard. "The Selling of the Free Clinics." *Health/PAC Bulletin*, February 1972, pp. 1-8.

Bazell, Robert J. "Health Radicals: Crusade to Shift Medical Power to the People." *Science* 173 (August 1971): 506-509.

California Medical Association. "Free Clinics in California, 1971." *California Medicine* 116 (April 1972): 106-111.

Corner, Rosemary; Carlyle, M. Kay; Bunce, Harvey, III; and Micks, Don W. "Appraisal of Health Care Delivery in a Free Clinic." *Health Services Reports* 87 (October 1972): 727-733.

Health Policy Advisory Center. "Clinic Council." *Health/PAC Bulletin 34* (October 1971): 11.

_____. "Free Clinics." *Health/PAC Bulletin* 34 (October 1971): 1.

_____. "Gimme Shelter." *Health/PAC Bulletin* 34 (October 1971): 6-7.

_____. "What Does It Cost to be Free?" *Health/PAC Bulletin* 34 (October 1971): 10-14.

_____. "With a Little Help From Their Friends." *Health/PAC Bulletin* 34 (October 1971): 2-9.

_____. "Women's Clinics." *Health/PAC Bulletin* 34 (October 1971): 14-16

Schwartz, Jerome L. "First National Survey of Free Medical Clinics, 1967-69." *HSMHA Health Reports* 86 (September 1971): 775-787.

Smith, David E., and Shubart, Peter. "A Regionalized Medical Clinic in the Haight-Ashbury." *Hospital Topics* 46 (March 1968): 25-26.

Stoeckle, John D.; Anderson, William H.; Page, John; and Brenner, Joseph. "The Free Medical Clinics." *Journal of the American Medical Association* 219 (January 31, 1972): 603-605.

Turner, Irene R. "Free Health Centers — A New Concept?" *American Journal of Public Health* 62 (October 1972): 1348-1353.

Index

AMA, 16, 60, 113
AMA Association News, 179
"Acres of Diamonds" address, 126
Administration, 157–73
Albert Einstein College of Medicine, 179, 257
Alford, Robert, 15–16
Alinsky, S.D., 33
American Academy of Pediatrics, 84
American Dental Association, 60
American Hospital Association, 180
American Medical Association, *see* AMA
American Public Health Association, 62
Alviso, Calif., 125
Anderson, Arne, and Gerald Sparer, 179–88

Baltimore, Md., 84
Bamberger, Lisbeth, 123; *and see* Schorr, Lisbeth Bamberger
Bathgate Avenue, Bronx, 127
Beckhard, Richard, and Irwin M. Rubin, 291–303
Bellaire, O., 80
Bellevue Hospital, NYC, 144, 149
Bellin, Seymour S., and Bernard M. Kramer and Robert M. Hollister, 13–23; and H. Jack Geiger, 197–98, 199–212, 213–229; and Count D. Gibson, 308, 309–316
Bernstein Institute, NYC, 326, 328
Beth Israel Hospital, NYC, 144, 149, 308, 326, 329–30, 31
Beth Israel Medical Center, NYC, 328
Biggs, Herman, 34
Black militancy, 96
Black Nationalists, 120
Blacks, 57, 60, 93–94, 116, 124–25, 138–42
Blossom Street Health Center, Boston, 34
Blue Cross-Blue Shield, 315
Bograd, Harriet, and Harold B. Wise, E. Fuller Torrey, Adrienne McDade, Gloria Perry, and Harriet Bograd, 277, 278, 281–90
Boston, Mass., 34, 54, 73, 80, 81, 134,
209, 309; *and see* Blossom Street Health Center; Boston City Hospital; Children's Hospital Medical Center; Columbia Point Neighborhood Health Center; Tufts University College of Medicine
Boston City Hospital, 200, 204, 227, 308, 309, 310–12, 313
Bureau of the Budget, *see* Office of Management and Budget

California, 55, 80, 84; *and see* Alviso; Los Angeles; San Francisco; South Central Multipurpose Health Services Center
Callen, Des, 129; and Oliver Fein, 109, 143–55
Candib, Lucy M., and John D. Stoeckle, 27, 28, 29–40, 121
Care, quality of, 255–73
Charney, Evan: and Bruce Hillman, 198, 243–52, 278; and Louis Hochheiser and Kenneth Woodward, 308, 317–24
Chicago, Ill., 73, 81, 123, 126, 127; *and see* National Opinion Research Center; University of Chicago
Chicanos, 125
Child health centers, Milwaukee, 32
Child health stations, NYC, 30–31
Children and Youth Projects (HEW), 71, 78, 79, 260, 261, 264, 270, 272
Children's Bureau (HEW), 59, 164, 260, 261, 270, 272
Children's Hospital Medication Center, Boston, 208
Chile, 36
China, 36
Churchill, Winston, 77
Cincinnati, Ohio, 33, 73
Civil rights movement, 17–18
Coleman, James, 119, 120
Colombo, T.J., *et al.*, 168
Columbia Point Health Association, Boston, 110n, 137–38, 200, 314
Columbia Point Neighborhood Health Center, Boston, 53, 57, 123, 134–38, 139, 184–85, 186, 197, 199–211, 213–29, 308, 309–316
Committee on the Costs of Medical Care, 15

Community action agencies, 52–53
Community Action Program, 1, 18, 45, 47, 53–53, 54, 55, 56, 57, 61, 62, 69, 92–93
Community Conflict, 119
Community control, 105–55
Comprehensive Health Services Program, (OEO), 70, 74, 198, 231–41
Consumer participation, 105–55
Conwell, Russell, 126
Coser, Louis, 119
Cost Finding System for Comprehensive Health Service Projects, 181
Costs and Financing, 83–86, 175–93
Council of Economic Advisors, 112
Counseling, 77–78
Covell, Dr. Ruth, 58
"Cycle of poverty" concept, 18

Daniel Yankelovich, Inc., 201, 215
Davis, Michael, 33; and R. Tranquada, 112
Day care, 86
Dayton, Ohio, 73
Dental care, 77
Decentralization, 20–21
Denver, Colo., 57
Denver Health Center, 59
Department of Community Health, Albert Einstein College of Medicine, 80, 257
Department of Health, Education and Welfare, *see* HEW
Department of Housing and Urban Development, 73
Department of Hospitals of the City of New York, 326
Department of Labor, 94
Department of Preventive Medicine, Tufts University, 134
Division of Socio-Economic Activities, (AMA), 60
Dixon, Bertha, 148
Donaldson, Rose D., Mildred A. Morehead, and Mary R. Seravalli, 255, 257–73

Economic Opportunity Act, 1, 45, 47, 51, 67, 94
Eligibility, 56–58
Elinson, Jack, and Conrad E.A. Herr, 107, 123–31
English, Joseph T., and Lisbeth Bamberger Schorr, 43, 45–50
Evaluation Unit, Department of Community Health, Albert Einstein College of Medicine, 257, 260, 265

Family health care groups (FHCGs), 199–200, 209
Family Health Insurance Plan (FIHS), 3n
Fein, Oliver, and Des Callan, 109, 143–55
Fein, Rashi, 177–78, 189–93
Feingold, Eugene, 67, 91–98, 163
Functions of Social Conflict, The, 119
Funding, 56–58, 58–60; *and see* Costs and financing

Geiger, H. Jack, 55, 56, 133–42, 109–110, 114–15, 123; and Seymour S. Bellin, 199–212, 213–30; and Bellin and Count D. Gibson, 308, 309–316
Genesee Hospital, 318–19, 320, 323
Gibson, Count D., 53, 123; and Seymour S. Bellin and H. Jack Geiger, 308, 309–316
Gordon, Jeoffry, 109, 111–22, 164
Gouverneur Ambulatory Care Unit, 326-27, 327–28
Gouverneur Hospital Services Program, NYC, 185, 308, 328–29, 330, 331
Great Britain, 36
Greenleigh Associates, 260
Group Health Association, 184, 186

HEW, 1, 2–3, 8, 9, 19–20, 58, 59, 62, 70–71, 72, 73, 76, 80, 83, 86, 94, 107, 112, 175; *and see* Children and Youth Projects; Children's Bureau; Health Services and Mental Health Administration
HIP, 80, 186, 252
Harpers Magazine, 127
Hawaii, 260
Head Start, 52, 54, 86
Health Committee, NENA, 144, 146, 147–50
"Health crisis," 15–16
Health Maintenance Organization (HMO), 102–103, 180, 240, 241
Health/PAC Bulletin, 67–68
Health Services and Mental Health Administration (HEW), 69
Health workers, 275–304
"Healthrights" program (OEO), 69–70, 111, 112, 120–21
Herr, Conrad E.A., and Jack Elinson, 107, 123–31
"Hill-Burton" health facilities program, 72
Hillman, Bruce, and Evan Charney, 198, 243–52, 278
Hochheiser, Louis, Kenneth Woodward, and Evan Charney, 308, 317–24
Hollister, Robert M., 1–12; and Bernard

M. Kramer and Seymour S. Bellin, 13–23
Hospital Review and Planning Council
of Southern New York, 326
Houston, Tex., 73
Hudson, Dr. Charles, 60
Hunt's Point Multiservice Center,
Bronx, 129

Indians, 55
Institute of Rehabilitation Medicine,
NYC, 329
Insurance, health, 189–93; *and see*
Blue Cross-Blue Shield; Family Health
Insurance Plan; Group Health Associa-
tion; HIP; Kaiser Health Plan

Johnson, Joyce, and Gerald Sparer, 68n
Johnson, Lyndon B., 19
Judson Health Center, NYC, 327, 328
Judson Memorial Church, NYC, 128

Kahane, Stanley B., and Kovner, An-
thony R., Gerald Katz, and Cecil G.
Sheps, 167, 308, 325–32
Kaiser Health Plan, 58, 184, 186
Kaiser-Permanente Medical Care
Program, 80
Kansas City, Kan., 73
Kark, S.L., 36
Katz, Gerald, and Anthony R. Kovner,
Stanley B. Kahane, and Cecil G. Sheps,
167, 308, 325–32
Kennedy, Edward, 1, 47, 54
Kennedy, Robert, 45
King City, Calif., 183, 184
Kovner, Anthony R., Gerald Katz,
Stanley B. Kahane, and Cecil G.
Sheps, 167, 308, 325–32
Kramer, Bernard M., Robert M. Hollister,
and Seymour S. Bellin, 13–23

Lashof, Joyce, 123
Legal Services, 86
Levitan, Sar A., 43, 51–63
Los Angeles, Calif., 73
Louisville, Ky., 84, 86
Lower East Side, NYC, 143–55; *and see*
NENA

Madison, Donald L., 43n
Maine, 80
March, J., and H. Simon, 117
Martin Luther King Health Center,
Bronx, 109, 179, 277, 278
Maryland, 84
Massachusetts, 84
Maternal and Infant Care Programs, 260,

261, 263–64, 270, 272
McDade, Adrienne, and Harold B. Wise,
E. Fuller Torrey, Gloria Perry, and
Harriet Bograd, 277, 278, 281–90
Medicaid, 2, 47, 57, 60, 61, 62, 63, 80,
83–84, 85, 95, 183–84, 191, 204,
243, 315
Medi-Cal, 179
Medical Committee on Human Rights, 60
Medicare, 47, 83, 84, 204, 310, 315
Mental health services, 78
Milbank Memorial Fund, 123
Mile Square Health Center, 81
Milk stations, NYC, 30–31, 32
Milwaukee, Wis., 32
Minnesota, 55
Mission Rebels, San Francisco, 116
Mississippi, 134, 138–42
Model Cities Program, 108, 164
Montefiore Hospital, Bronx, 127, 179
Montefiore Hospital Medical Care
Demonstration, 47, 183, 184, 185,
281–82, 289–90
Moore, Wanda, 144
Morehead, Mildred A., 128, 179, 186;
and Rose D. Donaldson, 184; Morehead,
Donaldson, and Mary R. Seravalli,
255, 257–73
Mothers for Adequate Welfare, Boston,
116
Mound Bayou, Miss., 53, 127–28
Mount Sinai Hospital, Chicago, 126
Mount Sinai School of Medicine of the
City University of New York, 328, 329
Mountin, J.W., 34

NENA Health Center, 109, 143–55
Nashville, Tenn., 73
National Association of Neighborhood
Health Centers, 83
National Association of Retail Druggists, 62
National Dental Association, 60
National Health Services Corps, 72
National Medical Association, 60
National Opinion Research Center (NRC),
Chicago, 238
Neighborhood health centers: adminis-
tration of, 157–73; costs and financing
of, 83–86, 175–93; demonstrations,
1–12; eligibility requirements, 56–58;
evaluation of, 65–103; evolution of in
the 1960s, 41–64; patients' use and
response to, 195–52; precursors of,
25–40; relations with other health
institutions, 305–32; as a social movement, 13–23; *and see* Care, quality of;
Health workers; Pediatrics

New Haven, Conn., 80
New York City, 30–31, 32, 78, 79, 161, 183–84; *and see* Bellevue Hospital; Bernstein Institute; Beth Israel Hospital; Gouverneur Health Services Program; HIP; Institute of Rehabilitation Medicine; Judson Memorial Church; Judson Health Center; NENA; Reform Democratic Club; Sixth Street Mothers
New York Infirmary, 145
New York Milk Committee, 30–31
New York Times, 179
New York University Medical School, 144, 149
Newark, N.J., 116
Nixon, Richard M., 3n, 94
North East Neighborhoods Association, *see* NENA Health Center
North Lawndale, Chicago, 127
Northern Bolivar City, Miss., 134, 138–42

OEO, 1, 2, 3n, 8, 9, 16, 17, 18, 19–20, 33, 43, 46, 53, 54, 55–56, 57, 58, 59, 60, 61, 62, 63, 67, 71, 72, 73, 74, 76, 80, 83, 85–86, 94, 96, 107, 108, 111, 112–13, 115, 116, 117, 123, 124, 125, 126, 127, 139, 140, 145, 161, 163, 168, 175, 179, 180, 181, 186, 189, 198, 199, 231, 233, 255, 262, 263, 270, 271, 281, 317, 326–27; *and see* Program: Comprehensive Health Services; "Healthrights" program; OEO Act; Office of Health Affairs; Office of Planning and Evaluation; Program Guideline
OEO Act, 85
Obstetrics, 268; *and see* Maternal Infant Care Programs
Office of Health Affairs (OEO), 10, 57, 69
Office of Management and Budget, 8, 19, 73
Office of Planning and Evaluation, OEO, 257, 260
Oklahoma City, Okla., 73
Oregon, 80; *and see* Portland, Ore.
Outpatient departments (OPDs), 99

Parker, Alberta W., 278n
Partnership for Health legislation, 1, 2, 75, 112
Patients, response to and use of neighborhood health centers, 195–252
Peace Corps, 56
Peckham experiment, 36
Pediatrics, 269, 317–24; *and see* Maternal and Infant Care Programs

Pennsylvania, 84; *and see* Philadelphia, Pa.; Pittsburgh, Pa.
Perry, Gloria, and Harold B. Wise, E. Fuller Torrey, Adrienne McDade, and Harriet Bograd, 277, 278, 281–90
Personnel, *see* Administration; Health Workers
Pharmacists, 61–62
Philadelphia, Pa., 73, 126, 127, 179; *and see* Temple University
Phillips, Wilbur C., 30–31, 32, 33
Pholela Health Center, 36
Physicians' Forum, 60
Pittsburgh, Pa., 73
Polio immunization, 216
Pomeroy, J.L., 35
Portland, Ore., 58, 81
Preventive care, 35–36
Program Guidelines, OEO, 70–71, 74–75
"Project Grants for Health Services Development," 1
Public Health Service (PHS), 53, 58 59, 62, 112, 113, 145
Puerto Rico, 36, 124

Recruitment, 160; *and see* Administration
Reform Democratic Club, NYC, 146, 148
Robertson, L.S., *et al.,* 211
Rochester, N.Y., 73, 198, 317–24; *and see* St. Mary's Hospital; Strong Memorial Hospital
Rochester Action for a Better Community, 243, 317
Rochester General Hospital, 318, 319
Rochester Neighborhood Health Center, 243–52, 278, 308, 317–24
Rosen, George, 5, 28n
Rouse, Dr. Milford O., 60
Rubin, Irwin, and Richard Beckhard, 277, 278, 291–303
Russia, 36

St. Mary's Hospital, Rochester, 317, 319
Salt Lake City, Utah, 86
San Francisco, Calif., 73
Sanders, Marion, 127
Schon, Donald, 4
Schorr, Lisbeth Bamberger, and Joseph T. English, 43, 45–50
Sears, Roebuck, Chicago, 127
Seattle, Washington, 80
Senate Appropriations Subcommittee, 54–55
Seravalli, Mary R., Mildred A. Morehead, and Rose D. Donaldson, 255, 257–73

Sheps, Cecil G., Anthony R. Kovner, and Gerald Katz, 167, 308, 325–32
Simon, H., and J. March, 117
Sixth Street Mothers, NYC, 144, 146
Socialized medicine, 60
South Africa, 36
South Central Multipurpose Health Services Center, University of Southern California, 124–25
Sparer, Gerald, 123; and Joyce Johnson, 68n; and Arne Anderson, 177, 179–88; and Mark A. Strauss, 198, 231–42
Staffing, 81–83; and see Administration; Recruitment
Standard, S., 167
Stoeckle, John D., and Lucy M. Candib, 27, 28, 29–40, 123
Strauss, Mark A., and Gerald Sparer, 198, 231–42
Strong Memorial Hospital, Rochester, 318, 319, 320, 323
Suffolk City, N.Y., 80
Sundquist, James, 93
Temple University, 126, 127
Temple University Hospital, 127
"10 Point Program of Health Revolutionary Unity Movement," 128–29
Thomas, Dean Lewis, 144
Tilson, Hugh H., 160n
Title V, 71
Title XVIII, 162, 166
Title XIX, 162, 164, 166, 260
Torrens, Paul R., 160, 161–73, 278
Torrey, E. Fuller; and Harold B. Wise, Adrienne McDade, Gloria Perry, and Harriet Bograd, 277, 278, 281–90

Tranquada, R., and Michael M. Davis, 112
Tufts Comprehensive Community Health Action Program, 128, 200, 213; and see Columbia Point
Tufts University College of Medicine, 53, 134, 137–39, 141; Department of Community Health and Social Medicine, 201; and see Columbia Point

University of Chicago, 238
University of Rochester, 243, 245; School of Medicine, 317
Utah, 84; and see Salt Lake City, Utah

Vietnam War, 101

War on Poverty, 45, 70, 101, 112, 199
Watts, 56, 95
Welfare Reform, 86
White, William O., 31
White House Conference on Health, 47
Wilinsky, C.F., 34
Winston-Salem, N.C., 73
Wilson, J., 117
Wise, Harold B.; 127; and E. Fuller Torrey, Adrienne McDade, Gloria Perry, and Harriet Bograd, 277, 278, 281–90
Woods, Robert, 31
Woodward, Kenneth, Louis Hochheiser, and Evan Charney, 308, 317–24

Yerby, Alonzo S., 47
Yugoslavia, 31

Zwick, Daniel I., 67, 69–90

About the Editors

Robert M. Hollister is assistant professor in the Department of Urban Studies and Planning, Massachusetts Institute of Technology. He received the B.A. from Antioch College in 1966, the M.C.P. from Harvard University in 1971, and the Ph.D. from the Massachusetts Institute of Technology in 1971. He did research on consumer participation and community control of neighborhood health centers at the Joint Center of Urban Studies of M.I.T. and Harvard, where he was a Katherine Bauer Wurster Fellow. His most recent research concerns the politics of health care and health planning.

Bernard M. Kramer is professor and chairman, Department of Psychology, College II, University of Massachusetts at Boston. He received the B.A. from Brooklyn College in 1944 and the Ph.D. from Harvard University in 1950. He is a social psychologist whose fields of specialization are race relations, mental health, public health, and urban affairs. Dr. Kramer has taught at the Department of Community Medicine, Tufts University School of Medicine, and was active in the early development of the Columbia Point Health Center in Boston. He is the author of *Day Hospital* and coeditor of *Social Psychology and Mental Health* and *Racism and Mental Health.*

Seymour S. Bellin is professor and chairman, Department of Sociology and Anthropology, Tufts University. He received the B.A. from Brooklyn College in 1948 and the M.A. and the Ph.D. from Columbia University in 1948 and 1962. His work has concentrated on the evaluation of federal policies and programs relating to poverty, health, and welfare. His most recent research examines citizen participation in policymaking at neighborhood health centers and community mental health centers, and evaluates the operation and impact of health centers in achieving social change. He was formerly a professor in the Department of Community Medicine, Tufts University School of Medicine.